Mental Health in Historical Perspective

Series Editors
Catharine Coleborne
School of Humanities and Social Science
University of Newcastle
Callaghan, NSW, Australia

Matthew Smith
Centre for the Social History
of Health and Healthcare
University of Strathclyde
Glasgow, UK

Covering all historical periods and geographical contexts, the series explores how mental illness has been understood, experienced, diagnosed, treated and contested. It will publish works that engage actively with contemporary debates related to mental health and, as such, will be of interest not only to historians, but also mental health professionals, patients and policy makers. With its focus on mental health, rather than just psychiatry, the series will endeavour to provide more patient-centred histories. Although this has long been an aim of health historians, it has not been realised, and this series aims to change that.

The scope of the series is kept as broad as possible to attract good quality proposals about all aspects of the history of mental health from all periods. The series emphasises interdisciplinary approaches to the field of study, and encourages short titles, longer works, collections, and titles which stretch the boundaries of academic publishing in new ways.

More information about this series at
http://www.palgrave.com/gp/series/14806

Robert Ellis

London and its Asylums, 1888-1914

Politics and Madness

palgrave
macmillan

Robert Ellis
School of Music, Humanities & Media
University of Huddersfield
Huddersfield, UK

Mental Health in Historical Perspective
ISBN 978-3-030-44431-0   ISBN 978-3-030-44432-7 (eBook)
https://doi.org/10.1007/978-3-030-44432-7

Cover credit: Hi-Story/Alamy Stock Photo

This Palgrave Macmillan imprint is published by the registered company Springer Nature Switzerland AG
The registered company address is: Gewerbestrasse 11, 6330 Cham, Switzerland

Preface

This book deals with the impact of political parties and allegiances on the development of policies and procedures in the treatment of those deemed to be mentally-ill. It offers an analysis of how evidence from lunatic asylums was appropriated for election purposes but it also considers where initiatives and treatments sat in relation to broader political visions and ideologies. With its focus on the turn of the nineteenth century, this has very much been an original piece of work but it is one that builds on previous research. In 2013, I wrote an article about London County Council which explored the Surrey town of Epsom's response to what was seen, in some quarters, as an imposition of the large-scale asylums on its doorstep.[1] Here, there was a consideration of how the dispute was negotiated by local, regional and national authorities, and how that was played out in the press. Absent from it, however, was any real sense of the politics of the people and authorities involved, and, while it would not have affected its conclusions, subsequent research revealed a central role for the management of madness within election materials, including pamphlets and posters.

Before the late 1880s, the management of madness in England and Wales had been the responsibility of local magistrates who formed Visiting Committees to oversee the administration, building and

[1]Ellis, Rob. 2013. A Constant Irritation to the Townspeople. Local, Regional and National Politics and London's County Asylums at Epsom. *Social History of Medicine*. 26:4: 653–667.

maintenance of lunatic asylums. From 1808, legislation had existed that allowed magistrates to raise the funds to build such institutions and this was followed in 1845 by an Act that compelled them to do so. The 1888 Local Government passed that responsibility to the new County Councils it had created and, for the first time, the management of madness became the responsibility of democratically elected bodies. In London, the political landscape was dominated by two groups; the Progressives, or Liberals, who held power from the first election in 1889 and the Moderates and Municipal Reformers, or Conservatives, who replaced them following their victory in 1907. It is through this lens, that the management of madness in London will be viewed. Previous work on this period has tended to focus on lunacy legislation generally, and the 1890 Lunacy Act specifically. Instead, this book seeks to recast asylums as sites of political discourse and debate and to highlight their corresponding impact on both medical management and practice. It argues that, influential policies owed their success to the political allegiances of the individuals that were driving them, and places London at the fulcrum of transnational debates about the nature of care.

Huddersfield, UK Robert Ellis

Acknowledgments

The origins of this book stem from an article I wrote about the Epsom Cluster in 2013. The research I did then suggested that there was much more to be said about London's place in the history of mental ill-health. I would like to take the opportunity to thank the people and organisations that have helped me along in the development of the ideas that feature in the pages that follow.

At the very outset, I was fortunate enough to receive a small grant from the Wellcome Trust, which allowed me to conduct some initial archival research in London and to scope out a longer-term plan. This was followed by a period of research leave awarded to me by the University of Huddersfield. These funds and his time enabled me the space to wrangle some of my initial ideas into shape, and my thanks go to Paul Ward who was particularly supportive of my sabbatical application.

As my research progressed, I spent a lot of time in various archives and repositories and some initial research assistance from Steve Taylor helped me to identify some additional useful resources. On my visits to 'that London' and other places I have benefitted from the expertise of staff at the Bishopgate Institute, the British Library, the Guildhall Library, the John Rylands Library, the London Metropolitan Archives [LMA], the London School of Economics [LSE], the National Archives, Surrey History Centre, the Wellcome Institute and the West Yorkshire History Centre. Special mentions go to Daniel Payne and Anna Towlson at the LSE, and Richard Wiltshire at the LMA, for their help in arranging the various image permissions, and also to the Wellcome Institute for the images reproduced under its Creative Commons license. There were so many images that I might have used and I hope to revisit some of those that did not make the cut in later work. For the time being, I am grateful to the Centre for Health Histories at the University of Huddersfield for the funds to reproduce some of them in this volume.

As my ideas took shape, I presented them at various conferences and I have welcomed the friendly and supportive feedback that I have received in each case. At the University of Huddersfield, Keith Laybourn has gone 'above and beyond' in his willingness to read my earliest and roughest chapters. He has always been on hand to offer friendly advice and support, and to regularly remind me of the importance of consistent footnote formatting. Wise words, thanks Keith! I am also grateful to the friends and colleagues who have been generous with their time, feedback and support when reading one or more chapters. Their suggestions have been invaluable so drinks on me, Barry Doyle, Shane Ewen, Rebecca Gill, Louise Hide, Janette Martin, Heather Shore, Len Smith, Matt Smith, Jen Wallis, Wendy Webster and Rebecca Wynter. Katherine Lewis even chipped in with the occasional hot drink to ensure that I did not die of thirst when we were in the office together. I have also received consistently brilliant support from the team at Palgrave Macmillan. Thanks to Molly Beck, Maeve Sinnott, and the *Mental Health in Historical Perspective* series editors, Cathy Coleborne and Matt Smith, as well as their anonymous reviewers.

The final stages of the book drafting came at a time when I was awarded AHRC funding for an international Impact and Engagement project which, in turn, became the basis of a draft Impact Case Study. Balancing the two was not always easy and I would like to thank Rob Light, Sue Moffat and Rachel Reddihough for their patience, as well as their good company during this time. The final word goes to the 'civilians' at home—Joanna, Joe and Daisy for their ongoing support, love and understanding. I know, for certain, they cannot wait to get reading.

January 2020 Robert Ellis

Contents

Abbreviations

APPG	All Party Parliamentary Group
BI	Bishopsgate Institute
BL	British Library
GL	Guildhall Library
LCC	London County Council
LGA	Local Government Act (1888)
LGB	Local Government Board
LMA	London Metropolitan Archives
LMS	London Municipal Society
LSE	London School of Economics
MAB	Metropolitan Asylums Board
MBW	Metropolitan Board of Works
NHS	National Health Service
TNA	The National Archive
WYAS	West Yorkshire Archive Service

List of Figures

List of Tables

CHAPTER 1

Introduction: 'The Mere Scope of It Is Immense', London and Its Asylums in Context

Since the 1950s we have become familiar with pronouncements from political parties on the topic of mental ill-health.[1] Often, these seek to address issues around stigma or tackle what appears to be a 'crisis' in care, or its funding. Concerns about an ageing population and predictions of an apparently inexorable demand for dementia care services, coupled with an apparent growth in the numbers of young people living with mental ill-health, are merely the latest areas of concern to grab the headlines. These issues are not strictly political, and the All Party Parliamentary Group [APPG] which draws it membership from Rethink Mental Illness, a campaigning charity, and members of the Royal College of Psychiatry, as well as cross-party MPs and peers, is just one example of the other groups and individuals with a vested interest in this topic.[2] The fact that this is an issue for 'All-Party' members, seems to suggest that mental health is somehow above party-political disagreements but we know that wider political philosophies impact on other aspects of health care, not least its funding. Using this as a starting point, this book aims to explore the impact of politics on mental health in a period that

[1] For a good overview of key political interventions in the twentieth and twenty-first centuries see Turner, John et al. 2015. The History of Mental Health Services in Modern England: Practitioner Memories and the Direction of Future Research. *Medical History* 59: 599–624, 623.

[2] Rethink Mental Illness. n.d. APPG on Mental Health. https://www.rethink.org/get-involved/public-affairs/appg-on-mental-health. Accessed 3 July 2019.

R. Ellis, *London and its Asylums, 1888-1914*,
Mental Health in Historical Perspective,
https://doi.org/10.1007/978-3-030-44432-7_1

has been largely overlooked by scholars. In particular, it will focus on the London County Council [LCC] from its inception, following the passing of the Local Government Act [LGA] in 1888, through until the eve of the Great War in 1914.

This period is important, not least because the passing of the LGA introduced triennial elections and the management of asylums became the responsibility of democratically elected bodies of councillors for the first time. Joe Melling and Bill Forsythe have concluded that the 'elaborate system of County Council governance' that was ushered in by the LGA 'had a significant impact on the management of the asylum', but any discussion of the politics behind these changes is still to be unpicked.[3] This is probably because, in this case, the coalescing of groups of councillors around political allegiances was not as obvious as it was in London. It has meant that initial studies of the post-1888 period have been primarily inward facing—that is focussing on the committee structures of the new County Councils. Until recently, there had been only one article on LCC's role as an administrator of lunacy policy and while some work has been done on the north-west of England, the changes in the management structures brought about by the new LGA have remained largely unexplored.[4] As a result, it is less clear how, or indeed if, this was affected by the new democratic processes instigated by the LGA. Furthermore, we have little or no idea of the role of the new democratically elected council chamber in debating, and vetoing or approving mental health policies.

The chapters that follow go beyond the continuities, or otherwise, of pre- and post-1888 managements, to explore more fully the internecine battles and external negotiations to consider how mental health policy was affected by London's new political landscape and how the new political landscape affected it. For these reasons, a study of London is

[3] Melling, Joe and Forsythe, Bill. 2006. *The Politics of Madness*. London: Routledge: 45.

[4] Cochrane, David. 1988. Humane, Economical and Medically Wise: The LCC as Administrators of Victorian Lunacy Policy. In *The Anatomy of Madness, Vol. III: The Asylum and Its Psychiatry*, eds. W.F. Bynum, Roy Porter and Michael Shepherd, 247–72. London: Routledge. Hayes, Bob. 2007. Lancashire Public Asylum Provision: Regional Co-operation. Local Rivalry and Factional Interest, 1889–1914. In *Urban Politics and Space in the Nineteenth and Twentieth Centuries, Regional Perspectives*, ed. Barry Doyle, 80–98. Newcastle: Cambridge Scholars Publishing. See also Melling and Forsythe, *The Politics of Madness*, 2006.

Table 1.1 London County Council Asylums

Name	*Location*	*Built by*	*Opened*
Hanwell	Hanwell	County of Middlesex	1831
Colney Hatch	Colney Hatch	County of Middlesex	1851
Banstead	Sutton, Surrey	County of Middlesex	1877
Cane Hill	Purley, Surrey	County of Surrey	1883
Claybury	Woodford Bridge, Essex	LCC but antecedents with the County of Middlesex	1893
Bexley Heath	Bexley Heath, Kent	LCC	1898
Horton Manor	Epsom, Surrey	LCC	1899
Horton	Epsom, Surrey	LCC	1902
Ewell Epileptic Colony	Epsom, Surrey	LCC	1903
Long Grove	Epsom, Surrey	LCC	1907
West Park	Epsom, Surrey	LCC	1924

particularly apposite because its development under the LGA was not just about the creation of a new county or a new unitary authority, it was about the creation of a new administration for the world's premier city. This offers a chance to consider the role of asylums in wider debates relating to electioneering and political rhetoric, but also to consider the place of mental health within wider political visions for the management of the capital. Here, it will be argued that although there was not necessarily a distinct political vision for mental health in this period, the discourse and debates surrounding it became an important feature of how the political parties in this period were represented, both in power and in opposition, as well as during election campaigns. It shows that the rhetoric around mental health was important in defining what political parties stood for—even if in some cases the focus of that rhetoric was on key individuals, rather than the parties themselves. Beyond this rhetoric, this work seeks to show how wider political philosophies impacted on the management of madness and demonstrate that the discussions of mental health were not somehow cut adrift from other political currents, debates and realities.

Table 1.1 lists the asylums managed by LCC in the period covered by this book and within it are the familiar names of places such as Hanwell and Colney Hatch. These already feature in specific as well as broader studies of institutional provision, and in more recent work that explores life in asylums in the period covered by this book.[5] Both Louise Hide's recent monograph, which takes an ethnographic approach to the everyday life for patients and staff at Bexley and Claybury, and Jane Hamlett's exploration of the material life in a range of institutions that include LCC's Long Grove Asylum, are evidence of an ongoing interest in these places.[6] Rather than replicate these excellent studies, I will shift the gaze from a straightforward overview of London's individual institutions to place LCC's management of them, and its municipalisation of madness, within their longer-term histories. The aim here is to consider the whole of London's stock in relation to the spatial and political understanding of what London represented.

A Spatial Understanding of London

Strictly speaking, before the passing of the 1888 Local Government Act [LGA] 'London was officially the City of London (that is the area administered by the Corporation) and nothing else'.[7] *The Times* claimed in 1855 that 'there is no such place as London at all' and the framing and understanding of London as a single metropolis was to be influenced as much by cartographers, statisticians, census enumerators and social reformers, as it had been by a demarcation of 'official' boundaries and legislation.[8] Culturally too, London had already expanded beyond the square mile and it was, for example, on the road to London

[5] See for example Suzuki, Akihito. 1995. The Politics and Ideology of Non-restraint: The Case of the Hanwell Asylum. *Medical History* 39: 1–17. Hunter, Richard and Macalpine, Ida. 1974. *Psychiatry for the Poor: 1851 Colney Hatch Asylum - Friern Hospital 1973*. London: Dawsons of Pall Mall. Barham, Peter. 2007. *Forgotten Lunatics of the Great War*. New Haven: Yale University Press. Scull, Andrew. 1993. *The Most Solitary of Afflictions*. New Haven: Yale University Press.

[6] Hide, Louise. 2014. *Gender and Class in English Asylums, 1890–1914*. Basingstoke: Palgrave Macmillan. Hamlett, Jane. 2015. *At Home in the Institution, Material Life in Asylums, Lodging Houses and Schools in Victorian and Edwardian England*. Basingstoke: Palgrave Macmillan. See also Hide Louise. 2013. From Asylum to Mental Hospital: Gender, Space and the Patient Experience in London County Council Asylums, 1890–1910. In *Residential Institutions in Britain, 1725–1970*, eds. Jane Hamlett, Lesley Hoskins and Rebecca Preston, 51–64. London: Pickering and Chatto.

[7] Porter, Roy. 1994. *London, A Social History*. London: Hamish Hamilton Ltd.: 10–11.

[8] Ibid: 10–11. Davies, John. 1988. *Reforming London: The London Government Problem, 1855–1900*. London: Clarendon Press: 4–5.

that Walter Harcourt first met the eponymous heroine of *The Woman in White* (1859), and it was the roads to and from the capital that played an important role in Dickens' *Barnaby Rudge* (1841). More concrete developments in the care and control of madness contributed to the framing of London beyond its square mile borders too. This included the introduction of the Metropolitan Commissioners in Lunacy, created in 1828 to license and inspect the already prevalent private madhouses in the London area. In turn, its powers were extended in 1842 so that it became a national inspectorate before it was renamed the Commissioners in Lunacy in 1845.[9]

This broadly defined and amorphous 'London' had other important and well-known institutions. These included Bethlem which had moved from the City to Southwark in 1815, and St Luke's on Old Street. In addition, there were a number of private asylums and the Metropolitan Asylums Board's [MAB] hospitals at Caterham and Leavesden. To this, we can add the significant numbers of people who were 'cared' for in the community—whatever that may have meant in terms of individual experience. Leonard Smith has summarised the options available in the public, private and voluntary sectors under a modern term; 'the mixed economy of care'.[10] Institutionally speaking, however, it was the growth of the County Asylum sector that would ultimately eclipse all of these options, in terms of both their patient numbers and their

[9] Bartlett, Peter. 1999. *The Poor Law of Lunacy: The Administration of Pauper Lunatics in Mid-Nineteenth Century England*. London: Leicester University Press: xii.

[10] Smith, L.D. 1999. The County Asylum in the Mixed Economy of Care. In *Insanity, Institutions and Society, 1800–1914*, eds. Joseph Melling and Bill Forsythe, 33–47. London: Routledge. For details of how the Poor Law administered care options including workhouses and the MAB asylums at Caterham and Leavesden see Murphy, Elaine. 2002. The Lunacy Commissioners and the East London Guardians. *Medical History* 46: 495–524. Murphy, Elaine. 2003. The Administration of insanity in England 1800–1870. In *The Confinement of the Insane International Perspectives, 1800–1965*, eds. Roy Porter and David Wright, 334–49. New York: Cambridge University Press. Murphy, Elaine. 2006. Workhouse Care of the Inane, 1845–90. In *Mental Illness and Learning Disability Since 1850*, eds. Pamela Dale and Joseph Melling, 24–45. London: Routledge. Stef Eastoe's recent research has shown that lunatics were also admitted to the Caterham and Leavesden Asylums. Eastoe, S. 2016. Idiocy, Imbecility and Society in Victorian England: Caterham Imbecile Asylum, 1867–1911. Unpublished PhD thesis, University of London, Birkbeck. See also Ayers, Gwendoline M. 1971. *England's First State Hospitals and the Metropolitan Asylums Board 1867–1930*. London: Wellcome Institute of the History of Medicine.

reach. Important acts of parliament passed in 1808 and 1845 allowed unelected magistrates in the counties of England and Wales to first build and administer new asylums, and then compelled them to do so. Even before the passing of the LGA, the institutions that would eventually come under LCC's control hosted many more of London's lunatics than Bethlem ever could. The then new Middlesex County Asylums at Hanwell (1831) and Colney Hatch (1851) were already bigger than it by the middle of the nineteenth century and the second Surrey Asylum, which opened at Brookwood in 1867, drew many of its patients from 'the workhouses of poor south London areas such as Bermondsey, Camberwell, Rotherhithe, Lambeth and Southwark'.[11] Even if we accept the claim that Bethlem was home to 429 patients in 1840, many more insane Londoners were being distributed within the burgeoning County Asylum network.[12] Thus, while contemporaries were not necessarily as pedantic as *The Times*, it is clear that London's 'mad' were, more often than not, the county of Middlesex's mad. It was these county boundaries that opened the door to their admission to the institutions at Hanwell, Colney Hatch, and later, Banstead and not the fact they were 'Londoners'.[13]

For the people in those institutions and elsewhere, the introduction of the LGA, and the birth of the new county of London appeared to change little—at least not in the first instance. As one commentator pointed out, the Act 'converted' the metropolitan areas in and around the city into 'a fictional unit' and treated the new county as 'if it possessed corporate interests and a common life' when it did not.[14] The implication here was that things carried on much as they had done before but politically and spatially, 121 square miles were now identified as the administrative county of London and this was to impact on how

[11]'Ten or twelve of the largest parishes in London [sent] all their pauper lunatics' to Hanwell at a time when it held 600 inmates and Bethlem held somewhere between 180 and 200. Grant, James. 1838. *Sketches in London*. London: W.S. Orr and Co: 259–61. Shepherd, Anne and Wright, David. 2002. Madness, Suicide and the Victorian Asylum: Attempted Self-Murder in the Age of Non-restraint. *Medical History* 46: 175–96, 182.

[12]Earle, Pliny. 1841. *A Visit to Thirteen Asylums in Europe*. Philadelphia: Dobson: 65.

[13]Young, Ken and Garside, Patricia L. 1982. *Metropolitan London, Politics and Urban Change, 1837–1981: Studies in Urban History 6*. London: Edward Arnold: 14–15.

[14]Jeyes, Samuel. 1906. *The Earl of Rosebery*. London: J.M. Dent and Co: 116–7.

the capital was represented both generally and in relation to its asylum provision.[15]

The *Spectator* may have actively encouraged the teaching and dissemination of a civic pride in a London, and a history that pre-dated 1888, but, for others the LGA represented year zero.[16] The other counties, as Jackson points out, 'had been in existence for centuries' whereas 'London was not a county at all'.[17] The redrawing of historic boundaries in 1888 meant the appropriation of lands from the counties of Middlesex, Kent and Surrey and a fresh start. In the debates leading to the introduction of the LGA, William Gladstone had told the House of Commons that 'the local government of London ... ought to be the crown of all our local and municipal institutions'.[18] The installation of county government, it was claimed, was 'little short of a revolution' while Woodrow Wilson, a then future president of the United States, described London before the passing of the LGA as 'the unresolved problem, the unregenerate monster of local government in England'.[19] Thus, while London had, for a long time, been the political hub of empire, here was an opportunity for its new county government to offer an exemplar—not just to the country but to the whole world. London's exceptionalism on these terms was important—what mattered in London mattered to the rest of the world, and the scale of its new geography featured heavily.

It was only after the first election of councillors in 1889, that London was recognised for what it was: a single metropolis, 'the largest the world had ever seen'.[20] The maps of poverty that were framed within the new County's boundaries and accompanied Charles Booth's *Life and Labour*

[15] Jones, Robert. 1905. The London County Council and the Care of the Mentally Afflicted. *Westminster Review* April: 409–21.

[16] Anon. 1907. Civic Pride. *Spectator*, 28 September.

[17] Jackson, W. Eric. 1965. *Achievement, A Short History of the LCC.* London: Longmans, Green and Co.: 5.

[18] Smellie, K.B. 1946. *A History of Local Government.* London: George Allen and Unwin: 178.

[19] Firth, J.F.B. and Simpson, Edgar R. 1888. *London Government Under the Local Government Act, 1888.* London: Knight and Co: i. Wilson, Woodrow. 1889. *The State: Elements of Historical and Practical Politics.* Boston: D.C. Heath and Co: 435–6.

[20] Weightman, Gavin and Humphries, Steve. 1985. *The Making of Modern London, 1845–1914.* London: Sidgewick and Jackson: 171.

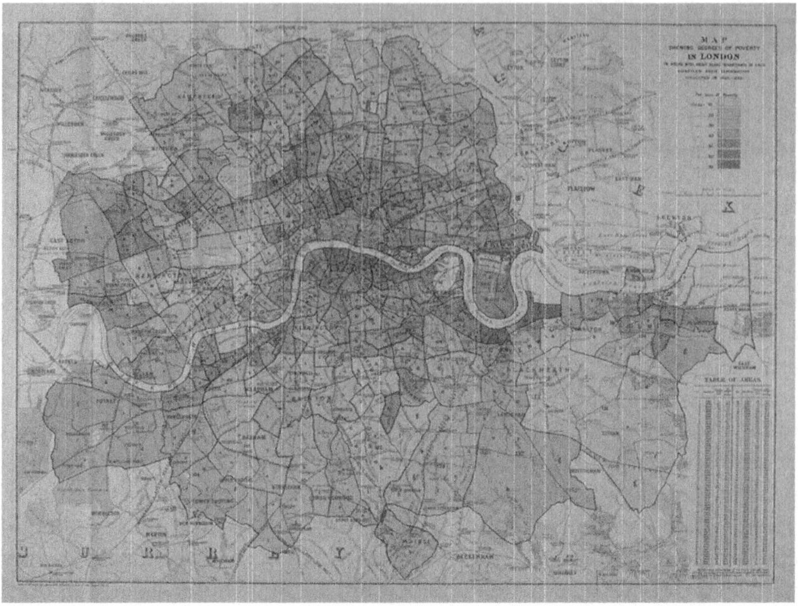

Fig. 1.1 Descriptive map of London poverty, 1889. (From Charles Booth's Life and Labour of the people of London.) Wellcome Library, London (Reproduced with permission. Wellcome Collection. CC BY)

of the People of London provide a visual representation of that (Fig. 1.1) but there were a number of other indicators that commentators were able to draw on. As a magnet for migrants, a significant proportion of England's total population lived there and it was home to the country's largest concentration of industry.[21] Its population in 1901 was larger

[21] Philip Waller's inclusion of London in his study on English Towns and Cities 'require[d] no lengthy defence' on the grounds of its scale. He has shown that London's population was on an upward trend, reaching a little over four and half million by 1901 with a slight decrease by the time of the 1911 census. Waller, P.J. 1983. *Town, City and Nation. England 1850–1914*. Oxford: Clarendon Press: 24, 45. See also Fraser, Derek. 1976. *Urban Politics in Victorian England*. Atlantic Highlands, NJ: Leicester University Press. Fraser, Derek, 1979. *Power and Authority in the Victorian City*. Oxford: Basil Blackwell. Fraser, Derek, ed. 1982. *Municipal Reform and the Industrial City*. New York: Leicester University Press.

than that of Scotland, Ireland, Switzerland and Norway.[22] The London Municipal Society [LMS], a Conservative-supporting pressure group, proudly boasted that by 1913 the Council's expenditure was exceeding that of a long list of countries that included Denmark, Norway, Greece and Switzerland. 'The magnitude of London County's Council's expenditure in itself' was, they boasted, 'sufficient to prove conclusively that there are scarcely any cities in the world which for the purpose of local government are in any sense comparable to London and certainly none in any part of the United Kingdom.[23] At the heart of this was London's place in the world. Jonathan Schneer describes it neatly as the nexus of Empire; the crossroad of people, things and attitudes.[24] Significantly too, as Waller points out, the dimensions and organisation of LCC meant something very different to the other administrative bodies such as the Metropolitan Board of Works [MBW], established in 1855 and the square mile of the City Corporation.[25]

More specifically, this spatial and political modelling and understanding of London was to impact on asylums policy and practice, and that included an enumeration of the task at hand. Like other County Councils, LCC had inherited the responsibility for the management of asylums from the County Justices and, in line with the LGA, had appointed an Asylums Committee for that purpose.[26] The 'mere scope' of this Committee's work, explained the *Daily Chronicle*, was 'immense' and it is easy to see why. With five asylums under its charge and another in the course of construction, the Committee was responsible for 11,000–12,000 patients and 1300 officers. There was, the article explained, no other authority in the world responsible for such numbers and it was little wonder that its duties 'afflict[ed] the nerves and trie[d] the temper' of its members.[27] Members of the MAB, the body appointed

[22] London School of Economics (Hereafter LSE), JS/57–60. c.1907. *Our London! What London Is and How It Is Governed*. London: Morning Leader Pamphlet Department.

[23] Guildhall Library (Hereafter GL), LMS110. 1913. *London County Council, Election 1913, Facts and Arguments*. London: London Municipal Society: 4.

[24] Schneer, Jonathan. 1999. *London 1900: The Imperial Metropolis*. New Haven: Yale University Press: 39.

[25] Waller, *Town, City and Nation*: 25.

[26] Local Government Act, 51 and 52, Vict., c.41., s.3 and s.86. Legislation.Gov.Uk. http://www.legislation.gov.uk/ukpga/Vict/51-52/41/enacted. Accessed 4 July 2019.

[27] *Daily Chronicle*. 1895. The Council and the Asylums: For Sick Minds and Bodies. *New London: Her parliament and Its work*. London: Edward Lloyd Limited: 50.

in 1867 to manage London's non-able bodied paupers, may have quibbled over numbers across its institutional services as a whole, but the evidence suggests the average number resident in its mental institutions was 'only' 5952 in 1899.[28] By contrast, estimates at the time suggested that LCC was responsible for over a fifth of all pauper lunatics in England and Wales and by 1913, the number of LCC's mental institutions had doubled and, so too, almost, had its patient population.[29]

LCC, Its Asylums and Historiographies

LCC's asylums were not the only places where lunatics in and around London were sent but the numbers straightforwardly challenge any implication that Bethlem had somehow become synonymous with the treatment of the capital's insane population.[30] Given the 'immensity' of its responsibility, coupled with such prodigious growth in a relatively short space of time, it is surprising that studies of LCC and its asylums policy have been largely overlooked. While one LCC anniversary publication wrote of 'the expenditure of millions of pounds of public money' and of the improvements in buildings and care, David Cochrane's short but useful chapter, was, for a long time, the only substantive modern analysis.[31] Other authors have used indicative data from the post-1888 period to inform broader or more general studies, or to compare and contrast data from their own more focussed research. As Mathew Thomson pointed out some time ago, 'such neglect would be justified

[28] Ayers, *England's First State Hospitals*: 324. See also Eastoe, Stephanie. 2017. Idiocy, Imbecility and Society.

[29] Anon. 1900. London Lunacy. *Journal of Mental Science*. Archive.org. https://archive.org/stream/journalmentalsc05assogoog#page/n141/mode/2up/search/%22london+county+council%22. Accessed 4 July 2019. Bibby, George H. 1896. *The Planning of Lunatic Asylums*. London: Bradley T. Batsford: 55. Harris, Percy. 1913. *London and Its Government*. London: J.M. Dent and Sons: 82.

[30] Arnold, Catharine. 2008. *Bedlam: London and Its Mad*. London: Simon and Schuster. Chambers, Paul. *Bedlam: London's Hospital for the Mad*. Birmingham: Ian Allan Publishing. Research on the origins of patients in the seventeenth century has shown that it was indeed a predominantly a 'local' institution. Andrews, Jonathan, Briggs, Asa, Porter, Roy, Tucker, Penny and Waddington, Keir. 2013. *The History of Bethlem*. London: Routledge.

[31] London County Council. 1949. *LCC Hospitals, A Retrospect*. London: Staples Press: 96. Cochrane, Humane, Economical and Medically Wise: 256.

if mental health care was a peripheral and insubstantial sector, but it was not'.[32] Thomson's article, even now, remains one of only a handful of studies to explore LCC and its responses to mental health in any great detail but his focus was primarily on its responses to mental deficiency.[33]

Moreover, there remains a continued oversight of the work of the Council and its Asylums Committee and this includes those with interests in local government, London, and its politics. Both Harold J. Laski *et al's Century of Municipal Progress* and K.B Smellie's *History of Local Government* included some details of the MAB and, while Susan Pennybacker's study of LCC included a section on its 'appetite for managing other people's lives', any references to the Asylums Committee were absent.[34] Similarly, Andrew Saint's edited collection, published to coincide with LCC's one-hundredth anniversary included a chapter on general hospital provision but this did not extend to any detailed analysis of the development of its mental health services.[35] Even Roy Porter's social history of London, which took its inspiration from H.J Dyos's study of Victorian Camberwell, neglected to look at this in any detail. The omission in this case seems unusual given Porter's well-known interest in and seminal contributions to the histories of 'madness' but Dyos's work, described as an 'inspiration' by Porter, is particularly important here.[36] The steps from his study of Victorian London (Camberwell) to the publication of *The Study of Urban History* have been cited as being influential in the 'resurgence of interest in urban history'.[37] Indeed, Dyos

[32] Thomson, Mathew. 1993. Social Policy and the Management of the Problem of Mental Deficiency in Inter-war London. *London Journal* 18: 129–42, 130.

[33] This covered 'the so-called idiots, imbeciles and the feeble-minded who were administratively divided from the mentally ill by the 1913 Mental Deficiency: 130. See also Thomson, Mathew. 1998. *The Problem of Mental Deficiency, Eugenics, Democracy and Social Policy in Britain c.1870–1959*. Oxford: Clarendon Press.

[34] Laski, Harold J., Jennings, W. Ivor and Robson, William, eds. 1935. *A Century of Municipal Progress: The Last Hundred Years*. London: George Allen & Unwin Ltd. Smellie, *A History of Local Government*. Pennybacker, Susan. 1995. *A Vision for London, 1889–1914: Labour Everyday Life and the LCC Experiment*. London: Routledge.

[35] See, for example, Sheldrake, John. 1989. The LCC Hospital Service. In *Politics and the People of London: The London County Council 1889–1965*, ed. Andrew Saint, 187–98. London: Hambledon Press.

[36] Porter, *London, A Social History*: 10–11.

[37] Young and Garside, *Metropolitan London, Politics and Urban Change*: 1.

described the latter as having 'put British urban history on the map'[38] but while urban historians too have cast their gaze over the development of London's other services—including those editions edited by Dyos before his death in 1978—consideration of the impact of London's mental health policies is also absent.[39]

Overall, LCC's Asylums' policy has represented a blind spot for historians with a range of interests that include London, mental health politics and policy, and urban and local governance more generally. Just as the story of London and LCC is absent from the histories of mental health, so too is the story of mental health absent from the stories of London and LCC. In terms of the historiography of madness, this can be explained, in part at least, by the 'convenience' of archive collections which are often centred around individual institutions.[40] Beyond this convenience, however, there have been shifts in the focus of studies to consider the impact of mental health policies on the people who lived with their consequences, primarily patients and their families. Some of this was in response to Michel Foucault's *Madness and Civilisation* in which he had challenged the Whiggish and progressive histories of psychiatry which were often written by (former) doctors. Instead, Foucault saw the development of asylums as an extensions of bourgeois morality, operating as systems of surveillance and control.[41] These were themes developed by Andrew Scull, whose own *Museums of Madness* has been described as 'arguably the most influential monograph on the history of psychiatry in Britain'.[42] Scull commented that those writing in the 1960s were influenced by the contemporary disenchantment with institutionalisation that led to a 'portrait, which amounted to a virtual mirror

[38]Unnamed reviewer cited in H.J. Dyos's foreword to Hennock, E.P. 1973. *Fit and Proper Persons: Ideal and Reality in Nineteenth Century Urban Government.* London: Edward Arnold: vii. For further analysis of the impact of Dyos see Cannadine, David and Reeder, David, eds. 1982. *Exploring the Urban Past, Essays in Urban History by H.J. Dyos.* Cambridge: Cambridge. University Press.

[39]Wohl, A.S. 1977. *The Eternal Slum: Housing and Social Policy in Victorian London, Studies in Urban History 5.* London: Edward Arnold. Young and Garside, *Metropolitan London, Politics and Urban Change.*

[40]Bartlett, Peter and Wright, David. 1999. Community Care and Its Antecedents. In *Outside the Walls of the Asylum*, eds. Peter Bartlett and David Wright, 1–18. London: Athlone: 2–3.

[41]Foucault, Michel. 1991 (1967). *Madness and Civilization.* London: Routledge: 227.

[42]Bartlett and Wright, Community Care and Its Antecedents: 1.

image of the old Whiggish picture' and instead sought to explain the origins and growth of asylums in more detail.[43] Here, he drew connections between a maturing market economy, a declining tolerance of kin, unwilling or unable to care for family members, and a corresponding growth and dominance of the medical professions, which, via their 'ownership' of the definitions and treatments of madness saw a growth in the numbers of those identified as mentally ill.

In the early 1980s, Roy Porter encouraged scholars to better understand patient-doctor roles in the past and get 'inside the heads of the "mad"' while Michael Ignatieff warned in 1983 of the 'dry as dust narratives' of by-gone bureaucratic battles.[44] Ignatieff's warnings were directed at those studies that failed to include the interrelations between asylums and the world beyond its walls. This helps to explain why, as Melling et al. point out, 'there is now much more scepticism about the ideological power of psychiatric physicians'.[45] This is not to say that an understanding of the political landscape has been ignored altogether but while the politics of provision in the nineteenth century is well served in the historiography, it is only relatively recently that there have been attempts to understand how this was impacted by the 1888 LGA.

Instead, there has been an understandable assumption that the LGA was less important than the 1890 Lunacy Act which, in Section 169, 're-enacted' the provisions of the LGA, and re-iterated the power of the County Councils to administer asylums.[46] As Melling and Forsythe point out, 'we still know far more about the formative years of the county

[43] Scull, Andrew. 1979. *Museums of Madness*. London: Allen Lane: 256.

[44] Ignatieff, Michael. 1983. Total Institutions and Working Classes: A Review Essay. *History Workshop Journal* 15: 167–73, 168.

[45] Much of this analysis focusses on the role of families in their role as carers and in the decisions taken both to send individuals to institutions and, in many cases, take them back. See for example Melling, Joseph, Adair, Richard and Forsythe, Bill. 1997. A Proper Lunatic for Two Years: Pauper Lunatic Children in Victorian and Edwardian England. Child Admissions to the Devon County Asylum, 1845–1914. *Journal* of Social History 31:2: 371–405, 393. Wright David. 1997. Getting Out of the Asylum: Understanding the Confinement of the Insane in the Nineteenth Century. *Social History of Medicine* 10: 137–55. Walton, John. 1985. Casting Out and Bringing Back in Victorian England: Pauper Lunatics, 1840–70. In *The Anatomy of Madness, Vol. II, Institutions and Society*, eds. W.F. Bynum, Roy Porter and Michael Shepherd, 132–46. London: Tavistock Publications.

[46] London Metropolitan Archives (Hereafter LMA), LCC/CL/PH/01/273, Procedure and Precedent book, 1890–1910.

asylums after the 1845 legislation than the period which immediately preceded and followed the law of 1890'.[47] The reference here is to the 1890 Lunacy Act which introduced new guidance on the reception of lunatics into asylums following years of concerns about the wrongful confinement of 'sane' individuals. Given the interest in the histories of mental health policies, the focus on 1890, and what Kathleen Jones dubbed the 'triumph of legalism',[48] this is understandable but, in both cases, there is a recognition that the responses to the problems of lunacy in the 1890s are still there to be explored. Indeed, Turner et al. have asked if,

> …the copious records of the Victorian and Edwardian civil service [could] yield a more nuanced account of the interaction of laymen, professionals, politicians and officials in the 'triumph of legalism' in the 1890 Lunacy Act or the more contestable triumph of eugenic thought in the 1913 Mental Deficiency Act, and the institutional changes which followed those pieces of legislation?[49]

Clearly, a study of the post-1888 landscape, rather than just the period that followed the 1890 Act, is timely and allows for an understanding of how lunacy legislation was interpreted and managed on a local level. This is important, not least because until the introduction of the National Health Service [NHS] in 1948, it was local authorities that were responsible for the provision of mental health services.

London and Its Politics

Early histories of urban politics focussed on what might be described as the northern powerhouses of Leeds, Manchester and Liverpool but London was different from all of these places. For one thing it was bigger but it attracted a 'degree of publicity unprecedented in British municipal history and attracted a cluster of celebrity councillors rare in local government'.[50] On the former point, this was certainly how *The*

[47] Melling and Forsythe, *The Politics of Madness:* 55.

[48] Jones, Kathleen, 1960, *Mental Health and Social Policy, 1845–1959*. London: Routledge and Kegan Paul: 7–42.

[49] Turner et al. The History of Mental Health Services in Modern England: 623.

[50] Davies, John. 1989. The Progressive Council, 1889–1907. In *Politics and the People*, ed. Saint, 27–48: 27.

Times saw it, reporting on LCC's elections and no other county authority but it did so in terms of its understanding of political allegiances.[51] At the outset, the hopes of nineteenth-century local government reformers had been for a non-partisan government acting solely in London's interests. The expectation was that candidates for the new council would rise above petty rivalries and, it has been argued, the first election was conducted on non-party lines against a slogan of 'No politics in municipal affairs'.[52] In the context of local politics in this period, the absence of organised political parties and allegiances was not that unusual.[53] Dunbabin has shown that in at least fourteen counties, the effect of political allegiances on results was absent or rare and this could change over time.[54] In Lancashire, for example, only 38.1% of divisions were contested in 1889 and this number dropped to 1.9% in 1907.[55] In London, by contrast, while many of the new Council's candidates appealed to the electorate on the grounds they were 'Municipal Reformers', they soon organised around two groups of Moderates and Progressives.[56]

John Davies has argued that that most of those returned in 1889 were party candidates but the local prominence of individuals could bring about the success at the ballot or, indeed, an offer from both parties to be their representative on election day.[57] Nevertheless, the *South London Press,* estimated that only six of the 36 candidates in south London were 'untainted by party affiliation' while the *Evening News* published a list of Conservative candidates encouraging its readers to vote on party

[51] Dunbabin, J.P.D. 1965. Expectations of the New County Councils, and Their Realization. *Historical Journal* 8:3: 353–79, 375.

[52] Smellie, *A History of Local Government:* 179. See also Pennybacker, Susan. 1989. The Millennium by Return of Post. Reconsidering London Progressivism, 1889–1907. In *Metropolis London, Histories and Representations Since 1800*, eds. David Feldman and Gareth Stedman Jones, 129–62. London: Routledge: 132.

[53] Keith-Lucas, Bryan and Richards, Peter G. 1978. *A History of Local Government in the Twentieth Century.* London: George Allen and Unwin: 111.

[54] Dunbabin, Expectations of the New County Councils: 353.

[55] Hayes, Lancashire Public Asylum Provision: 89.

[56] LMA, ACC/1632/001, Minutes of the Progressist [sic] Party of the London County Council, 1890–1895. Young, Ken. 1975. *Local Politics and the Rise of Party. The London Municipal Society and the Conservative Intervention in Local Elections, 1894–1963.* Leicester: Leicester University Press: 38.

[57] Davies, The Progressive Council, 1889–1907: 30–31.

lines 'wherever this is possible'.[58] Ken Young describes the Moderates as 'clearly aligned with the Conservative Party, while the Progressives included all shades of Liberal, from staid Liberal Unionist to Fabian "permeator"'.[59] In both cases, the breadth of opinion represented within these groups has been described as 'heterogeneous' meaning that the story of LCC cannot be told straightforwardly in party outline.[60] Similarly, Shane Ewen's study of the politics of policing in the Midlands shows that the prevalence of sub-committees further diluted any partisan influences on policy making.[61]

Nevertheless, London County Council elections were held triennially and, unlike other councils, all of the 118 councillors had to stand down at the same time. This meant that the whole council was subject to a complete change every three years.[62] In turn, the councillors elected nineteen aldermen who each served for a term of six years.[63] These nineteen individuals represented an approximate sixth of the Council, rather than the third that was the case in other local authorities.[64] As Table 1.2 shows, the appointment of Aldermen could be decisive, as it was in 1895, and this meant that the Progressives won the first six triennial elections, losing to the Moderates in 1907, who by this time had rebranded themselves as Municipal Reformers. It is worth pointing out at this stage, that other sources offer different figures for those presented in Table 1.2.[65] Usually, 1895 is seen as a 'dead heat' with both parties returning 59 candidates each and this and the appointment of aldermen

[58] Windscheffel, Alex. 2007. *Popular Conservatism in London, 1868–1906*. Woodbridge: Boydell Press: 141.

[59] Young, *Local Politics and the Rise of Party*: 39.

[60] Waller, *Town, City and Nation*: 60.

[61] Ewen, Shane. 2009. Policing Party Politics in the Midlands, c.1900–1938. In *Urban Politics and Space in the Nineteenth and Twentieth Centuries, Regional Perspectives*, ed. B. Doyle, 64–79. Newcastle: Cambridge Scholars Publishing: 72.

[62] Hasluck, E.L. 1948. *Local Government in England*. Cambridge: Cambridge University Press: 166.

[63] Ball, Michael and Sunderland, David. 2001. *An Economic History of London, 1800–1914*. London: Routledge: 409.

[64] Wilson, *The State: Elements of Historical and Practical Politics*: 436.

[65] See for example, GL, PAM 3462. 1911. Sixteenth Annual Report of the London Reform Union for 1910. London: London Reform Union. Butler, David and Butler, Gareth. 2011. *British Political Facts*. Basingstoke: Palgrave Macmillan: 516.

Table 1.2 Party representation on LCC, 1899–1913[a]

	Progressive		*Moderate/MR*		*Independent*	*Labour*
Year	*Councillors*	*Aldermen*	*Councillors*	*Aldermen*	*Councillors (C) and Aldermen (A)*	*Councillors (C) and Aldermen (A)*
1889	73	18	45	1		
1892	83	17	35	2		
1895	58	13	59	6	1 (C)	
1898	70	13	48	6		
1901	87	14	31	5		
1904	83	15	35	4		
1907	38	9	79	10	1 (C)	
1910	55	2	60	15	2 (A)	3 (C)
1913	50	3	67	14	2 (A)	1 (C)

[a]Gibbon, Gwilym and Bell, Reginald W. 1939. *History of the London County Council*. London: Macmillan and Co.: 677

is, perhaps, indicative of how difficult it is to align some candidates to specific party allegiances.

Despite these caveats, contemporaries often focussed on what they saw as pejorative common denominators. Writing just after the first election, held on 17 January 1889, in which the Progressives won 73 of the 118 seats, *The Times* proclaimed that 'the majority appeared desirous of throwing off the non-political mask and of proclaiming their adherence to the Radical Party'.[66] Indeed, it was the Progressive majority that allowed the party to secure 18 of the 19 aldermen on 'their ticket'. Packing the aldermanic bench in this way drew the condemnation of *The Times* which described it as an 'aggressive and uncompromising tactic'.[67] The LMS wrote of an LCC that had been founded by the Conservative Party and 'captured' by the Progressive Party. The immediate point being that the original Bill to create County Councils had been introduced by Gladstone's Liberals in 1886 but had been re-introduced and passed by Lords Salisbury's Conservatives in 1888.[68] It was, according to

[66]Smellie, *A History of Local Government*: 179.

[67]Haward, Harry. 1932. *The London County Council from Within: Forty Years Official Recollections*. London: Chapman and Hall: 19.

[68]Keith-Lucas, *English Local Government in the Nineteenth and Twentieth Centuries*: 22.

the LMS, the Progressives who had said '"We won't have any politics in these Municipal matters" .... And we poor innocents fell into the trap'.[69]

For Davies, such bi-partisan rhetoric deflected attention away from intra-party differences that might have challenged party unity.[70] More importantly, while the municipalities in the provinces saw much less political division after elections, most of those who served in LCC saw their work as intrinsically political.[71] Thus, while the scale of the new London was there for all to see, the working of the Council, its achievements and the pride in them was coloured by the politics the day. While the fifth Earl of Rosebery, the first Progressive Chairman of the LCC and the LMS may have shared a pride in the new London and its place on the world map, their politics were very different and it is important to recognise that how London was governed was still subject to debate and disagreement in the years after 1888.[72]

To the scholars of Progressive and Moderate histories this much is obvious but there is still a sense that the Asylums Committee was divorced from this new political reality. Like all of LCC's committees, it drew its membership from the elected councillors and made regular reports to the Council, which were acknowledged and debated in the Council chamber. Despite this, there were suggestions in some quarters that the work of the Committee was somehow hidden away. 'The Asylums Committee of the Council comes little before the public', wrote one commentator, while another noted that the privacy demanded by the delicate work of the Committee meant 'that its work must go on quite unrecognised by the public'.[73] Then there were the demands of new and existing lunacy legislation which meant that the new Council, before and after the introduction of the 1890 Lunacy Act, had a statutory responsibility to build and maintain asylums. It is this that probably

[69] GL, LMS127, London Municipal Pamphlets and Leaflets, 1909. The Progress of Municipal Reform. Municipal Reform Pamphlet: 47.

[70] Davies, The Progressive Council, 1889–1907: 37.

[71] Ibid: 27.

[72] In 1899 a new London Government Act was passed which created 28 metropolitan boroughs designed to act as a 'political and administrative counterweight to the possible prestige of a reforming' LCC. Smellie, *A History of Local Government* London: 178. See also Davies, Local Government 1850–1920: 51.

[73] Anon. 1892. *Three Years Good Work for the People*. London: National Press Agency: 19. Harris, *London and Its Government:* 82.

explained why, in London at least, the *Star* claimed it was the Asylums Committee 'over which the Council [had] least control'.[74]

Within this we can see evidence of a non-political civic pride in London and it is not hard to find such examples when it came to its mental health provision. On the elevation of John McDougall to the Chairmanship of LCC, Frederick A. McKenzie of the *Daily Mail* concluded that 'the work of necessity remains largely out of sight but none who know the facts that the monster asylums around London are now in many ways the Council's greatest glory'.[75] Such star-billing for asylums was not necessarily representative but it does reflect what others have indicated was a cross-party pride in both mental and general health services.[76] Latterly, however, the Labour Party in London was apt to make political capital of medical provision in the 1920s and 1930s, claiming that once in power it would make London's hospitals the best in the world.[77] More recently, at the very end of her book on gender and class in London's asylums, Louise Hide explained it was hard to understand how one anonymous commentator could describe the work of LCC as 'the most brilliant evidence of the dawn of a new era in the treatment of London Lunacy'.[78] 'Which particular prism', she asked, 'was he looking through?'[79] The answer to this, might be found in the politics of the post-1888 period and the fact that LCC 'was a brilliant opportunity to practice democracy in the new form'.[80]

Understanding these connections allows for an opportunity to build on the existing work on London's asylums and also on the forays into the *fin de siècle* political administration of institutions more broadly. In addition, while Michel Foucault has loomed large in the histories of psychiatry, an important criticism has been that there is an absence

[74] Anon, *Three Years Good Work for the People*: 19.

[75] Mckenzie, Fred A. 1902. The Triumph of Mr McDougall. *Daily Mail*, 12 March.

[76] Thomson, Social Policy and the Management of the Problem of Mental Deficiency: 137–8. Stewart, John. 2005. The Finest Municipal Hospital Service in the World? Contemporary Perceptions of the London County Council's Hospital Provision, 1929–39. *Urban History* 32: 327–44, 330–1.

[77] Stewart, The Finest Municipal Hospital Service in the world?: 332.

[78] Hide, *Gender and Class in English Asylums*: 180.

[79] Ibid: 180.

[80] Pennybacker, The Millennium by Return of Post: 130.

of institutional politics in the histories he presented.[81] This book, by contrast, poses questions about the impact of ideologies, interests, individuals and allegiances on asylum administration, how these were represented during elections, how they impacted on asylum management, and what happened with changes to majority political administrations.

Methodology and the Language of Lunacy Administration

As Porter pointed out, LCC's history is intricate and the struggles of its political cliques 'would fill volumes'.[82] A forensic analysis of the records of individual institutions would do little to shed light on their impact on the management of asylums. Instead, the starting point for this research has been on the top level of management, and the Committee and sub-committee records of what might described as 'head office'. This does not mean that institutional responses have been ignored all together, but the chapters that follow reflect the Council's overall control of, and impact on, London's burgeoning network of asylums. This new way of looking at mental health in this period has included analysis of political tracts, election campaign materials, party leaflets and propaganda, satirical cartoons, and newspaper leaders. Often missed in the stories of the development of services, each of these helps to illuminate the previously opaque links between political debates and disagreements, and the direction of policy. Included also, is some quantitative analysis of the impact of political economy on decision-making processes and propaganda.

This shift in the gaze has been a challenge, not least because the extant records are vast and, in a bid to manage the business of lunacy in the capital, a large number of sub-committees were created. For these reasons, I cannot claim to cover every single aspect of LCC's asylums administration but I hope that the choices I have made reflect the key issues at the time, and also build on and extend the work of other scholars who have gone before me. To achieve this, the chronology of this book will run from 1888 through to 1914, which broadly coincides

[81] Mellling, Joseph. 1999. Accommodating Madness. New Research in the Social History of Insanity and Institutions. In *Insanity, Institutions and Society, 1800–1914*, eds. J. Melling and B. Forsythe, 1–30. Abingdon: Routledge: 3.

[82] Porter, *London, A Social History:* 333.

with Hide's study of two of the hospitals in the Epsom Cluster. In making these choices, an obvious omission is the discussions that took place within the Council that led up to the passing of the 1913 Mental Deficiency Act but this already been explored in some detail in the excellent work of Mathew Thomson. Ending, the period in 1914 also misses the impact of the Great War but this remains an opportunity for another time. Given the period under consideration, this monograph will include archaic language which, on the face of it, may seem pejorative. However, the use of terms such as 'madness', 'lunatic', 'imbecile' and 'idiot' reflect the nomenclature of the time and are included only for the purposes of accuracy.

Chapter Themes and Structure

As a starting point, Chapter 2 will explore the immediate impact of the LGA in terms of the organisation and administration of asylums under the new County Council. This will necessarily mean an analysis of the politics of the new Council and how that was reflected in the composition of both it and its committees. In simple terms, LCC had three distinct eras of party dominance—that is, by the Progressives (Liberals) and others on the left from 1889 to 1907; by the Moderate Party, rebranded after 1906 as Municipal Reformers; and then the Labour party after 1934; the latter of which is beyond the scope of this monograph.[83] In each case, the rhetoric behind the successes and criticisms of the Council was based on political allegiances and this chapter will unpick how and why these related to the Asylums Committee. And, while this book does not focus on patients per se, it does consider how political decision-making impacted on their lives.

Moreover, it will build on the work of Cochrane and others to consider in more detail the individual membership of the Asylums Committee. For Laski, a professor at the London School of Economics and experienced political activist, it was the committee system adopted by local authorities after the Municipal Corporations Act of 1835 that became 'the pivot of the system of local government'.[84] Due to

[83] Ibid.

[84] Laski, Harold. 1935. The Committee System in Local Government. In *A Century of Municipal Progress: The Last Hundred Years*, eds. Harold J. Laski, W. Ivor Jennings and William Robson, 82–108. London: George Allen & Unwin Ltd.: 82.

the size of local authorities and the scope of their business, Councils had become report-receiving bodies, 'which, like Parliament in relation to the Cabinet, may criticise, protest or encourage, but cannot hope to control the details of the policy pursued'.[85] With Laski concluding that it was the committees where Council policy was made, this chapter will consider how the Asylums Committee worked in practice and which Councillors were pivotal to its operation.

The role of councillors and committees will be reiterated in Chapter 3 but the analysis will be extended into discussions around finance. While this has been a feature of studies of general health, it is only recently that there has been any attempts to understand this in relation to mental health in the period.[86] In Devon, it has been argued that the County Council's Finance committee was so powerful, that the Asylum Visiting Committee became increasingly answerable to it'.[87] This book builds on that analysis to consider how and why, in London at least, this relationship was coloured by its politics. In addition, it will reflect on how apparent concerns over spending on asylum infrastructure and operations were influenced by broader political views on public spending and private finance linked to the Progressive and Moderate visions of government generally, and the government of London more specifically. This will necessarily go beyond a study of interactions between committees, to demonstrate the role of asylums in election campaigns, and the links made by the parties to the wider electorate.

Chapter 4 will explain how Councillors and the medical profession sought to push the agenda in terms of the development of scientific and extra-institutional approaches to deal with London's burgeoning lunatic population. The decades around 1900, in particular, are seen as a crucial in the development of health care services and are often portrayed as a time of pessimism for the lunatic population with asylums degenerating into custodial warehouses or 'museums of madness'.[88] Moreover,

[85] Laski, The Committee System in Local Government: 82.

[86] For studies of general health see Gorsky Martin and Sheard, Sally, eds. 2006. *Financing Medicine. The British Experience Since 1750.* London: Routledge.

[87] Forsythe, Melling and Adair, The Politics of Lunacy: 83. Melling and Forsythe, *The Politics of* Madness: 42.

[88] Roelcke, Volker, Weindling, Paul J. and Westwood, Louise. 2010. *International Relations in Psychiatry.* Rochester: University of Rochester Press: 1. See Scull, Most Solitary. Scull, Andrew. 2015. *Madness in Civilization; A Cultural History of Insanity from the Bible to Freud, from the Madhouse to Modern Medicine.* London: Thames and Hudson.

Foucault saw the 'political critique' of eighteenth-century structures emphasising new models of confinement, rather than philanthropic or medical attention for the insane.[89] The political critique offered in this case was very different to the one under review here but this chapter considers the attempts to restrict long-term confinement and the reasons behind them. Recent studies have re-invigorated the study of asylum science but have tended to focus on institutions in general and on the West Riding Asylum in the north of England in particular.[90] This chapter will extend that analysis to London and contrast three key initiatives that attempted to arrest the rising numbers of patients, viz; A Hospital for the Insane, Receiving Houses divorced from the Poor Laws, and a Pathology Laboratory; and place the politics of the new Council at the heart of it. This chapter will not dismiss the importance of medical and expert opinion outright but it will consider the traction of 'insider' and 'outsider' experts in relation to committee membership and political allegiances.

Chapter 5 analyses London's role within long-standing international asylum and medical networks but also its reputation as the world's leading city and a new municipal behemoth. In doing so, it builds on studies of that have sought to uncover municipal networks and the sharing of ideas across transnational borders.[91] In particular, it will contrast London's status as the centre of Great Britain, of Empire and even of the world with its status as a newcomer in terms of its institutional management of madness, and consider the tensions between medical staff and lay councillors. Moreover, it will explain how notions of civic pride were informed by politics and, as a corollary how individuals, council committees and the Council itself impacted on transnational dialogues. Drawing on evidence from continental Europe and the USA, it will argue that much of the rhetoric behind LCC's status as an administrator of

[89] Foucault, *Madness and Civilization:* 227.

[90] Wallis, J. 2015. *Investigating the body in the Victorian Asylum*. London: Palgrave. Finn, M.A. 2012. The West Riding Asylum and the Making of Modern Brain Sciences in the Nineteenth Century. Unpublished PhD thesis, University of Leeds.

[91] Saunier, Pierre-Yves. 2008. Introduction: Global City, Take 2: A View from Urban History. In *Another Global City: Historical Explorations into the Transnational Municipal Moment 1850–2000*, eds. P.-Y. Saunier and S. Ewen, 1–18. Basingstoke: Palgrave Macmillan: 4.

asylums policy rested with its status as a world city, rather than its innovative practice in dealing with its rising lunatic population.

Chapter 6 is titled the 'Politics of Difference' and it focusses very much on LCC's responses to foreign nationals. Angela McCarthy and Catharine Coleborne argued recently that migration 'ought to be considered as a focus of a new generation of inquiries into mental health and institutional confinement'.[92] Significantly, their edited collection includes questions surrounding ethnicity and institutional confinement which, in turn 'contributes more broadly to the field of migration studies.[93] The responses to this issue have tended to be framed in medical terms but this chapter considers the impact of the Council chamber and the role of wider imperial policies on London's strategies for dealing with the issue. In particular, it will consider how the issue of 'Home Rule for London' and the introduction of the Aliens Act in 1905 impacted on the management of madness and how that influenced the Asylums Committees' relationship with other key stakeholders, including the capital's various Poor Law Unions. It will also consider how views about aged patents and also foreign nationals housed in asylums were further affected by Progressive and Moderate allegiances and how policies to deal with them were affected by majorities in the council chambers and in key committees. Ultimately, this chapter will show that the treatment of vulnerable migrant groups was influenced by wider political visions for London and Great Britain. A central feature of each of these chapters will be the change in party-political administration that followed the Municipal Reformers' success in the 1907 election.

These chapters cover themes that are important in recent and current debates in the histories of madness and psychiatry, but eagle-eyed readers will have noticed that a 'Politics of the Patients' chapter is absent. This is a deliberate choice based on the lack of voice that patients had in challenging the political rhetoric of the time. While the parties may have claimed to speak or advocate for them, their experiences were co-opted for political purposes and, instead, it has made sense for their responses to feature across the chapters more broadly where appropriate. Equally, London County Council was dominated by men and, without repeating

[92] McCarthy, Angela and Coleborne, Catharine. 2012. Mental Health, Migration and Ethnicity. In *Migration, Ethnicity and Mental Health, International Perspectives 1840–2010*, eds. Angela McCarthy and Catharine Coleborne, 1–14. New York: Routledge: 2.

[93] McCarthy and Coleborne, Mental Health, Migration and Ethnicity: 2.

the themes of Louise Hide's work on London's Asylums, it has been challenge to tease out what might later prove to be the hidden histories of women in relation to the management of madness. Having said that, there have been attempts to consider this more fully where possible and this includes the targeting of female voters in post-1888 elections.

Overall, a study of London speaks to more than a history of the capital, it helps illuminate the wider period and the concluding chapter represents London's mental health policy—not just as a series of internecine disputes but as one that was framed by themes of politics and civic pride. Across the whole period, the aim is to shift the gaze away from the capital's individual institutions to demonstrate the impact of politics on mental health policies. In doing so, the aim is to recast the capital's asylums as sites of political discourse and debate but rather than provide a 'dry as dust' institutional and insular narrative, show their wider connections to ideologies relating to welfare, intervention, and Imperial London's place in an increasingly globalised world. Finally, this book demonstrates the importance of London to our longer-term understanding of the impact of politics on mental health policies and procedures. By shifting the gaze it looks forward to a period in the later twentieth century when views about the role of mental health care became more firmly entrenched in party-political rhetoric.

CHAPTER 2

The Politics of Administration

Introduction

In 1895, Sidney Webb wrote of the 'silent devotion of the Asylums Committee, which never gets into the papers at all'.[1] Even if that was true at that stage, within a few years events at LCC asylums were headline news and they were to call into question the apparent success of the new administration. A scandal about the theft of provisions from the Horton Asylum in 1904 followed a huge fire at the Colney Hatch Asylum in the previous year, which had claimed the lives of 52 people. Thomas Bewley argues that these incidents highlighted concerns about 'the suitability of the actual asylum buildings and the probity of the management'.[2] The problems lay, according to Bewley, with 'the method of management in London County Council Asylums. It differed from that in other county asylums where the medical superintendent was fully in charge of all staff and had ultimate authority in the running of the establishment. In the city [*sic*] council institutions, medical superintendents had no such authority and could be undermined by

[1] Webb, Sidney. 1895. *The Work of the London County Council.* London: The London Reform Union, 1895: 5.

[2] Bewley, Thomas. 2008. *Madness to Mental Illness a History of the Royal College of Psychiatrists.* Trowbridge: Cromwell Press: 45.

R. Ellis, *London and its Asylums, 1888-1914*,
Mental Health in Historical Perspective,
https://doi.org/10.1007/978-3-030-44432-7_2

other asylum officials'.[3] There is plenty of evidence to show that, even before the introduction of the LGA, many medical superintendents did not quite have the autonomy suggested by Bewley.[4] More specifically, Hide has shown how LCC sub-committees at Bexley and Claybury were not prepared to simply rubber-stamp the demands of either of their Superintendents, Dr Robert Jones and Dr Thomas (T.E.K.) Stansfield, respectively, despite their unflinching leadership styles and their forthright opinions.[5]

Significantly, in wider studies of County Councils, it has been suggested that the committee structure created an oligarchy of chairmen with Beatrice Webb claiming it was government by a select minority.[6] Thomson too has argued that people serving in the 'bottom rung' committees had little power.[7] Beyond this, however, there is little sense of the relative powers and understanding of either the personnel involved in these Committees or their political affiliations, or how they impacted on access to and influence over decision-making processes. Melling and Forsythe point to more scrutiny of the work of the asylums committees in Devon from the County Council, which stemmed from a longer-term period of external criticism from bodies such as the Commissioners in Lunacy and Local Government Board [LGB].[8] Nevertheless, there is scope here to consider the connections across the committee structure and the elected chamber itself. Bob Hayes's short overview on Lancashire in the period after the passing of the 1888 Act is useful here. He has suggested that the stability of the political leadership, along with long-serving members of administrative staff, had much more potential to influence countywide provision than their relatively geographically and socially isolated counterparts in the medical profession, and this can be tested more fully here.[9]

[3] Ibid.

[4] Suzuki, The Politics and Ideology of Non-restraint: 2, 17. Scull, *The Most Solitary of Afflictions*: 247.

[5] Hide, *Gender and Class*: 4, 46–7.

[6] Davies, The Progressive Council, 1889–1907: 31.

[7] Thomson, Social Policy and the Management of the Problem of Mental Deficiency: 137.

[8] Melling and Bill Forsythe, *The Politics of Madness*: 42–3. Melling et al. Politics of Lunacy: 80–82.

[9] Hayes, Lancashire Public Asylum Provision: 91.

To begin with, there will be a consideration of the changes in administration and how that affected the management of London's institutions. In particular, there will be an exploration of LCC 'brand' of management, how this was represented in political terms and, as a corollary, how asylum management was used in political campaigns. Following on from this, the membership of the Asylums Committee will be unpicked. John Davies has described the 'mover and shakers' of the Council as its committee stalwarts and the aim here is to go beyond the broad catch-all term of 'Asylums Committee' to understand who the key players were and the networks in which they operated.[10] Similarly, it is important to recognise that nominations to committee chairmanships were determined by party machines and so were the posts of Chairman, Vice Chairman and Deputy Chairman of the Council itself.[11] In the final section, there will be a consideration of how wider political policies, including those related to temperance reform, impacted on the patient experience. Overall, this chapter will demonstrate the impact of key individuals and wider political views, not just on the management of the asylum, but also on its treatment regime.

The New Council and the Scale of Its Asylums Operation

It is important to recognise the different lenses through which London was viewed. 'There is no colony so distant that its children cannot see in imagination [*sic*] the lights of London glimmering across the wastes of ocean', wrote Jane Stoddart, Lord Rosebery's biographer, at the turn of the century.[12] London was the 'world's capital', the 'metropolis of the Empire' and it had to be a 'model for all her daughter cities', she proclaimed, but not everyone in those 'daughter cities', or indeed, closer to home, recognised the uncritical vision offered here.[13] For many, the model was not quite so positive and London's place at the centre of

[10] Davies, Local Government 1850–1920: 52.

[11] Ibid.

[12] Stoddart, Jane T. 1900. *The Earl of Rosebery K.G.: An Illustrated Biography*. London: Hodders and Stoughton: 94–5.

[13] Ibid.

Empire meant that it represented oppression on a grand-scale, not least in the treatment of those deemed to be mentally ill. This was a city that was riven with tensions related to its world status (see also Chapter 6) and this included many anti-imperialists in the capital who challenged the dominant and uncritical narrative of Empire.[14] Similarly, there were many deep-seated and ongoing issues closer to home that reflected a very different story. Industrial strife, including the Dock Strike of 1889, and the publication of the first volume of Booth's *Life and Labour of the People of London*, along with the maps of London's poverty in the following year, highlighted the disparities of wealth, opportunity and quality of life in the world's wealthiest city. Fears about foreign insurgents added to a volatile mix, as did the infamous Whitechapel murders, committed at the end of the same year that the LGA was passed.[15]

The focus on lunacy legislation draws the attention away from these wider issues but it was within this context that the challenge of asylums' administration very firmly sat. The disparities between London's East End and the more well-to-do boroughs in the west, only served to shine a light on what was seen as the muddle of its management. It is little wonder that in the decades before 1888, London was described as the 'worst governed city in the Empire'.[16] The immediate challenge for the Council was to develop a political and administrative infrastructure so that it might manage the capital more effectively. With the passing of the LGA, all County Councils inherited the power to administer bridges and entertainment licenses, as well as asylums from unelected bodies of County Justices.[17] In London, the new County Council also inherited the responsibility for parks, drainage and transport routes from the discredited MBW. Despite the huge list of responsibilities, it was the 'apportionment of the property, debts and liabilities' in relation to asylums provision that was described as the 'most urgent' order of business.

Following detailed negotiations with officials of the counties of Surrey, Middlesex and Kent, the nascent LCC took responsibility for four existing

[14] Schneer, *London 1900. The Imperial Metropolis.* New Haven: Yale University Press: 225–6.

[15] Walkowitz, Judith R. 1992. *City of Dreadful Delight: Narratives of Sexual Danger in Late-Victorian London*. London: Virago: 25.

[16] John Morley, cited in Walkowitz, Judith R.: 25.

[17] Inwood, Stephen. 2000. *A History of London*. London: Macmillan: 440.

County Asylums, at Banstead, Cane Hill, Colney Hatch and Hanwell, and another at Claybury which was in the course of construction. At this point, LCC decided to appoint one Asylums Committee 'for the management and control of all asylums' and, in line with the terms of the LGA, its membership was drawn from the body of elected councillors.[18] This contrasted with the situation in Lancashire, which introduced a joint board in 1891 to facilitate the purchase of provisions and in Yorkshire where a proposal for a joint Asylums Board was first made in 1912.[19]

The LGA empowered Councils with 'the provision, enlargement, maintenance, management, and visitation of and other dealings with asylums for pauper lunatics' but LCC's new administrative hierarchy brought important changes to how decision-making processes worked.[20] Under its new structure, asylum sub-committees were created, which met at, and were responsible for the individual institutional managements in each case. These mimicked the pre-1888 Visiting Committees, but, along with sub-committees created to consider specific issues such as accommodation, the appointment of new members of staff and rates of pay, they drew their memberships and delegated powers from the main Asylums Committee and reported to it.[21] In addition, there was an expectation that sub-committees would refer larger decisions up the administrative hierarchy, with the Asylums Committee retaining the right to subject them 'to any variation or alteration that it might determine as necessary'.[22] Along with the appointment of medical staff, this included the appointments of the Chaplain and the Clerk to the asylum, any alterations to any of the rules and regulations, the approval of repairs and improvements, and also the negotiation of contracts.[23]

While London may have 'lacked a county history and tradition', it could, like the other counties, draw on pre-1888 expertise during the

[18] LMA, LCC 18.6, London County Council, Minutes of Proceedings, January–December 1889, 26 February 1889.

[19] Hayes, Lancashire Public Asylum Provision: 84. British Library [Hereafter BL] *Municipal Journal*, 13 January 1912: 39.

[20] Local Government Act, 51 and 52, Vict., c.41, s.3.6.

[21] LMA, LCC 18.6, London County Council, Minutes of Proceedings, January–December 1889, 26 February 1889.

[22] LMA, LCC/CL/PH/01/276, Miscellaneous Printed Papers, Report of Sub-Committee appointed by Provisional Asylums Committee, 19 June 1889.

[23] Ibid.

transition of power.[24] Joe Melling and Bill Forysthe's ongoing study of Devon has been important here and they have shown that continued presence of County Justices on the County Council's Asylums' Visiting Committee meant that, in terms of personnel at least, 1888 hardly represented a revolutionary break.[25] These findings echo those of broader studies across the piece, which suggest that 'about half [of] the new councillors were magistrates; many of the others were their brothers or cousins'.[26] This meant that ideas and ideologies were shared in wider social networks as well as the relatively closed spaces of Council Committee rooms. In 22 of the counties, the new council Chairman had previously been the Chairman of the Quarter sessions and Keith-Lucas concludes that 'the new county councils must have looked remarkably like the old Quarter Sessions. The revolution had not taken place'.[27] By contrast, Steven Cherry's study of Norfolk's new asylums committee revealed that four of the seventeen members of the new committee had served under the previous system, providing an element, rather than a guarantee of continuity.[28]

In London, Philip Meadows Martineau, the Council's first Chairman of its new Asylums Committee, had previously served as a magistrate for the County of Middlesex and Richard Strong, his Vice Chairman, was Chairman at Cane Hill both before and after 1888.[29] Henry Hawkins' brief history of Colney Hatch also noted that the first chairman under the new regime (Mr Fletcher) had served on the former committee.[30]

[24] Jackson, *Achievement: A Short History of the LCC*: 5. Melling, J., Forsythe, B. and Adair, R. 1999. Politics of Lunacy: Central State Regulation and the Devon Pauper Lunatic Asylum, 1845–1914. In *Insanity, Institutions and Society, 1800–1914*, eds. J. Melling and B. Forsythe, 68–87. Abingdon: Routledge: 80. Cherry, Steve. 2013. *Mental Health Care in Modern England: The Norfolk Lunatic Asylum/St Andrews Hospital, 1810–1998*. Woodbridge: Boydell: 112.

[25] Melling et al., Politics of Lunacy: 80. See also Melling and Forsythe, *The Politics of Madness*: 55.

[26] Keith-Lucas, B. 1977. *English Local Government in the Nineteenth and Twentieth Centuries*. London: The Historical Association: 23.

[27] Ibid.

[28] Cherry, *Mental Health Care in Modern England*: 112.

[29] *Forty-Fourth Report of the Commissioners in Lunacy*, 1890: 218. Available at https://parlipapers.proquest.com/parlipapers. Accessed 24 July 2019.

[30] Hawkins, Rev Henry. 1901. *Some Notes on the History of the Colney Hatch Asylum, 1849–1901*. London: Potter, Batten and Davies: 9.

There is little wonder that the first reports at each asylum commended the magistrates for the maintenance of efficiency and the good order in which each institution had been handed over.[31] In their 1889 annual report, the Lunacy Commissioners, the national watchdog that had inspected the country's asylums since 1845, looked back to their past management in the hope that the new would be 'equally satisfactory'.[32]

More generally, there had been an expectation that the LGA would bring about a change in personnel. In other municipal authorities in this period there was an increase in the numbers of businessmen and labour representatives standing for election in the decades following its passing.[33] This was certainly the case in London with John Williams Benn, social reformer and radical, just one example of a self-made man who made his money in a publishing firm he founded with a partner.[34] John Burns, the radical Councillor for Battersea who was relatively well-known for his involvement in riots in 1886, the running battles with the police in Trafalgar Square, and the Dock Strikes of 1889, had previously served as apprentice engineer.[35] John McDougall, by contrast, stepped down from his role in his family's well-known flour business to seek election. In many respects, Martineau was very similar having trained as a barrister and worked in his family's sugar refining business. Despite his longer-term role in asylums administration, 1888 was cast as a turning point. In its first report to the Council, the Asylums Committee commented that its dealing with the populous portions of the old counties of Middlesex, Surrey and Kent had cast upon it 'a serious and difficult duty'.[36] In response, and with administrative power centralised to some degree in the hands of the Asylums Committee, it set about introducing uniformity across what were now metropolitan London's asylums.

[31] LMA, LCC 26.21. The First Annual Report of the Asylums Committee of the London County Council, for the year ending 31 March 1890. See also the individual reports of the Banstead, Cane Hill, Colney Hatch and Hanwell sub-committees in the same volume.

[32] *Forty-Third Report of the Commissioners in Lunacy*, 1889: 69.

[33] Dunbabin, Expectations of the New County Councils, and Their Realization: 353. Hennock, *Fit and Proper Persons*: 268.

[34] Brodie, M. 2008. Benn, Sir John Williams, first baronet. *Oxford Dictionary of National Biography*. https://www.oxforddnb.com/. Accessed 4 July 2019.

[35] Brown, Kenneth D. 2004. Burns, John Elliott. *Oxford Dictionary of National Biography*. https://www.oxforddnb.com/. Accessed 4 July 2019.

[36] LMA, LCC 26.21. The First Annual Report of the Asylums Committee of the London County Council, for the year ending 31 March 1890.

As part of a wider Council-wide programme of reform, LCC provided the Committee with a London office, first at 40 Craven Street and then at 21 Whitehall Place. Both offices were a short walk from the Council's headquarters at Spring Gardens, which were near Trafalgar Square, and they both served as the geographic centre of the new administration. When the new County Hall opened on the banks of the River Thames, asylum administrative staff took up residence on the fifth floor.[37] While the capital's asylums were in the relatively bucolic parts of north London, Essex, Kent, and later Surrey, those passing through those offices could not fail to notice its place at the heart of what was the administrative centre of, not just the nation, but also the British Empire.

The London offices allowed for a consolidation of the work of the new county in relation to what Martineau called its 'Lunacy business'.[38] From the outset, the Committee's offices became the 'gateway' into the four asylums with beds allotted to the various Poor Law Unions and parishes, depending on the space available at the individual asylums.[39] Wherever possible, vacancies at any particular asylum were given to cases which arose in the districts nearest to them but this was not always straightforward.[40] Table 2.1 shows that significant numbers of London patients were cast across England, and this national movement of 'out-county' patients was one that affected many authorities before and after the passing of the LGA.[41]

London's place within this larger national network was also reflected in the everyday logistical administrative operations needed to run the asylums. As well as administering the placing of patients, the central office served a second important function in that it became the place that was responsible for the purchase of supplies and sundries. Surplus produce cultivated at some LCC institutions was shared across the network but this could not meet all the requirements of a large and growing

[37] LMA, LCC/578, Signed Minutes, March 1912–October 1913: 19 March 1912.

[38] LMA, LCC 26.21. The First Annual Report of the Asylums Committee of the London County Council, for the year ending 31 March 1890.

[39] Ibid.

[40] Keene, H. F. 1907. *Memorandum as to the Procedure with Regard to the Admission and Discharge of Patients.* London: LCC.

[41] Ellis, Rob. 2008. The Asylum, the Poor Law and the Growth of County Asylums in Nineteenth-Century Yorkshire. *Northern History* 45:2: 279–93.

Table 2.1 LCC's 'out county' contracts for the accommodation of patients, 31 March 1891

Asylum	*Male*	*Female*	*Total*	*Date of commencement*
Gloucester	50	70	120	May 1887
Western Asylum	5	5	10	May 1887
Northampton	5	5	10	December 1888
South Weald (Essex)	25	40	65	October 1889
Exeter Borough	40	40	80	February 1890
Leicester Borough	40	40	80	March 1890
Wandsworth Asylum (Middlesex)	140	140	280	March 1890
Brookwood Asylum (Surrey)	150	200	350	March 1890
Birmingham Asylum	30	20	50	April 1890
Nottingham (Boro)	50	60	110	September 1890
Nottingham (County)	0	35	35	September 1890
South Weald (Essex)	50	0	50	December 1890
Lancaster	95	105	200	January 1891
Barming Heath (Kent)	284	366	650	January 1891
Total			2090	

Source LMA, LCC 26.31, The Report of the Asylums Committee of the London County Council for the year ended, 31 March 1891

institutional population.[42] Sample rooms were provided so the quality of goods could be tested and the scale of the purchases being made was enormous. At the Banstead Asylum alone, almost 50,000 lbs of condensed milk were consumed within one twelve-month period.[43] Tea was bought following a tender process at a fixed rate per pound and, from 1906, the Asylums Committee employed an expert tea taster who would choose the tea based on both its quality but also its suitability with each asylum's water supply. Thus, the ten asylums in 1908 (Banstead, Bexley, Claybury, Colney Hatch, Cane Hill, Hanwell, Horton, Manor, The Epileptic Colony and Long Grove) received their teas from three different suppliers.[44] One tender published in 1895 included goods that reflected international trade in this period such as cocoa, sugar, lemons,

[42]Thomson, *The Problem of Mental Deficiency*: 141.

[43]LMA, LCC/MIN/574, Signed Minutes, February 1907–February 1908, 10 December 1907.

[44]LMA, LCC/MIN/575, Signed Minutes, March 1908–February 1909, 12 May 1908.

oranges, tobacco, snuff and wines, as well as items that were sourced from closer to home. This included foodstuffs such as potatoes, carrots, butter, cheese and meats all of which it is often presumed were provided by in-house groups of patients and staff.[45]

While food was important, so too was the crockery, glassware and cutlery that was required to prepare, serve and eat it; the scales and weights that were required to measure it and the farm and gardening equipment, seeds and livestock, that helped produce it.[46] To this can be added the scientific and medical equipment, materials to clothe both patients and staff and the cleaning materials, such as soaps and turpentine to keep everyone and everything clean and tidy. With beds and bedding, carpets, and even birds and bird cages to make the asylum wards and day rooms seem homely, and the hymn books and sporting equipment to keep them occupied spiritually and physically, the list of goods coming into LCC's asylums were almost endless.[47] Of course, the choices being made here were not strictly neutral and much of the material culture making its way into London and other asylums reflected the gendered nature of their regimes. The everyday experience of men and women in these places was very different. This included the definitions and treatments of their madness but also the work and leisure activities that marked their daily routines.[48] Similarly, much of the vast stock lists emphasise the control of the everyday lives of both patients and staff; of keeping the days ordered and everyone busy.[49]

[45]Anon.1895. Contracts for Provisions and Necessaries. London County Lunatic Asylums. *The Times*, 20 September.

[46]LMA, LCC/MIN/574, Signed Minutes, February 1907–February 1908, 30 July 1907.

[47]LMA, LCC/MIN/574, Signed Minutes, February 1907–February 1908, 30 July 1907, 8 October 1907.

[48]Even within gendered categories, experiences could be very different. Hide, for example, suggests that there were differences in the ways that single, married and widowed women adjusted to life in the asylum, while Ellis has shown that participation in sporting activities was not open to all. See Hide, *Gender and Class in English Asylums* and Ellis, Rob. 2013. Asylums and Sport: Participation, Isolation and the Role of Cricket in the Treatment of the Insane. *International Journal of the History of Sport* 30: 83–101.

[49]Hamlett has shown how patients sometimes used institutional spaces and material culture for their own purposes, rather than for the purposes intended. Hamlett, *At Home in the Institution*.

By this time, asylums had become an important opportunity for businesses across the country and the purchasing power of LCC meant that its name added cachet to those it dealt with. The lock manufacturers Joseph Kaye and Sons, whose works were based at Hunslet, near Leeds and Charles and Frank Smith Limited, with works in Birmingham, both cited their work with LCC asylums in their advertisements, whereas Twyford Potteries claimed its 'practically unbreakable' closet basin was 'made to the requirements of the London County Council'.[50] The Leeds Fire Clay Company at Burmantofts near Leeds provided over 2,000,000 bricks for the Claybury Asylum—'the largest order of glazed bricks which has ever been given'.[51] An advertisement for 'Stuart's Granolithic Stone Paving' listed fifteen asylums in England and Scotland where the product 'had been used extensively and the company provided 20,000 yards of patent paving for the corridors of the Claybury Asylum alone.[52] Just as the Asylums Committee lent its name to particular products so too did it have a 'black list' for any individual or company supplying merchandise of an inferior quality.[53]

The sheer breadth of goods and people moving in and out of London's asylums should finally give lie to the assumption that institutions such as these were separate, self-supporting communities, not least because the numbers of patients made that an impossibility.[54] This offers a straightforward challenge to Foucault's contention that psychiatric power rested, in part, with the medical management and administration of asylums.[55] More prosaically, this publicly funded, publically administered organisation had an important impact on the finances of the country, as well as the finances of the capital.

[50] Bibby, *The Housing of Pauper Lunatics*: xxxvi.

[51] British Library, *London*, 23 August 1894, p. 72.

[52] Bibby, George H. 1985. *The Housing of Pauper Lunatics*. London: Drake, Driver and Leaver Ltd.: xlv. British Library, *London*, 23 August 1894, p. 72.

[53] LMA, LCC/MIN/575, Signed Minutes, March 1908–February 1909, 10 March 1908.

[54] For a discussion of the asylum and its place in wider society see Mooney, Graham and Reinarz, Jonathan. 2009. Hospital and Asylum Visiting in Historical Perspective: Themes and Issues. In *Permeable Walls: Historical Perspectives on Hospital and Asylum Visiting*, eds. G. Mooney and J. Reinarz, 7–30. Amsterdam: Rodopi.

[55] Foucault, Michel. 2008. *Psychiatric Power: Lectures at the Collège de France, 1973–1974*. Basingstoke: Palgrave Macmillan: 174.

In addition, the centralisation of procurement emphasised that this was a new municipal enterprise and outsiders recognised its Asylums Committee as gatekeepers to the wider network of institutions. Applications came from photographers asking to take pictures of buildings and grounds; from a phrenologist to visit the patients at Hanwell; from newspapers and magazines hoping to write journalistic pieces on the hospitals and from Henry S. Wellcome, the pharmaceutical entrepreneur, looking for 'rare and curious' objects he could exhibit at the International Medical Congress.[56] These examples represent just a small selection of the requests received and there were limits to what visitors could and could not see. In 1907, when the *Daily Mail* contacted LCC asking for permission to visit an asylum for information on an article on the housing of lunatics, it was granted but only at Long Grove and not any of the other, older institutions. [57] At the time, Long Grove was London's newest and, therefore, most modern asylum and there is a sense here that there was an attempt to manage what was and was not open to the public gaze.

LCC, Efficiency and Uniformity

In the first few years, the aim of establishing uniformity was to bring down costs. Some tenders remained in the hands of the various sub-committees, such as negotiations for the fitting up of the Horton Asylum with padded rooms.[58] Nevertheless, a London office meant that larger contracts and tenders for supplies could be negotiated centrally for all of LCC's asylums which would save both time and money. Contracts with the various fire insurance offices were renegotiated on more favourable terms.[59] In addition, a 'Common Fund' was created to ensure that expenditure was dealt with 'equitably' and, in 1901, one Treasurer was

[56]LCC/MIN/569, Signed Minutes, 1899–1901, 16 October 1899. LCC/MIN/569, Signed Minutes, 1899–1901, 13 November 1900. See also LCC/MIN/569, Signed Minutes, 1899–1901, 10 July 1900. LCC/MIN/569, Signed Minutes, 1899–1901, 9 October 1900. LMA, LCC/MIN/570, Signed Minutes, 1901–1902, 17 December 1901. LCC/MIN/570, Signed Minutes, 1901–1902, 18 March 1902. LMA, LCC/MIN/572, Signed Minutes, June 1904–November 1905, 23 May 1905.

[57]LMA, LCC/MIN/574, Signed Minutes, February 1907–February 1908, 26 March 1907.

[58]LMA LCC/MIN/570, Signed Minutes, 1901–1902, 8 October 1901.

[59]LMA, LCC 26.21. The Second Annual Report of the Asylums Committee of the London County Council, for the year ending 31 March 1891.

appointed to oversee the finances of all asylums.[60] Almost immediately, as the weekly charge for patients at Colney Hatch went up from 8s 9d to new LCC rate of 9s 4d, the charges at Cane Hill dropped from 9s 11d.[61] While it is tempting to see asylums as medical institutions, or even as Peter Bartlett has done as an extension of the Poor Law, there was also an entrenchment here of the centralised administrative power of LCC and the inclusion of asylums within its domain—the management of madness was being municipalised.[62]

The Asylums Committee's increasingly busy and important London office needed supplies such as telephones, typewriters and index cards, as well as the bound volumes that historians of mental health are so familiar with. It also needed the staff to run the office. In August 1892, Clifford Smith was appointed as engineer 'responsible for the supervision and control of engineering matters' at the Cane Hill, Claybury and Banstead asylums. Smith had his headquarters at the central office and would become responsible for similar duties at Hanwell and Colney Hatch when the 'present resident engineers cease to hold their appointments'.[63] At the time, Smith joined an existing office-based staff of eight but this would grow to fourteen.[64] This included the Clerk to the Asylums Committee, R. W. Partridge, who had served as clerk to the Middlesex Asylums before 1888 and R. F. Keene, his deputy who would eventually replace him in 1905.[65]

[60] LMA, LCC 26.21. The First Annual Report of the Asylums Committee of the London County Council, for the year ending 31 March 1890. The Thirteenth Annual Report of the Asylums Committee of the London County Council, for the year ending 31 March 1902.

[61] LMA, LCC 26.21. The Report of the Cane Hill Sub-Committee, for the year ending 31 March 1890. The Report of the Colney Hatch Sub-Committee, for the year ending 31 March 1890.

[62] Bartlett, Peter. 1999. *The Poor Law of Lunacy: The Administration of Pauper Lunatics in Mid-nineteenth Century England*. London: Leicester University Press: *passim*.

[63] LMA, LCC 26.21. The Fourth Annual Report of the Asylums Committee of the London County Council, for the year ending 31 March 1893.

[64] H12/CH/A3/2 The Eighth Annual Report of the Asylums Committee and Sub-Committees of Banstead, Cane Hill, Claybury, Colney Hatch, Hanwell, The Heath and Horton Asylums, 1897.

[65] LMA, LCC 18.6 Minutes of Proceedings, London County Council, January–December 1889, Report of the Asylums Committee, 3 December 1889. LMA, LCC/MIN/572, Signed Minutes, June 1904–November 1905, 21 March 1905.

These people joined an increasing number of 'experts' that local and municipal authorities were dependent on for advice.[66] The Clerk to the Asylums Committee would play a pivotal role in providing the intelligence on a number of issues in the form of reports for the Asylums Committee to consider. In an eighteen-month period at the beginning of the twentieth century, he produced 42 reports on matters as diverse at the appointment of a chaplain, the arrangements for Christmas holidays, the Colney Hatch fire and the establishment of a Pathology Laboratory.[67] The men in this position had a 'unique knowledge and experience'[68] of the work of the Asylums Committee and when, for example, the Asylums Committee dominated by the Municipal Reformers wished to reduce the balance within the Common Fund, it was the Clerk who warned that the County Council could request that the balance be paid thus reducing the Committee's funds and it was the Clerk who was asked to submit a full report with recommendations.[69] Whereas the County Councillors that served on the Council were local politicians subject to the whim of the electorate, it was the long-standing members of the administration team that provided the intelligence for them. This further emphasises the place of non-medical experts and it is little wonder that also based at Whitehall Place were five assistant clerks, an Inquiry Officer responsible for the settlements of pauper lunatics, and a messenger employed at 25 shillings per week.

These non-medical but specialist roles were replicated to some degree at the individual asylums and, when Long Grove opened in 1907, the five medical officers and their attendant staff were joined by a raft of individuals involved in the day-to-day running of the institution. Appendix 1 includes the non-medical but equally pivotal roles undertaken at Long Grove. Such roles were replicated across LCC's asylum

[66] Doyle, Barry M. 2001. The Changing Functions of Urban Government: Councillors, Officials and Pressure Groups, 1835–1950. In *The Cambridge Urban History of Britain*, vol. 3. Cambridge: Cambridge University Press, 287–313, 296–7).

[67] LMA, LCC/MIN/571, Signed Minutes, November 1902–May 1904, 14 May 1901.

[68] LMA, LCC/MIN/572, Signed Minutes, June 1904–November 1905, 21 March 1905.

[69] LMA, LCC/MIN/753. Minutes of Special Committees 1908–1914, 17 November 1908.

stock which by this time numbered ten institutions.[70] It goes without saying that each asylum was a significant employer of female nurses and attendants, but apart from a very short list of female officers, the opportunities for women in this period were limited. Some of this may have been an extension of the pre-1888 asylum system but, across the Council, employment roles were similarly gendered with women also being paid less and being forced to resign if and when they married.[71] Again, this emphasises the fact that this was not just a medical or a Poor-Law endeavour, it was a municipal one requiring a huge logistical and administrative operation. In terms of the range of staff involved in servicing the asylums, London was, perhaps, not that unusual but the novelty of the new administration meant an attempt to identify the transferred asylums as part of the new LCC domain.

The work of the individual asylums and the events that took place in them featured in LCC's *Staff Gazette*. This included magazine-style content and wider items of news from across the Council's departments that covered the retirements or deaths of staff members, staff letters, and updates on social activities such as LCC's Chess Club and Camera Club and on sports such as football and rugby.[72] The distance of the asylums to the centre of London must have precluded asylum staffs from active participation in many events and this and the longer-term tradition of sporting activities in asylums meant that football teams representing LCC faced teams based at individual asylums—such as the match in 1913 when the 'burley warders' of the Claybury Asylum beat LCC football team 4-1.[73] Nevertheless, individuals did represent the Asylums Department at events including LCC's Annual Sports Day held during the Summer[74] and being part of LCC entitled asylum staff to discounts on clothing and furniture from companies who advertised in

[70] LMA, LCC/MIN/574, Signed Minutes, February 1907–February 1908, 8 October 1907.

[71] Pennybacker, *A Vision for London, 1889–1914*: Chapter 1.

[72] See, for example, BL, *London County Council Staff Gazette* (1901), Vol. II, No. 14: 2. *London County Council Staff Gazette* (1901), Vol. II, No. 16: 42.

[73] BL, *London County Council Staff Gazette* (1913), Vol. XIV, No. 157: 3. BL, *London County Council Staff Gazette* (1913), Vol. XIV, No. 158: 40.

[74] See, for example, BL, *London County Council Staff Gazette* (1902), Vol. III, No. 31: 83.

the *Gazette*.[75] Moreover, along with other members of LCC staff, those who worked in asylums and their administration and had died in the Great War were included in the *Gazettes*' regular list of 'Our Fallen' during the war years of 1914–1918 and they, or their next of kin, were given a short history of the conflict in 1922, which included in an appendix the names of every member of the Council who had served.[76]

Some elements of uniformity took longer than others, and this reflected the relative autonomy of individual asylums, their sub-committees and their Medical Superintendents. Items such as standard patient clothing and standard forms for reporting diverse items such as patient property on arrival or *post-mortems* (see Chapter 4) came later in the period and, through a process of negotiation, were cherry picked from what was considered to be best practice at individual asylums.[77] Moreover, as the Clerk R. W. Partridge was to point out, the initial uniformity of many standard forms used in London asylums disappeared 'to some degree' and had to be revisited after the opening of newer LCC asylums.[78]

Despite this, the reorganisation of procurement and administration, along with new LCC rules and regulations for Asylums and their staffs, emphasised the Council's impact on the immediate and longer-term management of asylums. The rebranding of London's asylums as LCC institutions would have been recognisable to the patients but there were other changes too. It was the Asylums Committee and not the medical staff that increased the number of days that friends and relatives could visit patients. This included Sundays added to all asylums apart from Cane Hill where the 'necessary railway facilities' did not exist.[79] Moreover, its apparent strength allowed the Committee to petition

[75] See, for example, BL, *London County Council Staff Gazette* (1913), Vol. XIV, No. 157.

[76] See, for example, BL, *London County Council Staff Gazette* (1915), Vol. XVI, No. 182: 27. BL, LCC, *Record of Service in the Great War 1914–18 by Members of the Council Staff*, LCC, London, 1922, *passim*.

[77] LCC/PH/MENT/5/3, Minutes of Meetings of Asylum Officers, 10 December 1900. LMA, LCC/PH/MENT/05/003, Minutes of Meetings of Asylum Officers, 1899–1915, 10 December 1900, 7 October 1903.

[78] LMA, LCC/MIN/748, Pathologist Sub-Committee Minute Book, 1901–1908, 9 June 1904. LMA, LCC/MIN/748, Pathologist Sub-Committee Minute Book, 1901–1908, 5 April 1906.

[79] LMA, LCC/26.21, Annual Reports for LCC Asylums Committee for 1889–1892, The Second Annual Report of the Asylums Committee of the London County Council, for the year ending 31 March 1891.

railway companies about the possibility of reduced fares for the families of people in their asylums. In 1883, the Board of Trade had been given powers to compel companies to introduce workman's fare for the burgeoning network that served London.[80] Here, the Great Western Railway, which served Hanwell, and the Great Eastern Railway, which served Claybury, claimed their fares were already low enough but the South Eastern and Chatham, London Brighton and South Coast, and London and South-Western companies which served the Cane Hill, Banstead and Horton Asylums all offered vouchers for reduced fares.[81] When the Brighton and South Coast Railway increased its fares from London to Epsom, it was to the Asylums Committee that the relative of one patient wrote to. In this case the Asylums Committee ordered the Clerk to ring the railway company and, although no changes were made, they often saw themselves as the advocates of the patients and their families.[82] Similarly, in a bid to encourage staff to practice their own economies, arrangements were made for Post Office staff to attend each asylum on pay days so that they might receive cash from asylum staff wishing to make deposits in savings accounts.[83]

Significantly, the Asylums Committee also took advantage of its place within the new wider municipal network and the services provided by the other areas covered by the new LCC. Through negotiation with the Fire Brigade Committee, the chief officer of LCC's Fire Brigade inspected each asylum and made recommendations for improvements for the protection of the patients. The Parks and Open Spaces Committee provided 336 surplus ducks from the capital's ornamental parks which were then distributed across the, then, four asylums.[84] The Asylums Committee also paid the Council £100 for the services of its chemist and frequent analyses were made of standard samples and water from each of asylums

[80] Simmons, J. 1973. The Power of the Railway. In *The Victorian City: Images and Realities*, vol. 1, eds. H. J. Dyos and M. Wolff, 277–311. London: Routledge and Kegan Paul: 298.

[81] LMA, LCC/18.6, London County Council Minutes of Proceedings, May–August 1900, 17 July 1900.

[82] LMA, LCC/578, Signed Minutes, March 1912–October 1913, 26 November 1912.

[83] LMA, LCC 26.21. The Fourth Annual Report of the Asylums Committee of the London County Council, for the year ending 31 March 1893.

[84] LMA, LCC 26.21. The Second Annual Report of the Asylums Committee of the London County Council, for the year ending 31 March 1891.

was examined both 'chemically and microscopically'.[85] When it came to outbreaks of fever or other infectious diseases it used the services of London's Medical Officer of Health.[86] Costs incurred in using these services included not just seeds and animals but their carriage to the asylum and in the case of the latter tests for health.[87] Clearly, when consideration is given to the administration of the asylums in London, it is difficult to argue that this was a simple continuation of the pre-1888 period. The Asylums Committee had instigated a measure of uniformity and identity to create an LCC brand. This was framed not just about the service but it was also about London and its new administration.

Representing the Changes as a Progressive Success Story and Some Challenges

It is easy to see the changes taking place as somehow politically neutral; as purely administrative changes, rather than political ones but E. P. Hennock has shown that in Leeds, in the north of England, party-political debate and condemnations came to focus on efficiency and adequacy of services and it was the same here.[88] Commentators, politicians and newspaper editorials almost immediately highlighted the work of the Asylums Committee within their wider assessments of the new Council—good and bad. In the American *Yale Review*, George Fox commented on the Council's personnel and their high quality. The credit for its 'notable achievements', he concluded, rested with its Progressive majority and included here was the 'humane, beneficial and scientific' management of the capital's asylums.[89] More important were the debates and discussions that were taking place in London about the nature of its post-1888 government. Both the Liberal-supporting *Daily Star* and

[85] LMA, LCC 26.21. The Third Annual Report of the Asylums Committee of the London County Council, for the year ending 31 March 1892.

[86] LMA, LCC 18.6 Minutes of Proceedings, London County Council, January–December 1889, Report of the Asylums Committee, 3 December 1889.

[87] LMA, LCC/MIN/574, Signed Minutes, February 1907–February 1908, 19 February 1907.

[88] Hennock, *Fit and Proper Persons*: 253.

[89] Fox, George L. 1895. The London County Council and its Work. *Yale Review* May: 80–102: 83, 100, 101.

Daily Chronicle, which described itself as the 'organ of imperial and municipal progress', published first, a series of articles on the work on the Council and then re-published them for sale as edited collections. The *Star*'s collection was titled '*New London: Her Parliament and Its Work*', and the *Chronicle*'s 'Three Good Years' Work for the People'. Both emphasised the positive impact of the Progressive administration across the breadth of its responsibilities including health, housing, education and the management of Asylums. The administrative reforms that had followed the passing of the LGA had a part to play here and, commentating on the Asylums Committee, the *Star* proclaimed 'The organisation of it is excellent and it works without a hitch. The sub-committees have succeeded in carrying out considerable benefits for the patients, for the attendants and for the public. They have served every interest'.[90]

Politically speaking, this was contentious and *Three Good Years' Work for the People* was a direct riposte to those 'ignorant and mendacious opponents' of the Council who claimed that 'its members had failed in their administrative duties'.[91] Similarly, the *Star*'s piece on the Progressive management of Asylums was framed as a response to the 'reckless critics of the Council', including the Conservative-supporting *Spectator*, which had described the Progressives as 'meddlers', 'collectivist pedants' and 'ignorant theorists'.[92] Figure 2.1, shows a later critique with the Progressive Party satirised as a mixture of owlish Town Clerks, Irish Fenians and (Russian) Radicals. It is possible that the latter was a caricature of Peter Kropotkin, the Russian anarchist who had been 'cordially' welcomed to Britain in the late 1880s by socialists and radicals.[93] Either way, the image of a 'cheerful idiot' inviting members of the 'Radical Party' to join him in 'Barmyville Asylum' is indicative of how they and their policies were viewed by their opponents.

In these cases critics may not have necessarily attacked the Asylums Committee per se, but the results of the decisions it made were included in the marshalling of evidence in the defence, promotion or excoriation of the wider Council. Thus, the work of the Asylums Committee became

[90] Anon. *Three Years Good Work for the People*: 19.

[91] Ibid.: Preface.

[92] *Daily Chronicle*, The Council and the Asylums: For Sick Minds and Bodies: 50.

[93] Shpayer-Makov, Haia. 1987. The Reception of Peter Kropotkin in Britain, 1886–1917. *Albion: A Quarterly Journal Concerned with British Studies* 19: 3, 373–90, 375–6.

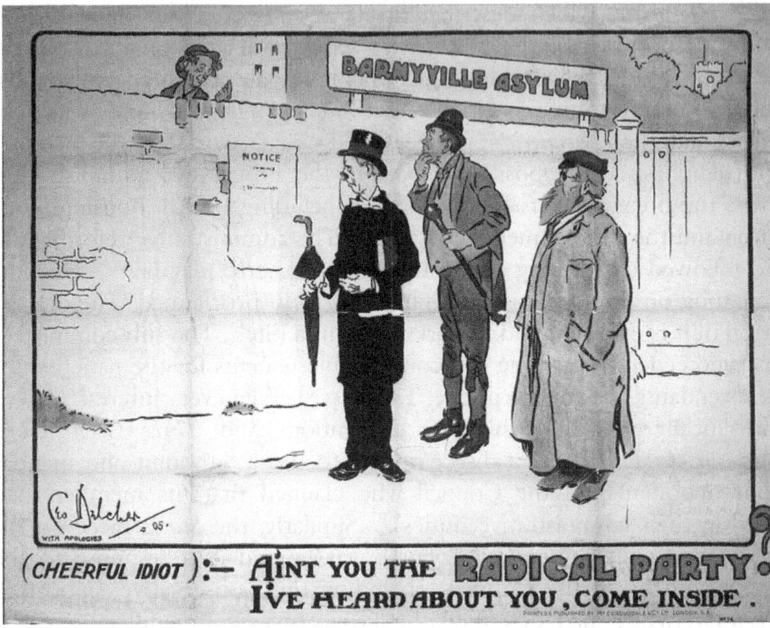
BARMYVILLE ASYLUM
NOTICE
Geo Belcher 05.
WITH APOLOGIES
(CHEERFUL IDIOT):— AINT YOU THE RADICAL PARTY?
I'VE HEARD ABOUT YOU, COME INSIDE.

Fig. 2.1 George Belcher. c.1906. 'Ain't you the Radical Party?' London: McCorquodale and Co. Ltd. London School of Economics, London. COLL MISC 0519/5 (Reproduced with permission of the London School of Economics under a Creative Commons Attribution-NonCommercial-ShareAlike [CC BY-NC-SA 3.0] license)

a feature of the political rhetoric that was directly linked to elections and electioneering. Indeed, *Three Years' Good Work* was updated for every election and in the 1907 version (*Eighteen Years Good Progressive Work for the People*) it reiterated what the Progressive administration had done 'to make London a better City to live in, and more worthy to be the Capital of the British Empire'.[94] The work of the Asylums Committee featured at Number 32 on a list of 39 'achievements', with the claim that that the Progressives had 'Improved the Asylums, facilitated the visits of patients' friends and relatives, and instituted investigations into the

[94]GL, PAM 3438, Progressive Leaflets, London County Council Election. 1907. *Eighteen Year's Good Progressive Work for the People*. London: Progressive Election Committee.

causes and cure of lunacy'.[95] The links between this and Britain's imperialism can sometimes seem opaque. Whereas some Councillors lobbied for changes to the names of streets, the erection of monuments and a new architecture that would form the basis of a new world identity, others such as John Burns (Progressive), pushed for improvements in health and living standards so that Londoners might play an active role in imperial affairs.[96]

In other cases, opponents hinted at the apparently inherent corruption of Progressivism and linked it to what was happening in the United States. Tammany Hall was the Democratic Party's political machine in New York and, under William 'Boss' Tweed, had become synonymous with bribery and other nefarious dealings in its control of the city. Captain H. M. Jessel, Chairman of the LMS claimed that 'The socialistic policy of the Progressives tends to create a second Tammany Hall and to produce in London a state or sordid political corruption similar to that rampant in New York'.[97] Similarly, Arthur A. Baumann had compared the LGA as a splendid temptation before the 'famished fingers of the Radical Party', with the day 'when Tweed ran his hawk's eye along Manhattan Island'.[98] Baumann stopped short of claiming that the Progressives in London were 'tyrants, or Tweeds' but they, nevertheless, established 'a propaganda for the spread of radical doctrines'.[99] More specifically, the *Sun* made what were ultimately unsubstantiated claims relating to the awarding of tenders and corruption at the Asylum Committee's central office and this was to be a recurring theme.[100]

In 1900, the *London Argus* urged John Burns to direct his attention to the 'hanky panky' that was going on in relation to certain items of

[95]GL, PAM 3438. 1907. Progressive Leaflets, London County Council Election. *Eighteen Year's Good Progressive Work for the People*. London: Progressive Election Committee.

[96]Schneer, *London 1900: The Imperial Metropolis*. New Haven: Yale University Press: 34.

[97]BL 8139B22, c.1907. *The Daily Mail and the Fight for London: A Handbook to the London County Council Election Giving both Sides*: 12.

[98]Bishopsgate Institute (Hereafter BI) 230/4, Baumann, Arthur A. c.1890. The London County Council, The Universal Review: 493–502: 493.

[99]BI 230/4, Baumann, Arthur A. c.1890. The London County Council, The Universal Review: 493–502, 493.

[100]LMA, LCC 18.6 Minutes of Proceedings, London County Council, July–December 1903, Report of the Asylums Committee, 27 October 1903.

consumption in London's asylums.[101] Burns was not a member of the Asylums Committee but he was a totemic member of the Progressive Party. As with the article in the *Sun*, the alleged 'hanky panky' related to the fees paid for items in relation to their supposed quality, but in other cases there were more direct examples of criminality taking place. T. Mynott, the Clerk of Cane Hill Asylum was sentenced to four months hard labour for embezzling £216 but one of the most important instances of this was the 'plundering' of the Horton Asylum stores by three members of staff including the Stores Clerk, Edward Morant.[102] While Morant claimed that extra portions were given to patients, or that foodstuffs such as bacon and sugar were disposed of in drains to help balance the books, it was found that many of the missing items were being sold in a nearby coffee house that he owned.[103] The defendants were imprisoned for periods ranging from three to eighteen months and the discovery of thefts led to new levels of scrutiny imposed by the Asylums Committee.[104]

In urban areas in particular, evidence of such scandals brought potentially new levels of public cynicism on the supposed probity of political elites.[105] A similar example in Lancashire had led the Commissioners in Lunacy to press its Asylums Board to place the auditing of their accounts on a more secure business footing.[106] In London, the scandals offered an opportunity to make political attacks on the majority administration. This included questions being asked about the probity of the administration in the aftermath of the disastrous fire at Colney Hatch, in which 52 patients lost their lives.[107] Following the arrest of six officers for the theft of foodstuffs, this time at the Claybury Asylum, an article appeared in the *Evening News*. 'London does not forget that the only scandals which have besmirched the fair name of the Council have occurred

[101] The *London Argus* cited in LCC/MIN/569, Signed Minutes, 1899–1901, 19 May 1901.

[102] LMA, LCC/MIN/575, Signed Minutes, March 1908-February 1909, 14 July 1908.

[103] *London Daily News*, 26 April 1904: 9.

[104] *Fifty-Ninth Report of the Commissioners in Lunacy*, 1905: 57.

[105] Garrard, John. 2003. Scandals: A Tentative overview. In *Corruption in Urban Politics and Society, Britain 1780–1950*, eds. James Moore and John Smith 23–40. Aldershot: Ashgate: 35.

[106] Hayes, Lancashire Public Asylum Provision: 89.

[107] Anon. 1903. Who is responsible? *Daily Mail*, 28 January.

under Progressive majorities', it claimed, 'we refer to the Horton Asylum Scandals, where criminal waste went on'.[108] Does this mean, asked Progressive member W. C. Johnson in response, that the Moderates were responsible for a shortage of the 103 tonnes of coal at the Banstead Asylum.[109]

The wider financial and political context of these attacks will be explored in Chapter 3 but it is safe to say that however much the work of the Asylums Committee was claimed to be separate from the Council, it was, in fact, at the heart of wider discussions about the merits, or otherwise, of the post-1888 government of London. Whether as supporters of London's Progressive administration or its opponents, commentators were apt to make political capital of its role and bring a new and different level of scrutiny to the ones already in place under existing lunacy legislation. In particular, the party machines understood the importance of what were described as the 'non-contentious' departments of the Council. Along with the supposedly non-political administration of sewerage, parks and drainage, the Asylums Committee was meant to be above party-political machinations. As the Municipal Reformers pointed out, however, it was:

> a favourite device of Progressive speakers to expatiate upon the details of one of the ordinary administrative work of one of the wholly non-contentious departments of the Council; to dilate upon the importance of the work, and upon the careful and conscientious way in which is it executed; and then to take all credit of it to the Progressive Party.[110]

This overview appeared in a much broader guide for Municipal Reform candidates and the messages relating to the non-contentious committees can be found in the election addresses of some candidates as a result. Henry Jarvis and Albert Waddell, Municipal Reform candidates in West Newington in 1907, explained to the electorate that the non-contentious work of the Council was a result of the hearty co-operation and united

[108] LMA, PH/Ment/3/5, Newspaper Cuttings, 'The Morning Leader', 14 March 1910.

[109] LMA, PH/Ment/3/5, Newspaper Cuttings, 'The Morning Leader', 14 March 1910. LMA, LCC/576, Signed Minutes, March 1909–July 1910: 9 October 1909. Anon. 1903. Colney Hatch Fire Verdict. *Daily Mail*, 13 February.

[110] GL, LMS107, *London County Council, Election 1904, Facts and Arguments*, London Municipal Society, London, 1904.

work of both parties.[111] Moreover, when Municipal Reformers tried to make political capital from the work of the Asylums Committee following their election victory in 1907, they were reminded by one Councillor (W. C. Johnson) that much of the work they were claiming credit for was initiated many months before they came into power.[112] In other places, such as Central Finsbury, Municipal Reform candidates in the 1907 election promised that the non-contentious services of the Council, including Asylums, would not suffer at their hands if elected.[113]

The Significance of the Council and Its Committee Structure

Despite some talk of some co-operation, as early as the 1898 election, the LMS was alerting voters to the fact that that members of the Moderate Party had had no opportunity of administering municipal business. This was despite the fact that the Progressives had allowed them to nominate Chairmen of some of the 'less contentious' committees of the Council.[114] This did not include the Asylums Committee but it reveals something important about the nature of Council business. Harold J. Laski suggested that the lack of time to deal with the vast array of Council responsibilities meant that 90% would be a conservative estimate of the resolutions that were passed without challenge.[115] While, Laski was making a general point about the nature of Committees across all Councils, and using a figure that did not appear to be borne of any scientific analysis, there is a sense that LCC's Asylums Committee operated outside of, or at least adjacent to the Council structure. The primacy of the lunacy legislation, and its imposition of a statutory responsibility to build and maintain asylums, appears to bear this out but closer analysis of the general committee structure undermines any claim for exceptionalism on the part of the Asylums Committee. As Davies explains, the

[111] LMA, ACC/3606/001 Election Literature and Newspaper Cuttings, 1906–1907, 'To the Electors of West Newington', February 1907.

[112] LMA, PH/Ment/3/5, Newspaper Cuttings, 'The Morning Leader', 14 March 1910.

[113] LMA, ACC/3606/001 Election Literature and Newspaper Cuttings, 1906–1907, 'London County Council Election', 1907, February 1907.

[114] GL, LMS132, London Municipal Society 1898. Election Leaflets and Pamphlets, 'Electors of London!', Leaflet No. 46.

[115] Laski, The Committee System in Local Government: 82.

Council 'lived and worked' in Committee with the Council's eighteen or so standing committees enjoying practical autonomy from the outset'.[116]

Moreover, it is important to recognise that, apart from the relatively impartial committees of 1889, the control of the Council rested with its party affiliations—the majority party appointed the Chairman of the Council but also the Chairmen of its various committees.[117] Barry Doyle has shown that the political management of health in Leeds in the interwar years was bound by strict rules of proportionality and slight majorities but here it was very different.[118] Following the 1907 election, for example, control of the Asylums Committee passed to the Municipal Reformers. Appendix 2 shows just how dominant they were with 23 of the 34 Councillors listed hailing from the Municipal Reform camp. It is also clear here that some members were more committed to attending the business of the Committee than others and this was already a recurrent theme. In the first year of operation in 1889, Martineau immediately and successfully petitioned LCC for an increase in the Asylums Committee membership from 40 to 60 in view of the urgency and the amount of its work.[119]

The Earl of Rosbery, one-time Liberal Prime Minister and leader of the first council, singled out LCC from other County Councils, District Councils and Parish Councils, describing its work as no less absorbing than the House of Commons, and quite as arduous.[120] In a review of that first year, however, he considered this in relation to the work and membership of particular committees. The Housing of the Working Classes Committee and the Parks Committee were the two most popular, wrote Rosebery, because 'almost every councillor feels an interest in those two subjects'.[121] Indeed, Rosebery argued that the better housing

[116] Davies, John. 1988. *Reforming London: The London Government Problem, 1855–1900*. Oxford: Clarendon Press: 147–8.

[117] Ibid.: 111–2.

[118] Doyle, Barry M. 2015. *The Politics of Hospital Provision in Early Twentieth-Century Britain*. London: Routledge: 144.

[119] LMA, LCC 18.6, London County Council, Minutes of Proceedings, January–December 1889, 5 March 1889.

[120] Geake, Charles. 1899. *Appreciations and Addresses Delivered by Lord Rosebery*. London: John Lane: 188–9.

[121] London County Council. 1890. *A Review of the First Year's Work of the Council in a Series of Addresses Delivered by the Chairman, the Earl of Rosebery*. London: LCC: 6.

of the poor was the 'primary task' of the Council and even though both committees had gradually been enlarged, he doubted they contained all those that were willing to serve on them.[122] By contrast, the Asylums Committee was described as being 'the most unpopular' of all the committees. It has, wrote Rosebery, 'more difficulty in getting suitable recruits than any other committee of the Council' and he could well understand the 'repugnance to which many feel to serving', it not being easy 'to contemplate human nature in its most degraded and pitiful form'.[123] For these reasons, he concluded, those who served on it deserved the gratitude of the Council and 'ours sincerest thanks'.[124] Likewise, Sidney Webb, influential in formulating Progressive Party Committee policies and one of its arch-propagandists, argued that London owed 'a special debt of gratitude' to all the members of the Asylums Committee.[125]

There were other more obvious reasons why there was a relative lack of councillors clamouring to be involved. Davies has described the work of the London councillor as arduous with four days of hard work for a committed and conscientious councillor.[126] For those on the Asylums Committee, there was the additional burden of its various sub-committees, including those for individual asylums. These met on site and involved the time and trouble it took to attend the meetings outside of central London. This, in itself, must have added to the sense in which the Asylums Committee seemed to be separate from the Council. Indeed, when asked for their thoughts on the creation of map for the use of both councillors and the public, the Asylums Committee pointed out that the institutions they dealt with were outside the boundary of the new County of London (see Chapter 1, Table 1.1).[127]

[122]Rosebery cited in Pennybacker, The Millennium by Return of Post: 133. London County Council, *A Review of the First Year's Work of the Council*: 6.

[123]London County Council, *A Review of the First Year's Work of the Council*: 9.

[124]Ibid.: 6.

[125]Webb, The Work of the London County Council: 130–52. Sidney Webb was first elected to the Council in 1892 as the Progressive member for Deptford, a working-class area in the south-east of London. Davis, J. 2008. Webb, Beatrice 1858–1943, social reformer and diarist. *Oxford Dictionary of National Biography*. https://www.oxforddnb.com/. Accessed 4 July 2019.

[126]Davies, The Progressive Council: 31.

[127]LMA, LCC/MIN/575, Signed Minutes, March 1908–February 1909, 8 December 1908.

Table 2.2 Asylum Committees and sub-committees 1888–1890

Committee and Sub-committee	*Membership*	*Meetings per year*
Asylums Committee	60	13
Banstead Asylum	13	25
Cane Hill Asylum	12	28
Colney Hatch	13	25
Hanwell Asylum	10	24
Claybury Asylum	13	15
Asylums Contract	14	8
To Consider Rates of Pay, Leave, &c., of staff	9	12
For Compiling Statistics for Annual Report	5	3
Additional Asylum Accommodation	10	4
Central Finance	10	4
Chairmen	6	6

Source Annual Reports of the Asylums Committee

In the first few years alone, the members of the Asylums Committee shared the responsibility on a variety of sub-committees (see Table 2.2) and the breadth of these increased over the course of the period.[128]

As well as changes brought about by elections, the demands of the Asylums Committee meant that its membership was not static. Time and again the issue of attendance affected both the membership and the ability of the Asylums Committee to meet its statutory and other responsibilities. Of the 61 members listed in 1891, thirteen of them did not attend any meetings and a further ten attended only one meeting. As a result, numbers were reduced at the beginning of the twentieth century to 40 and then to 35. When the Municipal Reformers won the election in 1907, it was reduced again to as low as 30 as they sought to rationalise the Council's business.[129] One of the key reasons behind these changes were the Council's standing orders which stated that a quorum of any committee could not be less than one-fifth of the number of its members, exclusive of *ex-officio* members.[130] With a membership of 60, getting

[128]LMA, LCC/26.21 Annual Reports for LCC Asylums Committee for 1889–1892, The First Annual Report of the Asylums Committee of the London County Council, for the year ending 31 March 1890.

[129]LMA, LCC/MIN/570, Signed Minutes, 1901–1902, 14 May 1901.

[130]LMA, GLC/DG/AE/ROL/82/001, LCC Standing Orders, 1891–3: 120.

twelve members to attend at times such as the autumn recess proved to be difficult and the Asylums Committee asked for special dispensation to reduce the numbers to five.[131] In the end, the Council agreed to reduce the number to nine by reducing the overall membership. This meant an end to the immediate problem of raising a quorate but it did not mean that all councillors immediately began to attend all meetings.[132]

Just as the Moderates were complaining about their lack of opportunities to be involved in Committee work, the Progressives began to use attendance figures for political purposes. In the run up to the 1898 election, the Progressives provided details of who and who had not attended all Committee meetings. Despite, the two parties being 'almost equal', it was shown that Progressive members attended 23,254 meetings compared to Moderates total of 13,658.[133] Significantly it was the Asylums Committee where more detailed information was provided. 'The Moderates shirk their work', proclaimed Progressive election materials but it was the Asylums Committee:

> that require[d] the hardest work and the greatest the greatest devotion. It should consist of 40 members. Its numbers have been, in 1895, 21 Progressives and 16 Moderates. In 1896, 21 Progressives and 10 Moderates. In 1897, 21 Progressives and 8 Moderates. Appeal after appeal has been made to the Moderate Party to fill these vacancies on the Committee but none will come forward. The Moderate Party have neglected their duty – disregarded their responsibility for 17,000 Lunatics whom Parliament has placed under the Council's care.[134]

These figures were updated and reiterated at subsequent elections but, despite what was being said here, attendance at Council and Committee meetings was seen by one author as part of the reason for the failure of the Progressive party at the 1907 election. After the 1906 General Election, 29 members of the Progressive Party were also Members of

[131] LMA, LCC/18.6, London County Council Minutes of Proceedings, July–December 1891, 14 July 1891.

[132] LMA, LCC/18.6, London County Council Minutes of Proceedings, January–June 1892, 5 April 1892.

[133] GL, PAM3472. 1898. Progressive Party Leaflets, 'Who Have Done London's Work?', Leaflet No. 9.

[134] GL, PAM3472. 1898. Progressive Party Leaflets, 'Who Have Done London's Work?', Leaflet No. 9.

Parliament. With constituencies sometime hundreds of miles away from the capital it was 'not easy for everyone to give adequate time to both'.[135]

This emphasis on attendance at meetings, and the problems in achieving the necessary quorum, reveal the importance of individual councillors in moving the business of asylums forward. According to Webb, there were four men whose 'incessant labours' were responsible for the vast improvements. Messrs John McDougall, Richard Strong, Philip Martineau and Arthur Leon spent a third of their days inspecting London's lunatic asylums and under their zealous care, they had become 'models for the world'.[136] All bar Leon had served as the Chairman of the Asylums Committee and McDougall was cited by the *Daily Mail*, along with Alderman Hubbard, as spending the best years of their lives watching the well-being of the inmates of asylums.[137] This was not unusual and, as Davies has pointed out, well-known Progressive councillors such as John Burns or John Williams Benn owed their 'celebrity' to the publicity that LCC received in first few years. Councillors were not as anonymous as those who served on the MBW but it was 'broadly true that the Progressives relied upon good works rather than great men to galvanise the metropolitan civic consciousness'.[138]

There is an obvious focus on men here and although the 1870 Education Act had enabled women to serve on School Boards it was not until the beginning of the twentieth century, and the passing of an act of parliament, that women were allowed to stand for election to the Council.[139] During this time, women's role in local politics was usually

[135] BI, 229/12, A. Emil Davies, The LCC 1889–1937: 13.

[136] Webb, The Work of the London County Council: 130–52.

[137] Anon. 1903. Housing the Insane. What the London County Council Has Done. *Daily Mail*, 29 January. Haward described Hubbard as a 'shrewd but bigoted Radical of the narrow-minded type, and an ardent worker in the Progressive cause'. Haward, *The London County Council from Within*: 23.

[138] Davies, Local Government 1850–1920: 52.

[139] Two women were elected to the LCC 1889 and another was appointed as alderman but this was challenged in the courts and they were unseated. The 1907 Qualification of Women (County and Borough Councils) Act of 1907 allowed women to be elected to councils in England and Wales. BI 229/12, Davies. Emil, A. 1937. *The LCC 1889–1937, a Historical Sketch*. London: Fabian Society: 6. See also Stokes, Wendy. 2011. Missing from the Picture. Women's Initiatives in English Local Government. In *Women and Representation in Local Government: International Case Studies*, eds. Barbara Pini and Paula McDonald, 95–108. London: Routledge: 97.

limited to domestic areas, such as health and, as Louise Westwood notes, in the history of psychiatry, women were far more visible as patients than practitioners.[140] This is particularly true of LCC where medically trained women such as Helen Boyle were limited to Assistant Medical Officer roles, although, as Appendix 1 again demonstrates, the number of female attendant staff continued to be significant.[141]

In the first election two female Progressive candidates, Lady (Margaret) Sandhurst and Jane Cobden had been elected and, along with Alderman Emma Cons, served until 1892 when a legal challenge effectively barred them from the election of that year.[142] Patricia Hollis has shown how this too was politically motivated with a direct challenge to Sandhurst coming from Beresford Hope, the opposing male candidate she had defeated in 1889. At the same time Cobden and Cons were advised to take a 12-month sabbatical following legal advice. On their return in February 1890, they faced additional challenges to their status from Moderate members which would ultimately preclude their participation in 1892. Cons's Aldermanic nomination from the Progressive party stemmed from her housing and social work and she, like Cobden, served as members of the Asylums Committee in their short time as Councillors.[143] Andrea Geddes Poole, argues that her work on the Mental After-Care Association gave Cons 'a far better understanding of the mentally ill than virtually any other councillor…' but the evidence of how that translated to LCC is patchy.[144] Cobden attended only one of the twelve Asylums Committee's meetings in the year ending March 1891, but Cons, having joined later, did not attend any of the five she might have done. Cobden was also attached to the sub-committees of the Banstead and Cane Hill Asylums and her attendance there was equally sparse.[145] This does not mean that either of them were without

[140] Doyle, *The Politics of Hospital Provision*: 144. Westwood, Louise. 2006. Separatism and Exclusion. Women in Psychiatry. In *Mental Illness and Learning Disability Since 1850*, eds. Pamela Dale and Joseph Melling, 91–111. London: Routledge.

[141] Milliken, Emma. 2006. Boyle, Helen 1869–1957. *Oxford Dictionary of National Biography*. https://www.oxforddnb.com/. Accessed 4 July 2019.

[142] Hollis, Patricia. 1987. *Ladies Elect: Women in English Local Government, 1865–1914*. Oxford: Clarendon Press: 310–17.

[143] Ibid.

[144] Ibid.

[145] LMA, LCC 26.21. The Second Annual Report of the Asylums Committee of the London County Council, for the year ending 31 March 1891.

influence. As a woman lacking the independent means to carve out a pioneering career in philanthropic work, Cons has been described as 'virtually unique' when compared to her more privileged peers.[146] This included social reformer Octavia Hill who wrote to her mother to describe the 'beautiful works' that Cons was doing on the Council while all the while 'keeping herself in the shade'.[147] Certainly, there is enough evidence to suggest that the work of both female Councillors was pivotal with proclamations of support and gratitude from both individual councillors and the Council as whole.[148] Indeed, the new all-male Progressive Council of 1892 passed a motion in support of women councillors but it was not until the Qualification of Women (County and Borough Councils) Act that female ratepayers were able to stand in 1907 and it was not until 1910 than any were elected.[149]

For those bidding to change the law on female suffrage and participation in County Council in the meantime, the management of asylums became the primary reason in their campaigns. Florence Fenwick Miller, the journalist and public lecturer, listed the reasons 'why women ought to be on County Councils'. The fact that 'they had the charge of the great lunatic asylums in which so great a number of the patients are women' was at the top of her list.[150] And, as the Women's Local Government Society [WLGS] pointed out, 'the care of Women Councillors is needed for these poor creatures ... Men Councillors cannot enter into the manner of bathing female patients, nor know much about their clothing; and a woman on the Council can give valuable help in planning occupations to pass the long hours and to brighten their lives.[151] The WGLS

[146] Geddes Poole, Andrea. 2014. *Philanthropy and the Construction of Victorian Women's Citizenship*. Toronto: University of Toronto Press: 97.

[147] Ibid.: 212.

[148] Ibid.: 211.

[149] Ibid.: 317. Gibbon and Bell, *History of the London County Council*: 80.

[150] Anon. 1903. A women's view of things. *London Daily News*, 10 August. Fenwick Miller practised medicine briefly after completing her medical degree at London's Ladies Medical College. She also served as an elected member on the London School board, representing the borough of Hackney. Ardsel, Rosemary T. 2004. Miller, Florence Fenwick, *Oxford Dictionary of National Biography*. https://www.oxforddnb.com/. Accessed 4 July 2019.

[151] BI LH P4168. 1913. Women's Local Government Society, LCC election, An appeal to women. See also BI P3422. 1913. Women's Local Government Society. Nineteen Reasons Why Women are Wanted on London County Council.

was a Liberal organisation that had supported Cons and Cobden and no doubt drew on their experience but this did not make things easier, even after 1907. As it pointed out, 'The party system and the party machinery make it very difficult for a woman to secure adoption as a candidate and there are also great though not insuperable difficulties in independent candidature'.[152] As a result, the numbers of successful female candidates was low. Henrietta Adler (Progressive) and Susan Lawrence (Municipal Reform) were elected as Councillors and Lady St Helier was appointed as an Alderman. Hollis explains that Adler and Lawrence said little at full Council meetings, but they worked hard on the Asylum and Education Committees.[153] Henrietta Adler attended 47 of 52 possible meetings which included the Asylums Committee and three of its sub-committees, while Lady St Helier appeared to be less conscientious, at least in terms of bare attendance figures.[154] It is possible that influential and titled women were also able to influence London County Councillors through informal means at luncheons, dinners and receptions. Along with politicians and diplomats, Councillors such as John Williams Benn were part of a lively social scene but, at the time of writing, any impact on the Asylums Committee remains hidden and an opportunity for future research.[155]

Often too, the appeals to women voters can be missed in the general messages in election propaganda. The Progressive poster in Fig. 2.2 is one example of the gendered nature of election materials in this period. At the heart of the image, is a working man making the choice between the Progressive Policy of the Welfare of the People, and the anti-municipal policies of the Moderates. Included here was Asylum Accommodation for 1400 patients. This is a typographical error which should have read 14,000, but the focus on the male voter obscures the significant numbers of women that had the right to vote in County Elections. Individual councillors were elected by those occupying rooms

[152] BI LH P4168. 1913. Women's Local Government Society, LCC election, An appeal to women.

[153] Hollis, Patricia. 1987. *Ladies Elect. Women in English Local Government, 1865–1914.* Oxford: Clarendon Press: 310–17.

[154] LMA, The Twenty-First Annual Report of the Asylums Committee of the London County Council, for the year ending 31 March 1910.

[155] See, for example, Schneer, *London 1900. The Imperial Metropolis.* New Haven: Yale University Press: 123–4.

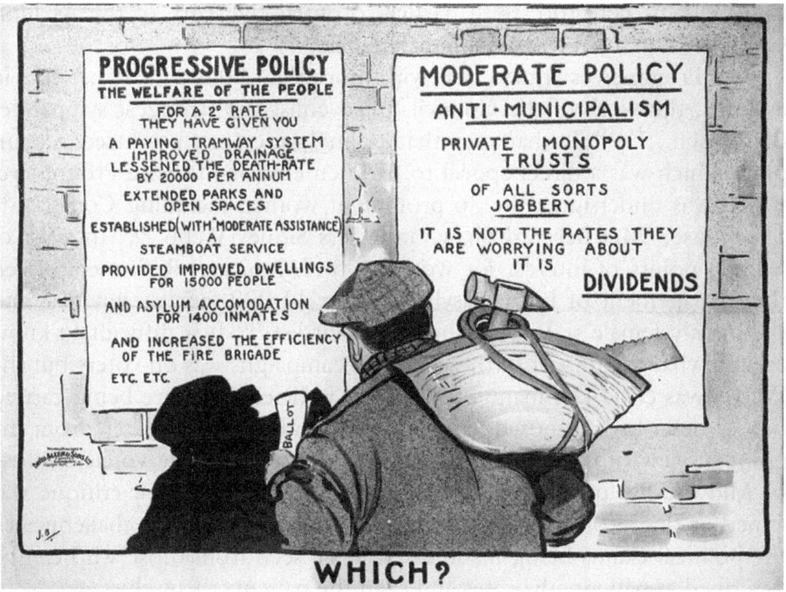
PROGRESSIVE POLICY
THE WELFARE OF THE PEOPLE
FOR A 2° RATE
THEY HAVE GIVEN YOU
A PAYING TRAMWAY SYSTEM
IMPROVED DRAINAGE
LESSENED THE DEATH-RATE
BY 20000 PER ANNUM
EXTENDED PARKS AND
OPEN SPACES
ESTABLISHED (WITH "MODERATE ASSISTANCE")
A
STEAMBOAT SERVICE
PROVIDED IMPROVED DWELLINGS
FOR 15000 PEOPLE
AND ASYLUM ACCOMODATION
FOR 1400 INMATES
AND INCREASED THE EFFICIENCY
OF THE FIRE BRIGADE
ETC. ETC.
MODERATE POLICY
ANTI-MUNICIPALISM
PRIVATE MONOPOLY
TRUSTS
OF ALL SORTS
JOBBERY
IT IS NOT THE RATES THEY
ARE WORRYING ABOUT
IT IS
DIVIDENDS
BALLOT
WHICH?

Fig. 2.2 Anon. 1907. 'Which?' London: David Allen and Sons Ltd. London School of Economics, London. COLL MISC 0844/21 (Reproduced with permission of the London School of Economics under a Creative Commons Attribution-NonCommercial-ShareAlike [CC BY-NC-SA 3.0] license)

or land to the value of £10 who resided in the county or within seven miles of it. The details of this household suffrage were laid down in a separate County Electors Act.[156] In a population of around 5 million people, 600,000 had the vote and 100,000 of them were women.[157] These figures were to rise and along with general messages to all votes, women were targeted by both parties. A pamphlet titled 'Why Women Should Vote Progressive' highlighted the fact that there were four areas deemed to be areas of special interest; rates, transit, education and

[156] Chandler, J. A. 2000. *Explaining Local Government, Local Government in Britain since 1800*. Manchester: Manchester University Press: 100.

[157] Pennybacker, *A Vision for London, 1889–1914*: 4–5.

housing but, here too, both parties co-opted the work of the Asylums Committee in a bid to attract female voters.[158]

The Progressives argued that with more than 8000 female patients in asylums, the work of the Council 'must enlist the strongest sympathies of women…' [159] To hammer that point home they produced a pamphlet which was a direct appeal to 'women electors' to vote Progressive, which was undersigned by 36 prominent women including Cons, Lady Hobhouse, 'Mrs Bernard Shaw' and 'Mrs Sidney Webb'.[160] In a list of 'special points of interest for women', the Municipal Reformers placed the management of lunatic asylums, their 11,000 females lunatics, and the mainly female staff at the head of their list.[161] It is difficult to know exactly what the impact of these specific campaigns was on voters but the WGLS was critical of many of the wider policies that were being carried out. It described proposed legislation 'as drafted so completely from the point of view of the artisan voter that the interest of the voteless Nurse or Midwife has quite been lost sight of'.[162] This particular critique was aimed at one group of working women, but some of the challenges to the political claims being made can also be seen from those who can be described as patient advocates and even the patients themselves.

Political Rhetoric and the Patient Experience

Although administrative efficiency was a recurring theme of political literature in this period, much of the rhetoric included some bold claims that emphasised an apparently positive impact on the patient experience. John Williams Benn, described by Andrew Saint as one of the 'ideological leaders' of Progressivism, again in a wider discussion of the Progressive administration, wrote of the 'Improved diet, more

[158] London County Council. 1910. Progressive leaflets. https://archive.org/stream/progressiveleafl00lond#page/n3/mode/2up. Accessed 4 July 2019.

[159] GL, PAM3556. 1907. Progressive Party Leaflets, 'A Letter to Women Electors?', Leaflet No. 18.

[160] Anon. 1901. *London County Council: A letter to Women Electors*. London: Alexander and Shepherd.

[161] GL, LMS72. 1910. London Municipal Pamphlets and Leaflets. 'The London County Council', Municipal Reform Leaflet A23.

[162] National Union of Women's Suffrage Societies, 'A word to midwives and trained nurses on pending legislation', 199. Cited in Pennybacker, *A Vision for London, 1889–1914*: 244.

cheerful social life, amusements and personal contact with patients are among the items in this ministry of London to 16,000 suffers'.[163] 'No part of the Council's work has produced more happiness', Benn continued, 'than its provision for these poor people'.[164] Rosebery, in a speech to the 'Progressive members of LCC', following his elevation to the post of as Prime Minister spoke of the Asylums Committee in glowing terms. The fact that the Asylums Committee had done so much for their patients and that was one of the 'brightest features in their record' was met with cheers from the partisan crowd, but even the *Daily Mail* recognised the work of the Committee in this regard.[165] 'It has improved the lot of every inmate', it concluded, 'it has increased their comfort'—and this was from a newspaper that regularly described the Progressives as 'wastrels'.[166]

In party-political terms, patients became important for the first time and the argument here was that Progressive changes to the administration and management of asylums brought about equally positive changes for the people within them. This was undoubtedly tied to Progressive notions of improving the lot of wider London society but the rhetoric did not always match the reality and the treatment of patients continued to attract a range of criticisms from key stakeholders. As part of their role, Councillors serving on individual committees were expected to tour their asylums, give the patients an opportunity to speak with them and listen to any grievances. John McDougall was said to know each of London's 15,000 patients personally but, beyond this hyperbole, were concerns from the Commissioners in Lunacy about the limited opportunities people had for 'ventilating their grievances' at a number

[163] Saint, Andrew. 1989. Technical Education and the Early LCC. In *Politics and the People of London: The London County Council 1889–1965*, ed. Andrew Saint, 71–92. London: Hambledon Press: 75. Benn, J. Williams. 1892. The Internal Working of the London County Council, *The Times*, 7 January 1892: 6.

[164] Benn, J. Williams. 1892. The Internal Working of the London County Council. *The Times*, 7 January. Although not mentioned here, Benn's father had been murdered by his brother, William, who was then sent to an asylum in 1883. I am grateful to Heather Shore for this information.

[165] The Earl of Rosebery. 1894. *Municipal and Social Reform*. London: Liberal Publications: 6.

[166] Anon. 1903. Housing the Insane. What the London County Council Has Done. *Daily Mail*, 29 January. BL 8139B22, *The Daily Mail and the Fight for London*: 5–6.

of asylums.[167] Then, there were the issues related to the ill-treatment of patients. Whatever claims were being made about LCC, its introduction did not prevent depressing and distressing attacks on patients, often by attendant staff. In these cases, the Commissioners in Lunacy lobbied for the prosecution of the individuals involved and the resulting court cases were played out in the press.[168]

Similarly, while some commentators and politicians spoke of 'efficiency', the Commissioners in Lunacy regularly raised concerns about overcrowding and the parlous state of staff:patient ratios in LCC's asylums.[169] They also questioned the small sums paid for low quality cloth which lead to 'shabby' uniforms for male attendants and the low quality of male patients' suits at Banstead and Colney Hatch.[170] Moreover, during a visit to the Cane Hill, they argued that the plans to introduce 'uniform clothing' at the asylum would 'destroy the individuality of the patients and lessen their self-respect' when they were currently

[167] *Forty-Seventh Report of the Commissioners in Lunacy*, 1893. 216. *Fifty Second Report of the Commissioners in Lunacy*, 1898: 312. *Fifty-Fifth Report of the Commissioners in Lunacy*, 1901: 300. *Fifty-Seventh Report of the Commissioners in Lunacy*, 1903: 318. *Fifty-Eighth Report of the Commissioners in Lunacy*, 1904: 322. *Fifty-Ninth Report of the Commissioners in Lunacy*, 1905: 344. *Sixtieth Report of the Commissioners in Lunacy*, 1906: 346. *Fifty-Seventh Report of the Commissioners in Lunacy*, 1903: 318.

[168] Following the death of a patient (W.S.) as a result of undue force at the Banstead Asylum, for example, the Commissioners recommended that the two attendants involved should be dismissed. Instead, the sub-committee at Banstead 'severely reprimanded' one attendant, while the other was only dismissed after a subsequent charge of using bad language towards a patient. *Fifty-Fourth Report of the Commissioners*, 1900: 28–9. *Fifty-Sixth Report of the Commissioners in Lunacy*, 1902: 309. In another case, an attendant was fined after an assault on a 'troublesome and violent patient' who was nicknamed 'Dummy' because he was deaf and dumb. In imposing the fine on the attendant for the assault, the bench noted that it did not consider it to be a bad case. Anon. 1908. Asylum Scene, *Daily News*, 17 April.

[169] *Forty-Fifth Report of the Commissioners in Lunacy*, 1891: 194. *Forty-Ninth Report of the Commissioners in Lunacy*, 1895: 264. *Fifty-Second Report of the Commissioners in Lunacy*, 1898: 316.

[170] The Liberal *Speaker* claimed the Asylums Committee had 'economised, improved, reformed, in every conceivable direction. Its sub-committees, sharing between them the control of 16,000 lunatics have set a new model for the management of public asylums'. Anon. 1892. Back to Vestrydom? *The Speaker*, 9 January. *Fifty-Second Report of the Commissioners in Lunacy*, 1898: 303. *Forty-Ninth Report of the Commissioners in Lunacy*, 1895: 270.

looking 'very well in various garbs of different hues'.[171] Significantly too, questions were asked about the warmth of clothing by both the Commissioners and the Poor Law authorities and, in 1893, after a visit to Hanwell, the representatives of the St Saviour's Union, wrote to express their concern at the treatment of one patient working in potato field who was improperly dressed and very cold.[172] Letters to the press escalated the complaint with the Guardians claiming that the building was 'entirely unfit for the curative treatment of the insane'.[173]

Not everyone was quite so critical and there is much evidence to show that individuals and groups preferred the apparent superiority of LCC accommodation, even if this was framed by concerns about the alternatives. When a group of patients arrived at LCC's Bexley Asylum, for example, the Commissioners in Lunacy commented that those transferred 'from other institutions spoke favourably of the change and the care bestowed upon them here'. [174] There is no evidence to explain where the patients in question had been but criticism of alternative accommodation usually meant private asylums. Fisherton House in Salisbury is particularly relevant here as it was used by LCC as alternative, over-flow accommodation to its own stock and to its out-county agreements. In one such example a Wandsworth woman became pregnant at the hands of an attendant there and, at a meeting of the Wandsworth Board of Guardians, 'indignant words were used' and calls were made for LCC to withdraw their lunatics from the asylum and for the Lunacy Commissioners to close it.[175] Similarly, when the Chelsea Guardians visited LCC's asylums and three other places where their inmates were sent, Fisherton featured heavily in their discussions. One Guardian stated that 'if he ever went barmy' he hoped he would not be sent to a private asylum but to an LCC asylum where he knew he

[171] *Forty-Fifth Report of the Commissioners in Lunacy*, 1891: 194.

[172] *Sixty-Fourth Report of the Commissioners in Lunacy*, 1910: 346.

[173] In their response, the Hanwell sub-committee, described the clothes as warm enough and they pointed to statistics of improving rates of cure, along with a diminishing death rates to deflect the criticism. They did, however, conclude, that as one of LCC's older asylums, Hanwell suffered from some defects that were undesirable to modern eyes. LMA, LCC/18.6, London County Council Minutes of Proceedings, January–June 1894, 24 April 1894. LMA, LCC/18.6, London County Council Minutes of Proceedings, January–December 1893, 21 November 1893.

[174] *Fifty-Fourth Report of the Commissioners in Lunacy*, 1900: 312.

[175] Anon. 1905. Asylum Scandal. *London Daily News*, 13 October 1905.

would be properly treated'.[176] Another Guardian agreed with the sentiment on the grounds that there had been a huge scandal at Fisherton House in the past. This probably referred to the transfer of patients to Fisherton from the Banstead and Claybury Asylums in 1903, in which five patients were wrongly identified. The families of these patients had been mistakenly told that their loved ones had passed away or, indeed, that they were still alive when they were not.[177] Similarly, an investigation into the St Pancras Union revealed the collusion of its relieving officers and doctors who profited from sending patients to private asylums, rather than LCC's public institutions. Moreover, while sane individuals were not detained, those who were cured remained incarcerated for the purposes of profit.[178] In this case, the *Municipal Journal* claimed that the scheme was practised in other London districts and was a 'legacy from the old days of Bumbledom', which resulted in the 'manufacture of lunacy'.[179] In the main then, the 'quality' of the patient experience tended to be an issue for other stakeholders, rather than a political point of debate. This did not stop politicians co-opting the voices of patients for political purposes. To emphasise this, and the impact of London's wider reformers further, links will now be drawn to the Progressive's focus on temperance.

The Progressives, Temperance and the Asylum Experience

In terms of treatment, rather than just administration of lunacy, one of the direct impacts that the Progressives had was in relation to drink. The first British temperance groups were formed in the 1820s but the highpoint of intervention came in the period covered by this book.[180]

[176] Anon. 1914. Chelsea Guardians. *Chelsea News and General Advertiser*, 26 June.

[177] *Sixty-Second Report of the Commissioners in Lunacy*, 1908: 77–85. This was something that was not undermined even when there was a case of mistaken identity at the Cane Hill in the same year. In that case, relatives were called to the bedside of a seriously ill-patient at the asylum only to discover the person in question was not their mother but a stranger with the same name. LMA, PH/Ment/3/5, Newspaper Cuttings, 'Evening News', 4 February 1907.

[178] Anon. 1900. What Will Follow St Pancras Inquiry. *Municipal Journal*, 13 July.

[179] Ibid.

[180] Yeomans, Henry. 2014. *Alcohol and Moral Regulation: Public Attitudes, Spirited Measures and Victorian Hangovers*. Bristol: Policy Press: 35, 98.

Following the first election in 1889, the Progressives removed beer from the asylum dietary. Election materials proudly proclaimed that

> The abolition of alcohol from the lunatic asylum as an article of diet is an admitted success, and many a drink made lunatic, by this non-alcoholic treatment, has been strengthened and encouraged in their struggle to overcome their appetite for strong drink. Most of the County Asylums are situated some distance from any refreshment house, except a public house. To meet this difficulty, arrangements have been made to supply the friends of patients on visiting days with tea, coffee, cake etc. of good quality at low prices. This is a boon appreciated by many thousands who visit several asylums. [181]

Barbara Taylor has described the decision to ban beer at the Colney Hatch asylum as one that was taken by a 'busybody subcommittee' of LCC and this fits in neatly with the tropes explored by other historians.[182] Akhito Suzuki, for example, has shown that the abolition of strait-jackets and other methods of restraint at nineteenth-century Hanwell was 'initiated, planned and executed by the magistrates'.[183] Similarly, Doyle has shown how elected officials in the twentieth century were often dependent upon or relied on managers and experts for providing the rationale for reforms.[184] In this case, however, a line can be drawn between the removal of beer at all London asylums with a wider campaigns against drink in the capital. The number of persons per pub may have been lower in London than any other city but the 1890s saw Progressive moves to close pubs and, more successfully, prohibit the sale of alcohol in music halls and theatres, and in the refreshment rooms of public parks.[185] This helps to explain why patients and

[181] GL, PM 3438. 1907. Progressive Leaflets, London County Council Election 1907, 'The Progressives and Temperance Reform', Progressive Election Committee.

[182] Taylor, Barbara. 2015. *The Last Asylum: A Memoir of Madness on Our Times*. Chicago: University of Chicago Press: 105.

[183] Suzuki, The Politics and Ideology of Non-restraint: 2.

[184] Doyle, Barry M. 2001. The Changing Functions of Urban Government: Councillors, Officials and Pressure Groups, 1835–1950. In *The Cambridge Urban History of Britain*, eds. D. M. Palliser, Peter Clark, and Martin J. Daunton, 287–313. Cambridge: Cambridge University Press: 296–7.

[185] Harrison, B. 1973, Pubs. *The Victorian City: Images and Realities*, vol. 1, eds. H. J. Dyos and M. Wolff, 161–90. London: Routledge and Kegan Paul: 162. Pennybacker, The Millennium by Return of Post: 131.

their visitors were said to appreciate the 'boon' of tea and coffee and it further blurs of the boundaries between asylum estates and wider society. The 'Rules for Visitors' expressly stated 'No Wine, Sprit, or Intoxicating Liquors of any kind are permitted to be brought into the Asylum or allowed under any pretext whatsoever to be given to any of the patients'.[186]

Jonathan Reinarz and Rebecca Wynter have charted changing attitudes to drink within European psychiatry and argue that it was this, along with ratepayer concerns about its costs, that led to the decline in its use as food and medicine in asylums more broadly.[187] This would have certainly found support among London's County Councillors but leading the charge in London were the relatively well-known councillors, John McDougall and John William Benn. The reforms were welcomed by the many temperance groups in the capital and beyond and, while there had always been concern about the impact of alcohol on individuals, the underlying discourse in this period was changing. Yeomans argues that debates about intemperance increasingly focused on the impact of the Boer War, concerns about national efficiency, and racial degeneration, which culminated in an Inebriates Act in 1898.[188] Such attempts to regulate the lives and bodies of drunks places London's asylums at the heart of much by wider political discourses and they came to be used in election propaganda for those purposes. As part of his election address in 1889, Benn had called for the regulation of liquor licenses.[189] As LCC Chairman, his speech on the work of the Council in 1904 included a tribute to the work of the Asylums Committee but also the positive impact in bringing back to a life of usefulness 'those afflicted with the drink disease'.[190] Lord Monkswell, another member of the Asylums Committee, addressed a large temperance meeting at Holborn Town Hall, and spoke of the exceptional opportunities he had

[186]LMA, H12/CH/B/46/63, Colney Hatch Female Reception Orders, 16451–16475: Rules for Visitors to Patients.

[187]Reinarz, J. and Wynter, R. 2014. The Spirit of Medicine: The Use of Alcohol in Nineteenth-Century Medical Practice. In *Drink in the Eighteen and Nineteenth Centuries*, eds. S. Schmid and B. Schmidt-Haberkamp. 127–40. London: Pickering and Chatto.

[188]Yeomans, *Alcohol and Moral Regulation*: 98.

[189]Brodie, M. 2008. Benn, Sir John Williams, first baronet. *Oxford Dictionary of National Biography*. https://www.oxforddnb.com/. Accessed 4 July 2019.

[190]BL, *Municipal Journal*, 14 October 1904: 72.

experienced in seeing the 'terrible consequences' of intemperance in the course of his visiting duties.[191]

Politically speaking, the attack on drink could be presented as an attack on working-class culture and Jon Lawrence has shown how the Tories used this to good effect to help them to defeat Radical-Liberal councillors in Wolverhampton.[192] Indeed, subsequent analysis has suggested that the Progressive's 'puritanical paternalism', which included the banning of park games on Sundays, played a part in their election defeat in 1907.[193] Of course, one person's puritanical paternalism was another's rational recreation, and it did not stop the Progressives using temperance as a device in election campaigns. A 1901 election leaflet listed the votes in which the Moderates had voted against temperance reforms in the Councils of 1895 and 1898 and, in this election at least, there were calls to mobilise electors via temperance groups as well as Friendly and Trade societies.[194] The Moderates [*sic*], it was claimed in 1909, 'thwart temperance' and in the run up to the 1913 election a conference of London's temperance organisations sought to secure the return of candidates, irrespective of party, pledging themselves to Temperance in light of the dismantling of 'old temperance policy of the Council'.[195]

In the interim, and according to the *Daily Mail*, much of the ire was directed towards 'The McDougall' whose work on temperance reform made him 'the best abused and most scorned man in London'.[196] Journalist Fred Mckenzie claimed it was McDougall who introduced an order to 'stop the supply of intoxicants to inmates, save when ordered by the doctors'.[197] The focus on McDougall is, perhaps, understandable given his well-known work on the Asylums Committee, but this

[191]Anon. 1898. Temperance Crusade. *The Times*, 26 October.

[192]Lawrence, J. 1993. Class and Gender in the Making of Urban Toryism, 1880–1914. *English Historical Review*, 108: 629–52.

[193]Ball and Sunderland, *An Economic History of London*: 411.

[194]Anon. 1901. *The London County Council of 1895 and 1898*. London: Alexander and Shepherd. Anon. 1901. *London County Council Election 1901*. London: Alexander and Shepherd.

[195]LSE, JS203–211. 1909. London Under the Moderates. LSE, ILP/6/22/1/84504. 1913. London County Council, An urgent appeal to Ministers and Churches.

[196]Mckenzie, Fred A. 1902. The Triumph of Mr McDougall. *Daily Mail*, 12 March.

[197]Ibid.

understates the importance of the Progressive dominance on it and the Council as a whole. Not all members of the Progressive Party welcomed the wider moves against drink it is true but, rather than a parochial assault on drink, John Griffiths sees initiatives designed to purify the city as part of a much wider progressive world movement.[198] Thus, the temperance policy was not limited or, indeed driven by what was happening in the asylums.

Once again, we can see the response of patients co-opted for political purposes. Election materials claimed that 'Fears of great dissatisfaction [about the removal of beer] among both patients and staff [were] 'groundless'. The Medical Superintendent of the Banstead asylum claimed that '[he heard] very little from the patients on the subject of beer' and that 'they have quietly acquiesced in its withdrawal'.[199] At Hanwell too, reports of the Commissioners in Lunacy reveal that only 'here and there did the patients complain about the withdrawal of beer'.[200] The Medical Superintendent at the Hanwell Asylum report the 'happiest results' with a decrease in 'squabbles and bickering among the patients'.[201] Hide notes that many other asylums had already banned alcohol, but this was a policy that put the Council at odds with the Commissioners in Lunacy and George Bibby advised that, in the near future at least, architects were likely to include plans for brewing establishments within many new asylums.[202]

In reality, the evidence from LCC's other asylums did not quite fit the claims made in relation to the acceptance of the changes. 95% of the attendants may have taken an increase in pay in lieu of beer but that did not prevent their ongoing prosecution for being drunk both on and off-duty.[203] At Colney Hatch, in particular, the patients were regularly vocal about the removal of the beer allowance with the Commissioners

[198] Griffiths, John. 2009. Were There Municipal Networks in the British World c.1890–1939. *The Journal of Imperial and Commonwealth History* 37:4: 575–597, 579.

[199] GL, PAM3556. 1907. Progressive Party Leaflets, 'What the Progressive Party on the County Council Has Done for Temperance in London?', Leaflet No. 13.

[200] *Forty-Fifth Report of the Commissioners in Lunacy*, 1891: 199.

[201] LSE, Coll. Misc. 904. No date. London Reform Union, Leaflet No. 57, 'What the County Council Has Done for Temperance Reform'.

[202] Hide, *Gender and Class*: 151. Bibby, *The Planning of Lunatic Asylums*: 67.

[203] *Daily Chronicle*. 'The Council and the Asylums: For Sick Minds and Bodies': 52. Hide, *Gender and Class*: 34–5.

in Lunacy reporting that the disuse of beer left the patients less contented.[204] The Commissioners lobbied on their behalf stating that:

> Having regard to the fact that the vast majority will never leave the Asylum, and that all these were brought here against their will, and that but a certain proportion of those ... have [become] insane through excess in drink, it does seem hard that the many should suffer for the sake of the few, and their possible, though not probable, amelioration in habits'.[205]

The asylum was not, they explained two years later, a reformatory but the response to such criticism were not confined to the pages of official reports and committee minutes. The Liberal-supporting *Daily Chronicle* described the Commissioners as 'not [an] especially progressive body' and their calls to reinstate alcohol as 'rather fatuous'.[206] Links were made to both the wider context of drink in London but also its impact on everyday life within the asylum. Numbers under the heading of *a potu*, the *Chronicle* pointed out were significant; almost 500, which accounted for many more cases that those which were due to 'misery and worry that came from domestic and business life'.[207] Cases of alcoholism, it continued:

> occur and reoccur and unless the patient is kept absolutely clear of the old habit, it fastens on him afresh. But that is not all. A single glass of beer might not do harm, but when you are victualling 2,000 patients a day you cannot be sure that each will have his glass and no more. The result of the old system was that patients often got two or three glasses, and were much the worse for them.[208]

For those prescribed alcohol for medical reasons nothing changed, but for the Commissioners total abstinence, rather than the avoidance of excess, was both an irritant and a disincentive to engage in that potent factor of recovery—work.[209]

[204] *Forty-Seventh Report of the Commissioners in Lunacy*, 1893: 214.

[205] *Forty-Sixth Report of the Commissioners in Lunacy*, 1892: 215.

[206] *Daily Chronicle*, The Council and the Asylums: For Sick Minds and Bodies: 52.

[207] Ibid.

[208] Ibid.

[209] *Forty-Eighth Report of the Commissioners in Lunacy*, 1894: 237.

As the pleas of their advocates fell on deaf ears, the patients took their own action and withdrew their labour with the Commissioners drawing a direct link between the removal of beer and the relatively low numbers of patients involved in employment.[210] This, they argued was seen as 'a potent factor in recovery and an effective remedy from some destructive habits' and the lack of drink as an inducement 'absolved Dr Seward, from any blame for the non-employment of his patients'.[211] When this was combined with the removal of another incentive of 'a trip out with an attendant', several patients complained. 'This complaint', the Commissioners reported, seemed 'to be worthy of attention, more especially as the patients who so complained were of intelligence, and know that work could not be demanded of them as of right'.[212]

Even at Banstead where the patients supposedly 'acquiesced' to the removal of beer, the number of working male and female patients was 32% and 39%, respectively, at a time when the average across all asylums in both cases was around 60%. These low numbers, the Commissioners concluded, resulted directly from the decision to remove beer as an incentive to work. At Hanwell, the Commissioners could not decide whether the relatively low number of patients undertaking useful employment was due to the broken-down nature of the patients or the lack of inducements. This did not stop those patients who could work complaining that apart from a small allowance of tobacco 'they obtained nothing for their services'.[213] Whatever we might think of asylum regimes in this period, patient employment was seen by the Commissioners 'a potent factor in recovery and an effective remedy from some destructive habits'. At a stroke, the Progressive Party's decision to remove drink from its asylums removed an incentive to work and, with nothing in place to replace it, actively contributed to our vision of the places of sites of inactivity and, perhaps even, as Museums of Madness.

[210] Ibid.

[211] Ibid.

[212] *Fifty-Second Report of the Commissioners in Lunacy*, 1898: 311. *Fiftieth Report of the Commissioners in Lunacy*, 1896: 300.

[213] *Fifty-First Report of the Commissioners in Lunacy*, 1897: 287. However, the rules of Colney Hatch revealed that small quantities of tobacco sent by relatives to patients was allowed. LMA, H12/CH/B/46/63, Colney Hatch Female Reception Orders, 16451–16475: Rules for Visitors to Patients.

Conclusions

Given the evidence presented here, it is difficult to see how contemporary commentators could claim that the work of the Asylums Committee was somehow hidden away or that it was somehow separate from the work of the Council. On a very basic level, the administrative reforms introduced and the centralisation of some services were presented as Progressive successes by commentators and election materials alike. This, however, was framed by the wider management of London and the work of the Committee was shaped by it and fed forward into wider debates. While there were critiques of the reality of the asylum experience from a number of stakeholders, the key points here were the claims and counter claims made by contesting political parties. Historians of mental health in this period are used to exploring the scrutiny of visiting committees, government watchdogs, and newspapers but in this period we can see the emergence of party-political scrutiny for the first time. Thus, the patient experience became useful evidence in the debates and propaganda, even if it did not necessarily match the claims that were being made on the ground. In this respect, the patients were largely voiceless and it is probable that for them political affiliation was less important than the ability to speak with those who claimed to be their advocates.[214] Either way, the parties co-opted their voices but were largely uninterested in the things they had to say as individuals.

To be sure, both the Council and the Committees had to meet the demands of a raft of lunacy legislation. However, the operation of this cannot be divorced from an understanding that Councillors stood on specific election platforms and subscribed to particular views about the ways in how London should be governed. Thus, when it came to elections, party-political organisations focussed on which Councillors were actively representing their electorate's interests. This does not mean that asylums policy was ever the number-one election issue, but it is representative of its place in wider understanding of political programmes of reform. As a result, the use of attendance at committee meetings was used for political purposes with the Asylums Committee held up to the electorate as an exemplar for all Councillors. This offers straightforward

[214]LMA, ACC/3606/001 Election Literature and Newspaper Cuttings, 1906–1907, 'Who have done London's work?', February 1907. 'Who does the work?', *Daily News*, 11 February 1907: 8.

evidence of the party division in relation to the operation of policy, rather than what have been described in some places as a cross-party pride in the development of the Council's mental health services. It is indicative of the contentious nature of its supposedly non-contentious work. Here then, while the work of the Committee became politicised it was a politicisation that was framed from the outset by both the membership of the Council and its committee structure.

Furthermore, more detailed analysis of attendance reveals that we cannot simply talk about this Committee or that Committee without seeking to understand who the people who served on it were. Their relative 'anonymity' makes some of this difficult but even the long-term absence of women on the Council tells us something about the role of the Asylums Committee in terms of wider debates about suffrage and participation. In terms of the Asylums Committee, both the negative, as well as the positive impact of 'the McDougall' can be seen here, but the citing of other key individuals such as Martineau or Strong, reveals that it was they who were responsible for driving areas of policy. When combined with details on Committee membership, and attendance more generally, this takes on more significance and challenges somewhat the party political rhetoric. Individuals may have been responsible for driving policy but political allegiances also had a part to play. In the chapters that follow, more thought will be given to individuals and the support their initiatives received from across broader party affiliations and, in the next chapter, the importance of political allegiances will be explored more fully.

CHAPTER 3

The Politics of Finance

Introduction

When LCC took office for the first time, it provided the capital with a directly elected authority which, unlike its predecessor the MBW, was accountable to a rate paying public.[1] The MBW had faced suspicion of its handling of the capital's affairs and, with more than a whiff of corruption, was known colloquially as the 'Board of Perks'.[2] Davies describes the immediate effect of its decline as the creation of a climate favourable to municipal enterprise.[3] In their discussion of the shift from the MBW to LCC, Ball and Sunderland argue that 'it satisfied the aspirations of both the economisers and those that saw metropolitan government as a way of radically improving urban social policy and creating a new London political identity'.[4] Despite this, there is a sense that the financial aspects of the work of the Asylums Committee were somehow untroubled by the changing political landscape. The only time it consulted the Council on expenditure, noted

[1] For an overview of the origins and achievements of the MBW, along with the developing case for its abolition, which included allegations of corruption, see Davies, Local Government 1850–1920: 47–56.

[2] Owen, David. 1982. *The Government of Victorian London, 1855–1889*. Cambridge, MA: Belknap Press: Chapters 8 and 9. See also Davies, Local Government 1850–1920: 47–56.

[3] Davies, The Progressive Council, 1889–1907: 27.

[4] Ball and Sunderland, *An Economic History of London*: 409.

R. Ellis, *London and its Asylums, 1888-1914*,
Mental Health in Historical Perspective,
https://doi.org/10.1007/978-3-030-44432-7_3

one contemporary, was when its forecasts included large capital projects, such as the building of new institutions.[5] Instead, its annual accounts were audited by the LGB and the overview of its operations were left to the Commissioners in Lunacy. Moreover, in more recent studies, the role of politics in the financial scrutiny and decision-making related to asylums in this period has been largely absent.[6] This might be explained by the fact that party allegiances in local politics were less well defined in provincial towns than in the capital but the costs involved could be huge. In London, the links between financial management and LCC were clear to see and, as was shown in the previous chapter, the sheer scope of the asylums' operation emphasised its expense. The wage bill alone in the early part of the twentieth century was £118,000 per annum and even from its earliest days, the broader issue of the economies of scale loomed large.[7]

Thus, to understand the significance of the debates over the governance of asylums, and particularly their finances, requires attention to both political priorities and also to party-political rhetoric. The relationship between the Asylums Committee and the Finance Committee, as explored by Melling and Forsythe, is important, as are the relationships between national 'watchdogs' and local administrators which have been explored in terms of general as well as mental health.[8] This chapter seeks to build on these studies to consider the issue of political allegiances and wider political visions to explore what impact, in any, they had on the financial decision-making processes of the Asylums Committee. Martin Powell's quantitative analysis of municipal health spending in the interwar period suggests that the role of politics in decision-making has been underestimated and that position will be tested here.[9] In particular,

[5]Donald, Robert. 1901. *The London Manual for 1901*. London: Edward Lloyd Limited: 75.

[6]Sheard, Sally. 2006. Reluctant Providers? The Politics and Ideology of Municipal Hospital Finance 1870–1914. In *Financing Medicine: The British Experience Since 1750*, eds. Martin Gorsky and Sally Sheard, 112–29. London: Routledge. Hayes, Lancashire Public Asylum Provision: 87.

[7]Donald, *The London Manual for 1901*: 75.

[8]Melling and Forsythe, *The Politics of Madness*: 45. Sheard, Reluctant Providers?: 112–29. Hayes, Lancashire Public Asylum Provision: 87.

[9]Powell, Martin. 1995. Did Politics Matter? Municipal Public Expenditure in the 1930s. *Urban History* 22:3: 360–79, 379. See also Levene, Alysa, Powell, Martin, Stewart, John and Taylor, Becky. 2011. *Cradle to Grave: Municipal Medicine in Interwar England and Wales*. Bern: Peter Lang.

attention will be paid to how the spending on asylums featured in election campaigns, and became part of the political rhetoric of the period. Questions will be asked about how and where spending aligned with the parties' broader political ambitions for the capital and how this was affected by majority administrations. Given that the focus of recent studies has been on the internecine disputes between various council committees, this chapter will first consider the relationship between the Asylum and Finance Committees using the development of the Epsom cluster as a case study. It will then go to explore the relationship between asylum finance and political ideology and how that linked to other initiatives. This will include a focus on staffing and also the Council's Direct Labour Organisation, the Works Department.[10] Using the 1907 election as a pivot, the aim here is to demonstrate that the relationship between Asylums and spending was ultimately defined by the politics and ideologies of those involved.

Asylum Committee Spending and the Finance Committee as the Council's Watchdog

In the first few years of the Council, as part of the transition process instigated by the LGA, various LCC officials and committees sought to interpret the role of the Asylums Committee in relation to financial matters and the demands of that legislation. Lord (Robert) Lingen, the chairman of the Council's first Finance Committee, was to play an important role in this and it was to him that the Council turned to provide its first regulations. Davis describes Lingen as 'untypical' of London Radicalism at this time and instead suggests that his appointment, along with that of Rosebery and Lubbock, was a nod to age and experience.[11] As permanent secretary to the national Treasury, Lingen had worked hard to impose financial control on the civil service. His biographer describes his style as 'abrasive', which emphasised his 'negative tone' when overseeing the national Treasury's scrutiny of the work

[10] Forsythe et al., The Politics of Lunacy: 83. Melling and Forsythe, *The Politics of Madness*: 42.

[11] Davies, *Reforming London*: 119. Haward also notes that Lingen was one of only three aldermen nominated to the first Council nominated to both sides, along with Lord Hobhouse and Quintin Hogg. Haward, *The London County Council from Within*: 19.

and spending plans of governmental departments.[12] Moreover, on his appointment as Chairman of the Finance Committee, he had stressed his objectivity, stating that he was unprepared 'to give any pledges', irrespective of the questions that would come before the council.[13]

From the outset, Lingen tried to implement a level of financial scrutiny on the work of the Council and, as a corollary, its Asylums Committee. It was noted that the Asylums Committee had the power to appoint a Treasurer and Clerk for each asylum and to set the terms of reference for their duties but, on the issue of large-scale spending plans, Lingen argued that the Finance Committee should play a key role.[14] It was, according to him, the Council in concert with the Finance Committee that should lead on the building of new asylums. Drawing on his reading of both the LGA and the 1853 Lunacy Amendment Act, his report stated that before the contracts for new buildings and land 'were completed or carried into execution', the Asylums Committee was responsible for reporting to the Council the amounts needed for its plans.[15] The Asylums Committee could procure and determine plans and estimates for new asylums only 'when authorised by the Council, on recommendation of the Finance Committee'.[16]

As Robert Millward and Sally Sheard have pointed out, the expansion in this period of other large-scale capital projects such as waterworks, town halls, roads and tramways was costly.[17] This included terms of the repayments and the interest accrued on the loans necessary to facilitate them and to this asylum projects can be added. LCC had inherited a cash balance of approximately £20,000 for each of the three Middlesex Asylums (Hanwell, Colney, Banstead) or £60,000 in total. By the end of 1908 that had risen to £103,000 but even then it could not cover

[12]Sutherland, G. 2004. Lingen, Ralph Robert Wheeler, Baron Lingen. *Oxford Dictionary of National Biography*. https://www.oxforddnb.com/. Accessed 4 July 2019.

[13]Cited in Davies, *Reforming London*: 119.

[14]The financial duties of the Treasurer and the Clerk were described in the Lunatic Asylums Act (1853) LMA LCC/CL/PH/01/276, Asylums Finance. 1899. Suggestions of Lord Lingen, LCC.

[15]LMA LCC/CL/PH/01/276, Regulations as to Asylums Finance. 1899. LCC.

[16]LMA LCC/CL/PH/01/276, Suggestions for Regulations as to Asylum Finance. 1889. LCC.

[17]Millward, Robert and Sheard, Sally. 1995. The Urban Fiscal Problem, 1870–1914: Government Expenditure and Finance in England and Wales. *The Economic History Review* 48:3: 501–35, 505.

the cost of new asylum.[18] Lingen's regulations were aimed at the large-scale capital projects that involved the financing and building of new ones but, over time, regulations were extended to include the smaller amounts involved in their maintenance. In 1895 and 1896, the Finance Committee, by then under the Chairmanship of Alfred Hoare, a banker and man of 'independent thought' had advanced monies from the county fund for the maintenance of several asylums.[19] Hoare suggested that this too was to be formalised in the Council's Standing Orders, the rules and regulations that governed the work of the Council. This included a responsibility on the part of the Asylums Committee to make it clear the amounts devolved to them by the Council and to provide clarity in terms of any expenditure already completed. There was also an expectation that, on the completion of any planned works, an account of receipts and expenditure would be provided and any 'unexpended balance' would be paid back into the county fund.[20]

All of this indicates detailed lines of financial reporting which were emphasised in a series of additional Standing Orders. Standing Order 262, for example, stated that 'No recommendation or proposal involving expenditure on the capital account shall be voted upon by the Council until an estimate of the costs, debts, or liability to be entered into has been submitted by the Finance Committee to the Council'.[21] Within this, the Asylums Committee had the power to 'order the execution of all necessary and ordinary repairs, and also of all necessary and proper additions, alterations and improvements to an amount not exceeding £400 at each asylum in any one year. Expenditure above £400 at any asylum required the sanction of the Council, and was, again, only given (under the Council's Standing orders) on the recommendation of the Finance Committee'.[22]

[18] LMA LCC/MIN/575, Signed Minutes, March 1908–February 1909, 22 December 1908.

[19] Haward, *The London County Council From Within*: 22.

[20] LMA LCC/18.6, London County Council Minutes of Proceedings, January–June 1896, 28 January 1896.

[21] LMA LCC/CL/PH/01/276, Heath Asylum, Bexley. 1899. Report by the Clerk of the Council, LCC.

[22] Keene, H.F. 1907. *Memorandum as to the Procedure with Regard to the Admission and Discharge of Patients*. London: LCC.

These examples emphasise the fact that the regulation of one committee by another was governed by Standing Orders which were agreed by the Council as a whole. As such, the regulation of finances was a concern of those on both sides of the political divide. The Progressives argued that theirs was not a 'slap-dash philanthropy' and, in 1898, Sir John Lubbock, Progressive Councillor and one-time Chairman of LCC, raised his own concerns in the run up to the 1898 election.[23]

> At present, if a Committee determines, with the assent of the Council on a certain purchase, on erecting a band stand, or a palm house, or some cottages, or appointing some new officials, the Finance Committee have no authority from the Council to consider, whether these buildings or officers are necessary, nor are the salaries refered to them. They merely consider whether the band stand or palm house, for instance, could be erected for less money. As I understand the Act, however, the intention of parliament was that the Finance Committee should exercise the same control as the Treasury does, with such great advantage over our national expenditure. … Unless such policy is adopted in London, and unless the ratepayers insist that their representatives shall abstain from any speculative and business transactions, I am firmly persuaded that the expenditure, and consequently the rate will rise indefinitely.[24]

Within this, it is easy to see the auditing of the business of the Asylums Committee as an administrative procedure, rather than a political one. And yet, the increasing clarity of the regulations only sought to shine a light on their ineffectiveness. In 1896, when the Finance Committee asked the Asylums Committee to estimate its expenditure for the next seven years, the response from the latter was that it regretted its inability to provide such information.[25] Three years later when the Finance Committee asked for a reduction in the repairs estimate, it was refused on the grounds that the original estimates had been carefully produced.[26]

[23] *Daily Chronicle*. 1895. The Council and the Asylums: For Sick Minds and Bodies. In *New London: Her Parliament and Its Work*. London: Edward Lloyd Limited: 51.

[24] GL, SL:30:03. 1898. A Collection of Tracts, Sir John Lubbock, 'On the Real Issues of the London County Elections', London: London Municipal Society.

[25] LMA LCC/MIN/567, Signed Minutes, 1894–1897, 14 July 1896, 13 October 1896.

[26] LMA LCC/PH/MENT/05/003, Minutes of Meetings of Asylum Officers, 1899–1915, 28 March 1899.

The first real test for the new financial regulations came with the planning of the Bexley Heath Asylum in Kent. Although the asylum at Claybury was the first of London's asylums to open as an LCC institution, its planning pre-dated the change of administration ushered in by the LGA. As a result, the first asylum to be planned and built by LCC was the one at Bexley Heath, which opened in 1898. Bexley would be LCC's sixth asylum and key to the discussions about the site and the design was finance. Both at Committee level and within the Council chamber, there were delays in first purchasing the site at Baldwyn's Park and also in advertising for plans and estimates from external contractors.[27] While the Asylums Committee may have had ambitions for the new institution, the reporting of it to the Council, in line with the new financial regulations, meant that it was open to the scrutiny of the elected chamber. It was the Council, rather than the Finance Committee that attempted to impose somewhat arbitrary spending limits in a bid to keep the costs down. Using their experience of Claybury, the Asylums Committee requested a fund 'not exceeding £350,000', which was to include the total cost of the site, furnishings and the architect's fees. However, a proposed amendment following a vote in the Council chamber reduced that figure to £300,000.[28] To be clear, many of those Councillors voting for the amendment were also members of the Asylums Committee and this was not a vote taken solely on party lines. While some members of the Committee voted to reduce the costs, other voted against, but as a whole, the Council Chamber sought to limit spending, in spite of the recommendations put forward by those with a specific interest and expertise in the administration of asylums.

Significantly, attempts to reduce the costs of the asylum by £50,000 were based on little other than an aspiration to keep costs down but this was to prove to be an academic exercise. Within a few months of the vote, the Asylums Committee went back to the Council to report that it was impossible to build an asylum for £300,000. This time, having been provided with estimates that had been scrutinised by the Finance Committee, the Council voted in favour of the original figure

[27] LMA LCC/18.6, London County Council Minutes of Proceedings, January–December 1893, 18 July 1893. LMA LCC/18.6, London County Council Minutes of Proceedings, January–June 1894, 19 June 1894.

[28] LMA, LCC/18.6, London County Council Minutes of Proceedings, January–June 1894, 26 June 1894.

of £350,000.[29] Within a year, the Asylums Committee was reporting that it was likely that even this would be exceeded which, in part at least, rested with the inability of its favoured chief architect, G.T. Hine, to provide detailed estimates.[30] Hine stated that he was happy to work with the Asylums Committee in the provision of an estimate for the Finance Committee, but he did so on the understanding that exact detail on costs was impossible because the asylum project was in its early stages. He was backed in this assertion by other members of his profession, with the *British Architect* similarly describing any attempts to identify exact costs at the outset as an 'impossible task'. Estimates could only ever be approximate, the *British Architect* argued, and the Works Department should not be surprised if they were sometimes 'a good bit off it'.[31] By October 1895, Hine was reporting that an additional £25,000 would be needed and by June of the following year it was reported that the cost would be somewhere between £390,000 and £400,000. By June 1899, the actual cost of the new Bexley Heath Asylum had risen to £420,000, which was £70,000 over the original estimate, and £120,000 over the figure originally voted for in the Council chamber.

During the course of the planning and building of the Bexley Heath asylum, the Finance Committee had regularly pressed for and failed to receive detailed estimates from the Asylums Committee. This was despite that fact that another Standing Order had been introduced in 1896 which stated that any additional requests for expenditure should be first scrutinised by the Finance Committee.[32] Indeed, the Asylums Committee used its relatively late adoption as an excuse to

[29] LMA, LCC/18.6, London County Council Minutes of Proceedings, July–December 1894, 3 November 1894.

[30] Although he had been the architect at Claybury, Hine was one of 69 architects who tendered their interest in the Bexley Heath Project. The Asylums Committee interviewed 28 of the candidates before settling on a shortlist of 6. At the end of the process Hine was appointed over Roland Plumbe and won the vote in the Asylums Committee by 15 votes to 10. LMA, LCC/18.6, London County Council Minutes of Proceedings, July–December 1895, 19 November 1895. LCC/MIN/00566, Signed Minutes, 1891–1894, 6 November 1894, 13 November 1894. LCC/MIN/00567, Signed Minutes, 1894–1897, 22 January 1895.

[31] Anon. 1896. Attempting the Impossible. *British Architect*, 27 November.

[32] Standing Order 266 stated that an excess of expenditure should be subject to supplemental estimates. LCC/CL/PH/01/276, Heath Asylum, Bexley. 1899. Report by the Clerk of the Council, LCC.

plead ignorance of the procedures. In similar circumstances in Devon, Forysthe and Melling have shown that the Finance Committee there took the opportunity to bring the Asylums Committee under its control by imposing the County Clerk on its membership.[33] Council members, and the LGB, were apparently not prepared to tolerate estimates for Asylum buildings which were increased from £35,500 to £45,500 within the space of four years, or the consistent excess of expenditure over estimates.[34] By contrast, when LCC came to build its next asylum at the Horton Manor Estate, near Epsom, similar issues to those at Bexley Heath were to arise.[35] It was under John McDougall, that the Asylums Committee recommended buying the Epsom estate at a cost of £40,900. Although the purchase was approved by the Council, the Finance Committee warned that there would be significant costs to follow. In addition to the outlay on the purchase, there were also be large payments for the erection and equipping of new buildings and, as the Finance Committee pointed out, no such estimates had, at that point, been submitted for consideration.[36]

These concerns were to fall on deaf ears and, with a pressing demand for accommodation, the Asylums Committee decided to utilise Hine's Bexley plans for what would be LCC's seventh asylum at Horton. This meant an immediate saving both in terms of time and money. On the one hand, it meant that the process of identifying and interviewing architects was not needed and, on the other, while Hine had received a £10,000 fee for the plans and project management at Bexley, this figure was reduced to £5750 for the new asylum. As a starting point, the Asylums Committee put forward an estimate for £350,000, despite its experience a few years earlier, and despite warnings that the sub-soil at the Horton estate was not as stable as the Bexley Heath site. With indications that there would be additional costs to offset this, it was little

[33] Neither the Local Government Board nor Council members were prepared to tolerate estimates for Asylum buildings which were increased from £35,500 to £45,500 within the space of four years. Melling et al., Politics of Lunacy: 80.

[34] Ibid: 80.

[35] Ibid: 80.

[36] The Horton site was purchased in August 1896. LMA, LCC/18.6, London County Council Minutes of Proceedings, January–June 1896, 16 June 1896.

wonder that the Finance Committee warned that the total cost would be nearer £410,000.[37]

The examples of both Bexley and Horton demonstrate that the ramping up of regulations and the provision of standing orders only served to highlight their toothlessness when it came to accurate financial reporting. Nevertheless, Cochrane has argued that it was the Finance and General Purposes Committee, in 1906, that obliged the main council to add a fifth asylum to the Horton estate.[38] By this time, however, Sir Harry Haward, erstwhile Comptroller of the Council, described any prestige that the Finance Committee may have had as in decline in this period (1904–1907), with the Council ignoring its warnings and advice and generally carrying on with large schemes of expenditure, contrary to any warnings. Thus, to understand the development of the Horton estate there has to be an understanding of a much wider context than simply the relationship between the Asylums and Finance Committees.[39]

The Horton Estate, Demand and Finances

The Horton estate was to play a significant role in the story of London's asylums. By 1903, the site in Epsom, Surrey, to the south of the capital, included three large institutions. The Manor Asylum (1899), the Horton Asylum (1902) and the Ewell Epileptic Colony (1903) were home to approximately 5400 inmates and 1000 members of staff.[40] It was little wonder that the Epsom cluster became known as a 'Suburb of Asylums' and by 1904 the Asylums Committee had decided that enough was enough.[41] With plans already in place for a fourth asylum on the Horton estate and a tenth asylum for London (Long Grove), the Asylums Committee expressed a preference for another new (eleventh) asylum on a new site. This was partly because of the large numbers of both patients and staff already on the site but the prospect of further additions had

[37] LMA, LCC/18.6, London County Council Minutes of Proceedings, July–December 1896, 15 December 1896.

[38] Cochrane, Humane, Economical and Medically Wise: 265.

[39] Haward, *The London County Council from Within:* 84.

[40] LMA, LCC 18.6, London County Council, Minutes of Proceedings, April–June 1906, 'Adjourned Report of the Asylums Committee', 22 May 1906.

[41] LMA LCC/MIN/711, Accommodation Sub-Committee Minute Book, 1905–1908, 28 March 1905, 9 April 1906.

provoked vehement opposition from some individuals and groups in the nearby town, notably Lord Rosebery and the Epsom Urban District Council.[42] From an administrative point of view too, a new site made sense as there were 'more patients chargeable in the north than in the south' of the capital.[43] A new asylum situated in the north of London would also have made it more accessible for the patients, their family and friends, as well as the parochial authorities.

Building institutions relatively near to the populations they served had a longer-term history. When the Finance Committee of the Kent County Council proposed that the East Kent Asylum at Chartham Down, near Canterbury, be sold to LCC for £260,000 in 1889, it was rejected by its Council which voted 49 to 25 in favour of retaining the asylum for Kent. It was Lord Harris, Kent's Vice Chairman, who urged the Council 'not to forget the hardship that would be entailed upon the poorer friends of the luckless patients' who would have to spend more money and travel further to visit those forced to move to Kent's other asylum at Barming. This, the *BMJ* stated, would inflict 'a great hardship upon a large number of poor people who deserve and who ought to receive every kindness and consideration'.[44] Harris reminded the Kent Council that 'this humane consideration was the *raison d'etre* for the erection of the asylum in the first instance'.[45]

As Cochrane has shown, the Asylums Committee 'saw itself as progressive and was uninspired by the prospect of building another 2000-bed institution' when it first became responsible for the capital's asylums. In 1890, it briefed a special Accommodation Sub-committee to examine ways of providing for over 2000 lunatics in several small asylums or in one or two of moderate sizes.[46] In the following year, the Asylums Committee advertised for a site to contain not more than 1000 individuals but by 1894 had settled on the 2000 bed institution that would

[42] Ellis, A Constant Irritation to the Townspeople: 653–67.

[43] LCC/MIN/711 Accommodation Sub-Committee Minute Book, 1905–1908, 28 Mar 1905, 9 April 1906.

[44] Anon. 1889. Proposal of the London County Council to Buy the East Kent Asylum. *British Medical Journal*, 20 July.

[45] Anon. 1889. The Proposed Sale of the East Kent Asylum to the London County Council. *BMJ*, 14 September.

[46] Cochrane, Humane, Economical and Medically Wise: 255.

become the Bexley Heath Asylum.[47] Cochrane puts this change down to a pressure to build that was being exerted by the Commissioners in Lunacy and also the mounting costs of boarding out London's patients in the various asylums up and down the country.[48] '[T]he greatest difficulty', the Commissioners argued, was 'experienced in finding room anywhere for the numerous pauper patients in the metropolis who daily are ordered to asylums, and who are consequently sent to the most various and distant parts of the country, far from their homes and friends'.[49] On a visit to the Nottingham Asylum they noted that London's patients were 'loud in their complaints' of being sent so far from home. 'We thought it was clearly understood', the Commissioners wrote in 1893, 'that no patients were to be sent to a distance from their homes if they were ever visited'.[50] Three years later they reiterated their concerns but shifted the focus away from the patients.

> The sending of patients to asylums at a long distance entails great hardship on the friends who desire to visit them, and many protests have been received both from friends and patients on this account, besides which the Common Poor Fund has to bear the burden of the increased cost of removals and of the visits of parochial and other authorities. It has also been practically impossible to allocate patients to the asylum nearest the parish from which they are sent, whereas if there were sufficient beds they would be sent to the asylum best situated for the visits of their friends.[51]

From the very first day that LCC took control of London's asylums, it was clear that there was an apparently inexorable demand on its services. In 1896, the architect George Bibby claimed that in the period between 1882 and 1896, five asylums the size of Claybury, which had opened in 1893, should have been built to meet the demand for services in

[47] LMA, LCC 26.21, The Third Annual Report of the Asylums Committee of the London County Council, for the Year Ending 31 March 1892. LMA, LCC 26.21, The Fifth Annual Report of the Asylums Committee of the London County Council, for the Year Ending 31 March 1894.

[48] Cochrane, Humane, Economical and Medically Wise: 256.

[49] *Forty-Fifth Report of the Commissioners in Lunacy*, 1891: 46.

[50] *Forty-Seventh Report of the Commissioners in Lunacy*, 1893: 229.

[51] LMA, LCC/18.6, London County Council Minutes of Proceedings, January–June 1896, 4 February 1896.

London.[52] With its focus on the total number of Lunatics, as well as the increase on the previous year, Fig. 3.1 demonstrates the ongoing awareness of this demand within the Council and the Asylums Committee. The following chapters will explore how first the Progressives and then the Municipal Reformers sought to manage that demand but, for the Commissioners, it was Claybury, and not smaller institutions, that they saw as the model that would help London meet its need for more accommodation.

The Commissioners' vision for the capital was based on Claybury's modernity, as well as its capacity, arguing that the consideration and revision they had given to its initial plans had led to the 'production of a very good asylum', with suitable accommodation and treatments for its 2000 acute, chronic and epileptic patients (See Fig. 3.2).[53] Thus, while it is easy to see the longer-term building programme as the Asylums Committee focussing on sequestration, as Cochrane has done, the Commissioners couched their concerns in terms of the innovation offered by the Claybury asylum; the positive impact that the building would have on the patients and their friends and families; and also the savings that could be accrued. Each of these themes can be seen in the positive claims made by the Progressive supporters of the Asylums Committee as shown in the previous chapter and this was not just a question of giving in to the demands of the Commissioners or the Finance Committee.

When it came to the considerations for the eleventh asylum, as usual, a special sub-committee was convened to consider the issue and within a few months had identified ten possible sites. All the sites were to the north of London with their relative distances to railway stations an important factor in the conveyance of people and goods (see Appendix 3). These sites reflected the demands from the Poor Law Unions and a little while later the Hackney Union complained that 45% of its lunatics had been submitted to asylums on the south side of the Thames. 'Although the population of the northern parishes is almost twice that of the southern parishes', the Asylums Committee reported, 'the accommodation in northern asylums is less than half of that in southern asylums'.[54] As well as their own costs and time, the Hackney Guardians wrote of the suffering

[52] Bibby, *The Planning of Lunatic Asylums*: 11–12.

[53] *Forty-Eighth Report of the Commissioners in Lunacy*, 1894: 233.

[54] LMA, LCC/MIN/713, Accommodation Sub-Committee Minute Book, 1910–1912, 21 February 1911.

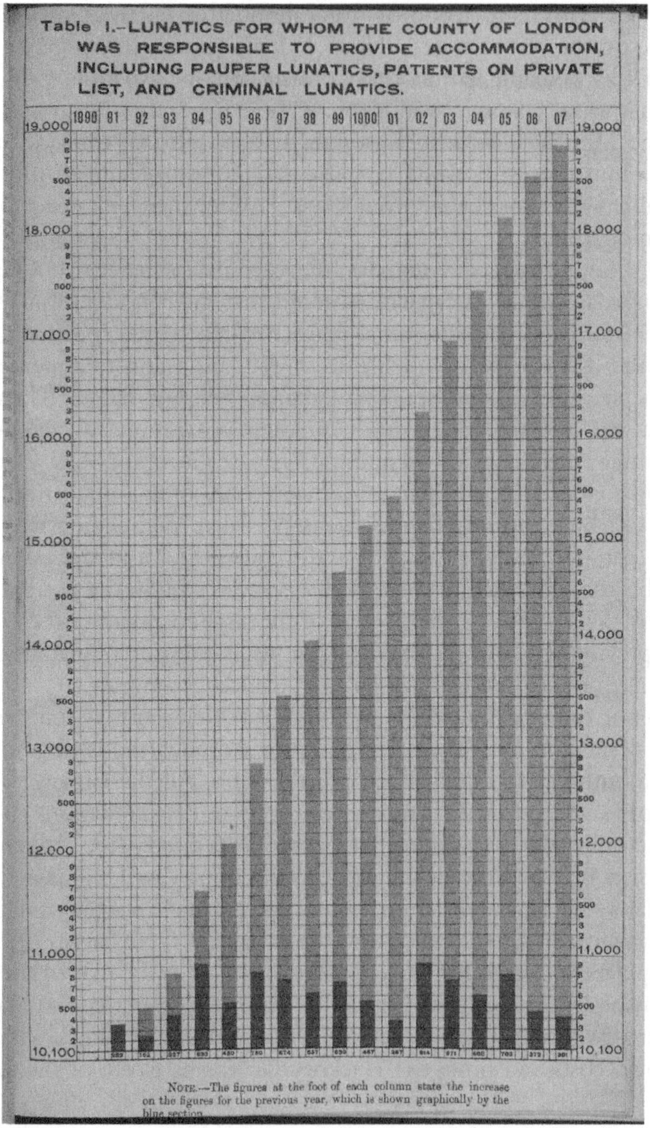

Fig. 3.1 Lunatics for whom the County of London was responsible to provide accommodation, 1890–1907. c.1907. LMA, LCC/MIN/711 (Reproduced with permission of London Metropolitan Archives, City of London)

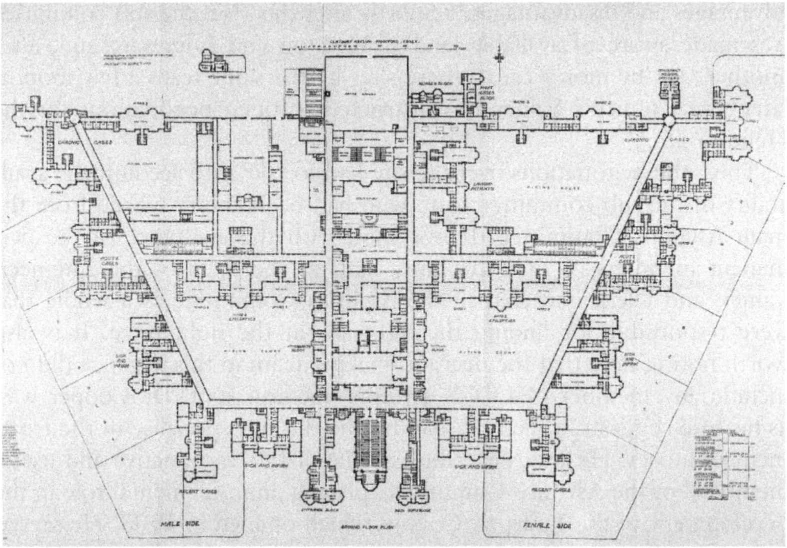

Fig. 3.2 Claybury Asylum, Ground Floor Plan. c.1890. Wellcome Library, London (Reproduced with permission. Wellcome Collection. CC BY)

for patients involved in longer journeys and also of the 'hardship to the patients and relatives, many of whom are very poor and find it very difficult to bear the expense or find the time necessitated by the long journeys involved in visiting'. [55]

Six of those north London sites were ruled out immediately, while others were added to the list over the course of the year and visited, in the first instance, by the Asylums Engineer and the Council's Assistant Valuer, Mr. Cook. After settling on a shortlist of two sites, councillors Dr Cooper, the sub-committee's Chairman, Mr. Hubbard and Mr. Hunter, the Chairman and Vice Chairman of the Asylums Committee, respectively, joined the Asylums Engineer and the Asylums Clerk and 'proceeded by Motor Car' to visit the two sites to assess their relative

[55] LMA, LCC/MIN/713, Accommodation Sub-Committee Minute Book, 1910–1912, 21 February 1911.

advantages and disadvantages.[56] Shortly after this visit, the sub-committee was made aware of available land at Hendon and Edgeware and, after another visit by motor car to these sites by the same team a few months later, the Council's Valuer was instructed to open negotiations for the Hendon site.[57]

Thus, the negotiations over the site had to take into account the availability of the sub-committee team who had been cherry picked from the main Asylums Committee. It was they, with the assistance of the permanent members of LCC Asylums' staff in the form of the Engineer, Valuer, and Clerk, rather than the Asylums Committee as a whole that were responsible for finding the right site at the right price. It is also worth noting here that the decision-making team in this instance did not include any member of LCC's asylums' medical staff. Dr Cooper was, as his title suggests, a medical man but he did not specialise in the treatment of lunacy. He was, nevertheless, one of the 'most active and useful members' of the Asylums Committee, playing an instrumental role in the development of the Epileptic Colony, which opened in 1903. He served as a Councillor from 1889 until he resigned when elected to the House of Commons in 1906.[58]

Despite this, the Finance Committee urged the Asylums Committee 'most strongly that, in view of the necessity for economy at the present time, no further land should be purchased until the surplus land at Horton had been used'.[59] If the preference for a new site was maintained, the Finance Committee asked, 'what steps [the Asylums Committee] propose to take to terminate the annual charge for interest and repayment of debt … in respect of the 350 acres at Horton at present unused'?[60] Shortly afterwards, the Asylums Committee officially abandoned the search for new land in favour of additional building work

[56]The Engineer recommended ruling out the Naphill site because it was too steep and difficult to get to, and also the Durrant estate because it was bisected by a highway. LCC/MIN/711, Accommodation Sub-Committee Minute Book, 1905–1908, 28 February 1905, 14 March 1905, 28 March 1905, 11 July 1905.

[57]LCC/MIN/711, Accommodation Sub-Committee Minute Book, 1905–1908, 28 March 1905, 11 December 1905.

[58]George Joseph Cooper, *BMJ*, 16 October 1909: 1200.

[59]LMA, LCC 18.6, London County Council, Minutes of Proceeding, April–June 1906, 'Adjourned Report of the Asylums Committee', 22 May 1906.

[60]LMA, LCC/MIN/711, Accommodation Sub-Committee Minute Book, 1905–1908, 18 February 1905, 9 April 1906.

on the existing site.[61] The Hackney Guardians, one of the Poor Law authorities that had pressed for the next asylum to be built north of the Thames were told 'that the Council already being in possession of a site at Epsom, there is no probability of the Eleventh Asylum being built in the North of London'.[62]

The timing of the abandonment seems to emphasise the power of the Finance Committee, but this ignores other salient factors. A longer-term consideration of extra-institutional and institutional alternatives played a part here and these will be explored in Chapters 4 and 5 but there were more immediate pressures too. Lord Rosebery, a former Prime Minister and former Chairman of LCC, had urged the Asylums Committee to sell any unused land on the Horton Estate and utilise the income to purchase land nearer to London.[63] As an Epsom resident, Rosebery had become of a critic of the Epsom cluster and its impact on the town and, by this point, other options for Epsom were already being explored. Figures provided by the Asylums Clerk indicated that commercial rents from the land would indeed leave the County with a profit.[64] This, however, was easier said than done and it proved to be a key sticking point with the will to provide more local institutions for the benefit of patients and their families seen as less important by the Finance Committee than the balancing of the books.

Negotiations to transfer some of the lands to the Education Committee fell through and by 1906 it had become 'increasingly apparent' that the commencement of the new asylum could no longer be delayed.[65] Significantly, this realisation pre-dated the demands from the Finance Committee to utilise the site. To the Commissioners in Lunacy, the need for additional accommodation had been obvious since

[61] LMA, LCC/MIN/711, Accommodation Sub-Committee Minute Book, 1905–1908, 28 March 1905, 9 April 1906.

[62] LMA, LCC/MIN/713, Accommodation Sub-Committee Minute Book, 1910–1912, 21 February 1911.

[63] LMA, PH/Ment/3/5, Newspaper Cuttings, 'Hospital', 9 March 1907. Ellis, A Constant Irritation to the Townspeople?

[64] LMA, LCC/MIN/711, Accommodation Sub-Committee Minute Book, 1905–1908, 28 March 1905, 9 April 1906.

[65] LMA, LCC 26.21, The Seventeenth Annual Report of the Asylums Committee of the London County Council, for the Year Ending 31 March 1906.

1903 when it first urged the Council to consider an eleventh asylum.[66] Moreover, while the decision to build another institution on the Horton site was not the Asylums Committee's first choice, the decision to do so offered financial benefits to all those who looked to safeguard the rates for their electors, irrespective of which party they represented. As the *Municipal Journal* pointed out, when the Epileptic Colony opened on the Horton site, it negated the need for additional costs on such items as farm buildings, laundry facilities, a chapel, *post mortem* facilities and a mortuary as these were all already available at the Horton Asylum.[67]

In this respect, it can be seen that the Finance Committee did eventually impose its will on the Asylums Committee but, as Haward, pointed out, 'a perfect system of standing orders' could not prevent the moral authority of the Finance Committee being weakened by a constant undermining of its advice.[68] Its 'power' in this case, followed a coalescing of a range of factors that included the demands of lunacy legislation and pressure from the Commissioners in Lunacy to build but, crucially also, the failure of the Asylums Committee to find alternative uses for its land. To understand this more fully there has to be some understanding of the politics of LCC and how this impacted on public spending in relation to its asylums.

The Asylums Committee and the Politics of Public Spending

One of the reasons why the finances of the Asylums Committee seemed to be disconnected from the politics of LCC were the Lunacy Acts which compelled county councils in England and Wales to provide asylum accommodation for paupers. However, the costs for new buildings, the preliminary equipment, extensions to existing stock, repairs and maintenance, along with any interest on monies borrowed for such came out of the Asylums' capital account. Alternatively, it was raised through a special county rate which, as the name suggests, was payable by county ratepayers.[69] In the case of the Horton estate, the county rate included

[66] *Sixty-Second Report of the Commissioners in Lunacy*, 1908: 356.

[67] British Library, *Municipal Journal*, 25 January 1901: 72.

[68] Haward, *The London County Council from Within*: 84.

[69] LMA LCC/CL/PH/01/276, Suggestions for Regulations as to Asylum Finance. 1889. LCC.

the costs needed to repay loans and associated interest on the original purchase of the land. The cost of maintaining individuals in asylums, its operating costs, which included staff, provisions, fuel, lighting and washing (often referred to as 'necessaries'), clothing, medicine, and food, was passed to the Poor Law Guardians of the various parishes and Unions who operated as one of the key gatekeepers into the asylums.[70] On the face of it, maintenance rates may seem unconnected with the setting of the county rate but the vast majority of those who voted in parochial elections for the election of Guardians also had the right to vote in County Council Elections.[71] Asylum committees had the power to ask Boards of Guardians to pay maintenance costs of up to 14s per week, per lunatic, and anything lower than that was seen as a mark of their financial prudence.[72] It is little wonder that the many economies and efficiencies, along with its kind and considerate treatment, played such an important part in the Asylums Committee's 'great reputation'.[73] As such, this was not a simple dichotomy of tax and spend by one group, or straightforward financial prudence by the other. There was political capital to be made out of the management of finances across the board, and whether the funds requested in the form of taxes and the money spent represented value for money.

Debates about the levels of public spending were not limited to London, and nor were the limited to local or county politics. In the 1870s, the municipalisation of Birmingham under Joseph Chamberlain had demonstrated what publicly funded intervention could achieve.[74] Moving first into the House of Commons, and then into the cabinet as President of the Board of Trade, allowed Chamberlain a platform to extol the merits of municipal intervention more widely.[75] On a national level, this was to take some time. The general election of 1906 produced a Liberal government that was largely a 'victory for traditional Liberal values

[70]Jephson, Henry, 2010. *The Making of Modern London, Progress and Reaction*. London: Bowers Brothers, London: 87.

[71]Donald, *The London Manual for 1901*: 11.

[72]Ibid: 75.

[73]Ibid: 75.

[74]Hammond, J.L. 1935. The Social Background, 1835–1935. In *A Century of Municipal Progress: The Last Hundred Years*, eds. Harold J. Laski, W. Ivor Jennings and William Robson, 37–54. London: George Allen & Unwin Ltd: 51.

[75]Hennock, *Fit and Proper Persons*: 175.

and the Campbell-Bannerman government was very much in the mould of Liberal cabinets of the nineteenth century…'[76] David Dutton argues, that the only indication of any impact on the part of Progressive politics was the introduction of the Trades Disputes Act of 1906.[77] This was to change when Herbert Asquith became Prime Minister in 1908 and this is an easy reference to mark the move from an 'old Liberalism' of laissez-faire to a 'new Liberalism' of social reform and progressive taxation.[78]

Back in London, LCC under the Progressives may not have achieved control of gas and water supplies in the same way that Birmingham's council had, but, as has been shown in the previous chapter, its intervention on its asylums was couched very much in terms of the good work it had done on slum clearances, new housing schemes and the provision of parks and open spaces. All of this pre-dated the new Liberalism at the national level but the costs of these interventions became important evidence in election campaigns as candidates sought to define the issue of the rates in terms of whether they represented value for money, or not. Indeed, there had been an expectation in some quarters that the introduction of the LGA would lead to increased expenditure and for Progressive candidates such as Frederick Dolman, the issue was obvious.[79] In the build-up to the 1907 election, he wrote to the *Daily Mail* to argue that any detailed retrospect would show that the work undertaken by its Progressive Council was worth the costs for what Londoners received in return.[80]

In some cases, direct links were made between the rates and the work of the Asylums Committee and was framed within the wider conception of what London's government represented. A.J.D. Gilbert, one of the two Progressive candidates along with Evan Spicer, standing in West Newington in 1907, argued that the quarter penny rise on the rates represented good value for money, considering the work carried out in

[76] Dutton, David. 2014. *A History of the Liberal Party Since 1900*. London: Palgrave Macmillan: 46–7.

[77] Ibid: 46–7.

[78] Howe, Anthony. 1996. Towards the "Hungry Forties": Free Trade in Britain, c.1880–1906. In *Citizenship and Community: Liberals, Radicals and Collective Identities in the British Isles, 1865–1931*, ed. Eugenio F. Biagini, 192–218. Cambridge: Cambridge University Press: 193.

[79] Dunbabin, Expectations of the New County Councils: 356.

[80] Dolman, Frederick. 1907. In Defence of the Progressives. *Daily Mail*, 8 February. Dolman was the author of *Municipalities at Work* (1895) and Progressive Councillor for Brixton. Saint, *Politics and the People of London*: 49.

London's asylums, on its fire brigade and its sewers, as well as the rather catch-all phrase of 'other works'.[81] Similarly, according to J.W. Clelland, the rate rise of a farthing included 'the better treatment of lunatics in [London's] asylums'.[82] Thus, the work of the Asylums Committee became useful ammunition in election campaigns and at the heart of these claims was the rhetoric around money well spent. This was partly on the grounds of prudence and good financial management, but also on the grounds they were interventionist in tone and linked to a wider belief in what Progressivism could achieve in and for the capital.

Such claims were not limited to one party. Whereas Progressive literature had made much of the efficiency of the new asylums' structure in terms of rationalisation, standardisation and economies of scale (see Chapter 2), the Moderates spoke of the great need for administrative reform in the direction of the additional savings that could be made. As excellent as the work of the Asylums Committee had been, election materials in 1898 proclaimed, more 'administrative reform in the direction of economy is greatly needed'.[83] Thus, while all candidates, irrespective of political persuasion were keen to stress value for money, the focus here was on the apparently profligate spending which spoke to wider concerns about the nature of the Progressive majority. Rather than commenting on the value of intervention, critics spoke of 'waste'. John Williams Benn was described as the 'wastrel Chieftain' by the LMS and the term wastrel on its own was often used more generally to critique the Progressives and their policies.[84] Following the defeat in the election of 1907, which ended eighteen years of Progressive rule, the *New York Times* described the result as 'The Wastrels' Waterloo'.[85] Thus, concerns about the spending of public money on asylums was linked to the contested nature of London's new political landscape. The Asylums Committee and its work became part of that discourse, and there were other issues to consider in two key areas of employment.

[81] LMA, ACC/3606/001, Election Literature and Newspaper Cuttings, 1906–1907, 'West Newington Progressive Candidates', 11 February 1907.

[82] Cleland, J.W. 1907. The Question of London's Rates. *Daily Mail*, 21 February.

[83] GL, SL:30:03. 1898. A Collection of Tracts, London Municipal Society, 'Election 1898, Facts and Arguments', London Municipal Society.

[84] GL, LMS133. n.d. London Municipal Society, Election Leaflets and Pamphlets, 'Truth Will Out!', Leaflet No. 12, Series A.

[85] BL, London and America, *Municipal Journal*, 8 March 1907: 200.

Asylum Staff and Their Conditions of Employment

Three years after the Municipal Reformers took power in 1907, Henry Jephson looked back on the work of the asylums committee under the Progressive administration in a publication sub-titled 'Progressive Rule and Moderate Misrule'. Along with what had become the usual focus on the work of the Asylums Committee in terms of Progressive administration and efficiency, Jephson wrote of the improvements to asylum staff remuneration and conditions.[86] In the first few years of LCC, the Asylums Committee added 126 new members of staff at the then four asylums and at its central office, which increased annual wage costs to the tune of £7600 with a further £2000 per year being spent on increased wages for existing staff.[87] The Commissioners in Lunacy were less convinced at any suggestions that this was necessarily having a positive impact on the service. While the attendant to patient ratios at the Banstead Asylum was described as 'sufficient', for example, the ratios at Colney Hatch were described as 'unsatisfactory' and this was to become a recurring theme.[88] Nevertheless, on an individual level, by 1895 the Commissioners in Lunacy were concluding that London's attendants had more 'advantages in the way of leave' than any other county and have 'their comforts studied in a way that would be much appreciated elsewhere'.[89]

These improvements, and the fact that attendants were municipal employees, were reflected in the number of organisations including unions which co-opted them as members. When it came to the negotiations over contracts, those that spoke with a collective voice on the behalf of attendants included the Asylum Workers' Association, the London County Council Employees' Protection Association, the London County Council Employees' Union, and the Municipal Employees' association.[90] The lack of

[86] Jephson, *The Making of Modern London*: 87.

[87] LMA, LCC 26.21, The Fourth Annual Report of the Asylums Committee of the London County Council, for the Year Ending 31 March 1893.

[88] LMA, LCC 26.21, Copy of Lunacy Commissioners, County of London Lunatic Asylum, Banstead, 14 June 1890. *Forty-Seventh Report of the Commissioners in Lunacy*, 1893: 214.

[89] *Forty-Ninth Report of the Commissioners in Lunacy*, 1895: 268.

[90] LCC/MIN/00567, Signed Minutes, 1894–1897, 15 January 1896, 13 October 1896. LCC/MIN/570, Signed Minutes, 1901–1902, 16 July 1901. LCC/MIN/569, Signed Minutes, 1899–1901, 12 December 1899. LMA LCC/MIN/572, Signed Minutes, June 1904–November 1905, 14 June 1904.

one trade union to represent all municipal staff in this is period is reflected elsewhere but we can begin to see attendants and others, not just in terms of a medical history, but also in terms of the place of their employment in wider shifts in labour relations and as part of a wider political vision.[91]

In this case, however, it is hard to see a significant change after the 1907 election and the change in administration, whatever point Jephson may have been trying to make. A 1911 survey of the working hours undertaken by asylum staff across the country found that the average working week was around 84 hours per week but this was gendered too. Across London's asylums, male attendants worked an average of 66 hours and female nurses worked 72. Despite these differences, these were the lowest hours of duty in the country, and LCC was described as being 'a body distinguished for its liberal policy in this respect'.[92] Only the Lancashire Asylums Board came anywhere close, but this was still short of what some members of the Progressive administration wanted. Under the heading of 'The Proper Treatment of Labour'—it was, again, the Fabian Society that asked councillors and candidates if they were prepared to insist that all persons employed by the Council worked 'a normal eight hours day'.[93] Clearly, the will to improve the conditions of working Londoners was stronger in some sections of the Progressive administration than others and this reflects the breadth of opinion within both the party and LCC. By contrast, the Municipal Reformers claimed it was they who were the friend of the worker. In election materials they pointed to positive changes they had made to the pay and conditions of employees across LCC, including those working in asylums.[94] In this case then, rhetoric around economy and efficiency was used by both parties in their propaganda, even if, on the face of it, there may have been little practical difference.

[91] See, for example, Nevers, Jean-Yves. 2003. The "Iron Triangle" of Municipal Government: Trade Unions, Bureaucracy and Political Parties in a French Town (Toulouse, 1910–1970). In *Municipal Services and Employees in the Modern City: New Historic Approaches*, eds. Michèle Dagenais, Irene Maver and P.-Y. Saunier, 159–76. Aldershot: Ashgate.

[92] *Report and Special Report From the Select Committee on the Asylums Officers (Employment, Pensions, and Superannuation) Bill.* 1911. London: Wyman and Sons: iv.

[93] BI 228/10. 1898. Fabian Society, Questions for London County Councillors. BI LH P2291. 1891. Fabian Society, Questions for London County Councillors.

[94] London Municipal Society. c.1912. *The Municipal Reformers and Labour, London County Council Election 1913, Facts and Arguments for Municipal Reform Speakers and Candidates.* London: George Berridge and Co: 101–2.

The Significance of the Works Department

The distinction between the parties was much clearer on the issue of direct labour and the employment of men to carry out the Council's work—rather than to tender work out to private contractors. Since the 1860s, the vestries had been employing direct labour and their growing politicisation meant that upwards of 60% of the labour undertaken by them was employed this way.[95] In Progressive Battersea, for example, direct labour was responsible for all works carried out there. Following these examples, the second Progressive County Council of 1892 passed what John Davies described as two of its most controversial measures. The first was to link LCC wages to the rates and the second was to convert the Stores Department into the Works Department and to make it responsible for all Council Building and Engineering.[96] The radical Councillor John Burns was the driving force for this change but he needed the support of his Progressive peers, which drew the ire of the opposition.[97] Critics on the Moderate side of the Council described the Works Department as a Progressive tactic for increasing the power of the Council, and 'to create at the expense of the ratepayers a labour paradise for a privileged body of working men'.[98] To achieve this, the LMS claimed that the Works Department was independent of any other department of the Council and supervised by a Works Committee under the complete control of the Radical labour members, and they had a point.[99] At a Council meeting after the 1904 election, Moderates attempted to address their lack of membership on the Works Committee claiming they had a right to be represented on every department of the Council's Work. In the debate that followed, Progressive members described the Moderates as 'wreckers' and Burns agreed that the

[95] Ball and Sunderland, *An Economic History of London, 1800–1914*: 377.

[96] Davies, The Progressive Council, 1889–1907: 34.

[97] Brown, Kenneth D. 2004. Burns, John Elliott. *Oxford Dictionary of National Biography*. https://www.oxforddnb.com/. Accessed 4 July 2019.

[98] GL, LMS106. 1898. *London County Council, Election 1898, Facts and Arguments*. London: London Municipal Society: 29. Ball and Sunderland, *An Economic History of London, 1800–1914*: 378.

[99] GL, LMS106. 1898. *London County Council, Election 1898, Facts and Arguments*. London: London Municipal Society: 29–31.

success of the Works Department rested with the fact 'that there were no Moderates on the Works Committee to put sand in its machinery and to thwart its works in many ways'.[100]

The issue of direct labour was one that was not limited to the capital,[101] but in London, the Works Department became one of the sticks with which the Moderate candidates could regularly beat the Progressive Administration in relation to value for ratepayers' money. The Works Department was, according to the LMS, created for 'theoretical and ulterior reasons', which meant it carried out work without regard for its capacity to do so.[102] Furthermore, employees of the Works Department were compelled to join a trade union, and evidence to a special committee supposedly suggested that they would never work with the same zeal as they would for a private contractor.[103] Overall, the LMS concluded, the whole concept of direct labour was flawed—the Works Department produced bad work slowly, while providing better conditions for the workmen and at the same time disadvantaging London's private contractors.[104] The Progressives met these claims with counter claims relating to the money saved and the good work undertaken.[105] Given the scale of the asylums' operation, and the role played by the Works Department on its stock, it is not surprising that the Asylums Committee became an important part of this discourse.

Along with Mains Drainage and Housing, the Asylums Committee was named as one of the Council's three main spending Committees where the use of the Works Department was described as an example of extravagance and of the Progressives 'pour[ing] money out like

[100] Anon. 1904. London County Council. *The Times*, 23 March.

[101] Moore, James R. 2006. *The Transformation of Urban Liberalism: Party Politics and Urban Governance in Late Nineteenth Century England*. Aldershot: Ashgate: 214.

[102] GL, LMS106. 1898. *London County Council, Election 1898, Facts and Arguments*. London: London Municipal Society: 32.

[103] GL, LMS106. 1898. *London County Council, Election 1898, Facts and Arguments*. London: London Municipal Society: 29–31.

[104] GL, LMS107. 1904. *London County Council, Election 1904, Facts and Arguments*. London: London Municipal Society: 144–7.

[105] LSE, Coll. Misc. 904. n.d. London Reform Union, Leaflet No. 49, 'The Truth About the Works Department'. LSE Coll. Misc. 904. 1896. London Reform Union, Leaflet No. 74, 'The Truth About the Works Department of the London County Council'.

water'.[106] Comparisons of estimates for work to be undertaken and the actual costs paid became useful ammunition in election campaigns and the almost £8000 spent beyond the estimate on the Bexley Asylum was included as part of a long list of 'squandering' by the Progressive administration.[107] The Asylum at Horton, which was meant to be completed by September 1900 but actually completed in June 1903, had a final estimate of £291,165, an actual cost of £329,044 and an excess of £37,878. The Asylum Station was over-budget by £1977 and the epileptic colony by £5019. Entrusting the building on the Horton estate to the Works Department had meant that final estimates were exceeded by £45,000, it was claimed.[108] It was, according to the *Daily Mail*, the building of the Horton Asylum that offered the most notorious example of rate burdening with Works Department costs running to 6½ times more than private contractor estimates.[109]

Even the smaller sums involved in the maintenance, rather than the building of asylums, became useful ammunition in the production of election materials. The pamphlet entitled 'Reckless Squandering of Ratepayers Money by the Progressives of London County Council', compared the additional £70 required by a contractor for 'small additional works' at the Banstead Asylum, with a deficit of £5442 at the Colney Hatch for work carried out by the Works Department.[110] This was not necessarily comparing works of a similar scale but at Colney Hatch the LMS described the difference between the estimate of £19,114 18s. 6d. for additional works with an actual cost of £22,942 3s. 10d. as an example of 'falsified accounting'. In addition, they employed an expert in the form of Mr. E.A. Gruning, a Fellow of the Royal Institute of British Architects, to comment on the quality of the work carried out. In Gruning's 'independent assessment', the quality

[106] GL, LMS107. 1904. *London County Council, Election 1904, Facts and Arguments.* London: London Municipal Society.

[107] GL, LMS132. 1898. London Municipal Society, Election Leaflets and Pamphlets, 'Squandering the Rates', Leaflet No. 55.

[108] GL, LMS107. 1904. *London County Council, Election 1904, Facts and Arguments.* London: London Municipal Society: 153–4.

[109] BL, 8139B22. c.1907. *The Daily Mail and the fight for London: A Handbook to the London County Council Election Giving Both Sides*: 33–4.

[110] GL, LMS132. 1898. London Municipal Society, Election Leaflets and Pamphlets, 'Reckless Squandering of Ratepayers Money', Leaflet No. 41.

of the work that had been done there was described as mixed. Some of the boards used for flooring, for example, were very good but 'the match-boarding throughout is the worst standard I ever saw ... [and] the workmanship was rough in the extreme'.[111] Moreover, the materials being used for the boarding, it was claimed, were not fit for purpose and suitable only for packing cases. Gruning had presumed that the aim of any works was to 'obtain better results as to quality' and 'to economise the funds with which the corporation is entrusted by the ratepayers', but his assessment concluded they had failed on both counts.[112] The use of matchboard was later implicated in the aftermath of the Colney Hatch fire but the style of the building was not the issue at stake here.[113] 'How long will the ratepayers of London suffer this costly fad of the Progressives to last?', the LMS asked and 'How long will the over-burdened ratepayer submit to this audacious jobbery?'[114]

Both parties were conscious of the potential condemnation from ratepayers that might result in election defeat or other interventions. The Progressives, in particular, had to be cautious with first a London Ratepayers Defence League and then The London League formed with a view to overturning its majority.[115] The Progressives responded with leaflets claiming that under the Municipal Reformers 'the contractor reigns and the ratepayer pays' with images of what could only be described as a cigar smoking, top hatted 'fat cat' business man with a bundle of private contracts in the inside pocket of a large fur coat.[116] This is reflected in Fig. 3.3 which contrasts the 'motive spirit' of the 'People's Welfare' with the greed of the Moderate and the private sector.

[111]GL, LMS107. 1904. *London County Council, Election 1904, Facts and Arguments*. London: London Municipal Society: 144.

[112]GL, LMS106. 1898. *London County Council, Election 1898, Facts and Arguments*. London: London Municipal Society: 34–5.

[113]Bewley, *Madness to Mental Illness*: 44.

[114]GL, LMS106. 1898. *London County Council, Election 1898, Facts and Arguments*. London: London Municipal Society: 36–7.

[115]Young, *Local Politics and the Rise of Party*: 51–3. See, also Fraser, Derek. 1980. Politics and Society in the Nineteenth Century. In *A History of Modern Leeds*, ed. Derek Fraser, 270–300. Manchester: Manchester University Press: 288.

[116]London County Council. 1910. Progressive Leaflets. https://archive.org/stream/progressiveleafl00lond#page/n3/mode/2up. Accessed 4 July 2019.

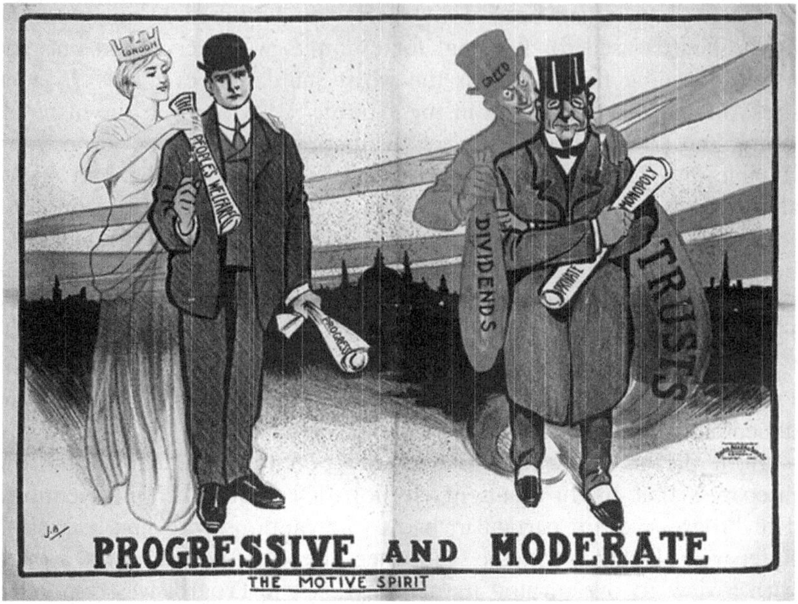

Fig. 3.3. Anon. 1907. *Progressive and Moderate—The Motive Spirit.* London: David Allen and Sons Ltd. London School of Economics, London. COLL MISC 0844/22 (Reproduced under a Creative Commons Attribution-NonCommercial-ShareAlike [CC BY-NC-SA 3.0] license)

One other commentator, while not necessarily representative, felt that the employment of direct labour needed to ring-fenced. A letter to the *Daily News* from 'a Socialist', brought the subject of patient labour to the attention of its readers. Using the Bexley asylum as an example, the author pointed to patients employed as carpenters, painters and bricklayers who were entrusted with sharp and heavy weapons in the form of chisels, bradawls, screw-drivers, hammer and mallets without supervision.[117] Whereas, patient labour was described by the asylum authorities as therapeutic, 'a Socialist' claimed that LCC was coolly exploiting patient labour, and the Boards of Guardians and the ratepayers

[117] Anon. 1903. Patient Labour in Asylums. *Daily News*, 23 October.

that paid for their upkeep. Moreover, work done by patients—work that was a skilled trade—such as the painting of corridors was done very badly indeed. The work of these unfortunate patients made 'blacklegs' by LCC was an issue for Mr. Crooks, Mr. Burns and the other ardent trade unionists on the council and was an issue that they would have to answer to at the March election. 'In the meantime it is curious to note such a pernicious system growing and developing under a Council in which Progressive and Labour men are in such a clear majority'.[118] More specifically, the Commissioners in Lunacy hinted at the advantages of having an 'in-house' team. In 1893, they raised concerns that the tendering process caused delays in the building of the extensions to the Banstead Asylum.[119] In the following year they noted that the repairs needed to 'staircases, ward offices, and water closets were not under constant observation. In an asylum of this size that kind of work needs to be constant and carried out by a sufficient staff of workmen'.[120]

After the 1907 election, control of the Works Committee, along with the control of the Council passed to the Municipal Reformers and they made good of their election promises in this regard. They immediately began the process of putting 'sand in the machinery' of the Works Department and reduced the work given to its department until Edward White, its Chairman, recommended its discontinuance and it was closed at the end of 1909.[121] 'The extravagant Works Department, which needed £400,000 worth of work each year to keep it going has been closed', proclaimed the Municipal Reformers, 'and contractors have in two years and a half carried out work for which the Departments charged under ordinary conditions £180,000 more than the contractors agreed to do it for'.[122] After that date Labour candidates called for the restoration of the Works Department, both as a useful check on private

[118] Ibid.

[119] *Forty-Seventh Report of the Commissioners in Lunacy*, 1893: 208.

[120] *Forty-Eighth Report of the Commissioners in Lunacy*, 1894: 230.

[121] Haward, *The London County Council from Within*: 324–5.

[122] GL, LMS123. 1909. London Municipal Pamphlets and Leaflets, 'The Work of Municipal Reform in London, 1907–1909', Municipal Reform Pamphlet 37. GL, LMS72. 1910. London Municipal Pamphlets and Leaflets, 'Why Was the Works Department Closed?', Municipal Reform Leaflet A7.

contractors and as a way of finding work for London's unemployed.[123] Central to this process of privatisation was the Asylums Committee and when the Works Department asked what work it might be expected to carry out in the forthcoming year in 1908, the Asylums Committee, now also dominated by Municipal Reformers, replied stating that there were no works of repair or construction that it was in a position to ask them to carry out.[124] Here, links can be seen between LCC's management of asylums and wider ideological views on the spending of public money and the employment of public services. Significantly also, we can see how party majorities affected the direction of policies in key areas and a change in that direction after 1907 was to impact more directly on the work of the Asylums Committee.

The 1907 Election, Finances and a Change in Direction

In the first meeting after the 1907 election, in which the Municipal Reformers took control of the Council from the Progressives for the first time, the Asylums Committee was reconstituted with Alfred (A.O.) Goodrich in the Chair and H.R. Taylor as Vice Chairman. Goodrich, a produce merchant, was one of two Municipal Reform councillors from Tower Hamlets (Stepney), whereas Taylor was one of two Progressive members for Camberwell (North).[125] As was shown in the previous chapter, this 'new' Committee was overwhelmingly made up of Municipal Reform councillors and this, and their majority on the Council, undoubtedly affected the direction of policy. As Ken Young has shown, it was only after 1907 that Councillors sat in party groups in the Council Chamber, and this only added to the sense of political polarisation.[126]

Shortly after the election victory, Goodrich had backed the decision to build an eleventh asylum on the Horton site because it would be cheaper than buying additional land but this was to be a short-term view.[127] Although the demand for another asylum was apparently

[123] LSE, ILP/6/22/1/84504. 1913. J. Gilbert Dale Labour Candidate.

[124] LMA, LCC/MIN/575, Signed Minutes, March 1908–February 1909, 12 May 1908.

[125] Anon. 1936. Wills and Bequests. *The Times*, 30 December 1936. Anon. 1907. *The Story of the London County Council*. London: George Edward Wright: 67, 75.

[126] Young, *Local Politics and the Rise of Party*: 100–1.

[127] LMA, PH/Ment/3/5, Newspaper Cuttings, 'Epsom Herald', 6 April 1907.

obvious, and there was ongoing pressure from the Commissioners in Lunacy, at the first meeting of the 'new' committee Goodrich hoped that 'the Progressive proposal to build a new asylum at a cost of £500,000 might be reviewed'.[128] This was something he reiterated at the opening of the tenth asylum at Long Grove when, as Chairman of the Asylums Committee, he stated his hope that it was the last asylum that the Committee would have to build.[129]

An editorial in the *BMJ* welcomed the decision to put an eleventh asylum in abeyance. Those in asylums, it argued, were 'largely senile', and were sent to asylums by their parishes because it was easy to do so. Instead, it hoped that LCC would move in the direction of treating acute cases while considering a simpler way of treating chronic cases.[130] This medical perspective on chronic and acute cases will be examined more fully in the following chapter but, for the time being, the message here was informed, in part at least, by Municipal Reform rhetoric. Goodrich had argued that many of the people going into the existing asylums were over 70 years of age. Edward Easton, another Municipal Reformer, argued that many of the women were over 80 and suffering from senile decay and were forced into asylums by the Poor Law Guardians. 'If the poor law unions – and particularly Hammersmith – would be careful not to send out-county patients to the asylums', Goodrich said, 'the figures with regard to lunacy in London would be greatly reduced'.[131]

Despite this, the Commissioners in Lunacy criticised the decision to postpone on the grounds it was a false economy and, reminding the Council of this fact and of its obligations under the lunacy legislation, urged the Asylums Committee to work with the Finance Committee in this regard.[132] By this time, the Finance Committee, just like the Asylums Committee, was part of a majority Municipal Reform administration. The Municipal Reform Councillors that served on those

[128] GL, LMS122, London Municipal Pamphlets and Leaflets, 1908, 'The Progress of Municipal Reform', Municipal Reform Pamphlet 26.

[129] 'Surrey', *Daily Mail*, 17 June 1907: 5.

[130] LMA, PH/Ment/3/5, Newspaper Cuttings. *British Medical Journal*, 23 May 1908.

[131] 'London County Council, Drink and Insanity', *Manchester Guardian*, 13 March 1908: 9.

[132] LMA, PH/Ment/3/5, Newspaper Cuttings, 'Pall Mall Gazette', 1 July 1908. LMA, LCC/MIN/575, Signed Minutes, March 1908–February 1909, 12 May 1908.

committees were part of the campaign that had made the twin track strategy of reducing both capital expenditure and public borrowing a central plank of the 1907 County Council election.[133] In their manifesto, published in December 1906, they asked

> Who are the Parties and what are their issues in the coming struggle? On the one side stand the Progressives, many of them the very men who have promoted the enormous and wasteful expenditure under which we groan. Of these, many are Socialists and will be supported by the Socialist vote except in the few cases where the Socialists run candidates even more reckless of the rates than the Progressives. On the other side stand the Municipal Reformers supported, let us hope, by all sensible business-like people of all Parties and of no Party who are sick of the way in which the Progressives have imported the worst form of party politics into local educational and financial administration.[134]

This focus on the wasteful nature of Progressive spending was hardly new and rising rates, and the apparent lack of steps taken by them to co-ordinate or control expenditure, were a recurring theme of previous election materials.[135] As Pennybacker points out, to limit the explanations of why the Progressives were 'trounced from office in 1907' to a discussion of the rates alone is to ignore other salient issues.[136] Davies has argued, that lower rates were a concern of middle-class ratepayers but that it was qualified by the benefits of cheaper municipal water, gas and transport. Nevertheless, just as in the twenty-first century, London was a high-rent city and with a rising rate burden, 'the politics of economy would always find a constituency'.[137] It is this that explains the focus of Municipal Reform election literature. In 1909, one of their posters asked

[133] GL, LMS124. 1909. London Municipal Pamphlets and Leaflets. 'What the Municipal Reform Have Done in Two Years!', Municipal Reform Leaflet 117.

[134] GL, LMS72. 1910. London Municipal Pamphlets and Leaflets. 'LCC Election 1907', Copy of Manifesto issued 4 December 1906.

[135] GL, LMS107. 1904. *London County Council, Election 1904, Facts and Arguments.* London: London Municipal Society: 156–7.

[136] 'Rate rises, expensive experiments in dubious forms of municipalisation, fissures and fractures amongst its own supporters, and the organizational revitalization of municipal Conservatism all signalled Progressivism's dissipation.' Pennybacker, The Millennium by Return of Post: 131–2.

[137] Davies, The Progressive Council, 1889–1907: 34.

'You must vote again for Municipal Reform. Why?' to which the first two answers were '1. Because Municipal Reform has reduced the rates' and '2. Because Municipal Reform has reduced the Borrowing of Money'.[138] These were seen as the key issues for election strategists and whatever the reasons for individuals voting in the way they did, it would nevertheless impact on how the Council's finances operated.

As a result, the ramping up of the Finance Committee's watchdog role across the whole of the Council's operations spilled out into the pages of the press. According to the *Daily Mail* 'the wastrels' on the Progressive Party had rejected Lingen's attempts improve financial scrutiny and reporting. This 'wise proposal which would have saved millions of money [*sic*], and while conforming to the letter of the law, so far as sending proposals to the Finance Committee, decided that they would merely have the advice, take it or leave it'.[139] Under the then 'current' Chairman, Lord Welby, 'The County Council's Finance Committee is perhaps the strongest Committee of its kind in the kingdom. It is mainly composed of bankers, financiers, directors, stockbrokers, and men having a thorough knowledge of public finance. And the majority on that committee belong to the Wastrel Party'.[140]

Following their victory in the election, the Municipal Reformers were keen to explain that they had 'passed rules for the first time [giving] the Council full control over its finances'.[141] Included here was the requirement for all plans above £5000 to be first referred to the Finance Committee. This Committee would then produce a report showing how the money was to be raised and whether the plans could be described as excessive. Only at this point could schemes be put before the Council for a vote.[142] As Henry Percy-Harris (Municipal Reformer and later Conservative MP) pointed out, in the past schemes were presented to

[138] GL, LMS124. 1909. London Municipal Pamphlets and Leaflets. 'You Must Vote Again for Municipal Reform. Why?', Municipal Reform Leaflet 127.

[139] British Library, 8139B22, *The Daily Mail and the fight for London: A Handbook to the London County Council Election Giving Both Sides*, n.d., c.1907, p. 15.

[140] BL, 8139B22. c.1907. *The Daily Mail and the Fight for London: A Handbook to the London County Council Election Giving Both Sides*: 15.

[141] GL, LMS133. n.d. London Municipal Society, Election Leaflets and Pamphlets, 'Municipal Reform v Progressive Socialism', Leaflet No. 17.

[142] GL, LMS122. 1908. London Municipal Pamphlets and Leaflets. 'The Work of Municipal Reform in London, 1907–1909', Municipal Reform Pamphlet 37.

the Council before they had been endorsed by the Finance Committee. This new system allowed any issues arising from such plans to be highlighted early and any extravagant schemes could be amended or stopped before any money was allocated. Percy-Harris claimed that the Finance Committee, which came into existence in March 1907, 'is the first which has been successful in carrying out its statutory duty, viz., in the words of the Act, to control and regulate the expenditure of the Council'.[143]

While some of this was political posturing, there can be little doubt that the Municipal Reform majority aided this new level of scrutiny and the election victory in 1907 had enabled the Finance Committee to come under their control. In the early twentieth-century, Laski advised that the best way to build-up a Finance Committee was to compose its membership of those who did not have similar responsibilities in other Committees.[144] By contrast, the reason the Finance Committee was so successful, the Municipal Reformers argued, was 'that they have behind them a majority on the Council who are in favour of economy' and this was reflected in its membership.[145] Haward described the new Finance Committee as being packed with 'men with knowledge of finance and business affairs ... No municipality', he argued, 'has ever been served by a more-able and distinguished body of men on its Finance Committee'.[146] Significantly, with the Municipal Reformers, A.F. Buxton in the Chair and the Right Honourable William St John Brodrick, his Vice Chairman, its majority enabled them to amend the standing orders of the Council and to formalise elements of its power.

As the first part of this chapter showed, there was nothing new in attempting to formalise financial regulations but, beyond the rhetoric, what this meant in practice was that the Asylums and Finance Committees, along with the Council as a whole, shared a desire to cut costs in the face of rising rates. At a meeting in May 1907, the Asylums

[143] GL, LMS108. 1910. *London County Council, Election 1910, Facts and Arguments Vol. 1*. London: London Municipal Society: 12–13.

[144] Laski, The Committee System in Local Government: 85.

[145] GL, LMS108. 1910. *London County Council, Election 1910, Facts and Arguments Vol. 1*. London: London Municipal Society: 13.

[146] Haward, *The London County Council from Within*: 89–90.

Committee read a memorandum from the Finance Committee, dated 24 April 1907. It 'urged that the most careful consideration should be given to every proposal involving capital expenditure, and that wherever possible, such proposals should be postponed pending a material improvement in the financial position'.[147] It was within this context that Goodrich and his colleagues were able to call a halt to the building of the eleventh asylum, at least in the short-term. Moreover, the Municipal Reformers made the cutting of 'waste' a feature of their campaigning materials. In 1908 a pamphlet titled 'The Progress of Municipal Reform – It's your money we save', listed seventeen key changes. The 'defeat' of the Progressive proposal to spend £500,000 [*sic*] on a new asylum was included at number two on a list of savings made, with only a reduction in the rates above it at number one.[148]

While the Municipal reformers made much political capital out of their postponement, the official reports on the issue couched it in terms of a declining demand. In the early 1980s, Edward Hare and Andrew Scull had a disagreement in print about the rising numbers of lunatics in the nineteenth century. While Hare, a psychiatrist at the Maudsley Hospital, emphasised a new epidemic of madness and a corresponding medical and humanitarian response, Scull responded with a sociological critique.[149] Although not a medical response, here too was an imperative to view the numbers through a political lens. The first Asylums Committee report published under the 'new' Moderate Council and completed on 9 July 1907 declared that, 'In view of the recent steady decline in the rate of increase of London Pauper lunacy', and the possibility that there may cease to be an increase, it is doubtful whether it will be necessary for us to take steps, at any rate for the present, towards the provision of an eleventh asylum'.[150] A little while later, Goodrich put the falling numbers down to the decrease of 'drink patients' which

[147] LMA, LCC/MIN/574, Signed Minutes, February 1907–February 1908, 14 May 1907.

[148] GL, LMS122. 1908. London Municipal Pamphlets and Leaflets. 'The Progress of Municipal Reform—It's Your Money We Save', Municipal Reform Pamphlet 102.

[149] Hare, Edward. 1983. Was Insanity on the Increase? *British Journal of Psychiatry* 143: 439–55. Scull, Andrew. 1984. Was Insanity Increasing: A Response to Edward Hare. *British Journal of Psychiatry* 144: 432–6.

[150] LMA, LCC 26.21, The Eighteenth Annual Report of the Asylums Committee of the London County Council, for the Year Ending 31 March 1907.

had resulted from a more sober London and also looked forward to the introduction of the old age pension which might keep out those described as suffering from senile decay.[151] Ironically, these were policies introduced by the Progressives in LCC and the Liberals in the British Parliament, respectively, but John McDougall criticised the decision to postpone a new institution on the grounds that, at the then current rate of increase, there would be 2000 patients ready for an asylum before one was built.[152]

Indeed, it is difficult to see what had changed in the short time since the Progressive administration had decided to go ahead with an eleventh asylum. In the first year after the election, figures suggested that there had been an increase of 408 pauper lunatics but the new Committee argued that 'It would seem that the increase in the lunacy statistics for London, which has been apparent of late years, is not due to a real increase of the incidence of the disease, but it is rather due to more comprehensive registration and accumulation and that this increase, such as it is will probably not persist'.[153] Moreover, in a bid to ramp up their argument, they re-iterated the plans that were already underway to explore new ways of dealing with the capital's lunatics. This included planned accommodation for aged patients, attempts to introduce receiving houses and the consideration given to a merger with the MAB.[154] These efforts will be explored in a subsequent chapter (Chapter 4) but these were longer-term discussions stretching back to 1896 and did not amount to new policy directions on the part of the new administration. When a report from the Asylums Clerk estimated that there would be over 1000 places needed for London's lunatics by 1912, the Committee's first response was to visit an existing MAB hospital at Carshalton. This was on the grounds that the MAB may have been willing to dispose of it and any potential costs to LCC would be much less than a new purpose-built institution.[155]

[151] Anon. 1908. Our Alien Lunatics. *Daily Mail*, 13 May.

[152] Anon. 1908. London County Council, Drink and Insanity. *Manchester Guardian*, 13 March.

[153] LMA, LCC/MIN/574, Signed Minutes, February 1907–February 1908, 11 February 1908.

[154] LMA, LCC/MIN/575, Signed Minutes, March 1908–February 1909, 14 April 1908.

[155] LMA, LCC/MIN/711, Accommodation Sub-Committee Minute Book, 1905–1908, 24 March 1908.

Unsurprisingly, the Commissioners in Lunacy continued to be unmoved by such claims and responded with a lengthy rebuttal. As a corollary, the Asylums Committee forwarded a letter to the Finance Committee 'with an intimation that in all probability it will be necessary for further asylum accommodation to be provided in the near future'.[156] Having made so much of the decision not to build an asylum, Jephson reminded Londoners that 'It should be borne in mind that the Council is not a free agent in the matter of accommodation. It has to provide accommodation for lunatics, and if it does not, it can be compelled to do so by the Commissioners in Lunacy'.[157]

Nevertheless, beyond the large capital expense involved in new asylums, there remained a will on the part of the Municipal Reformers to cut costs and to reduce what they saw as 'waste' in other areas. Working with the Clerk of the Committee and the Asylums Engineer, significant cuts were made to the projected costs of the male villa at Bexley (£1900), additional accommodation costs at the Horton Asylum (£15,000) and the erection of and equipment budget at Horton (£2000).[158] In other cases, as with the planned alterations to the Steward's House at Hanwell, where the work was not carried out, the £1000 allocated for it was returned to the central fund.[159] At the same time, capital estimates for 1908–1909 were rounded down from £99,780 to £90,000 on the understanding that the balance would be available if it was needed.[160]

While key members of the Progressive administration had tried and failed to get an asylum in the north of London off the drawing board, the Municipal Reformers were happy to maintain lunatics in distant out-county institutions. In a further bid to demonstrate the lack of demand for an eleventh asylum, the Committee argued that 'there were many vacancies in asylums in other parts of the country and as

[156] LMA, LCC/MIN/575, Signed Minutes, March 1908–February 1909, 12 May 1908.

[157] Jephson, *The Making of Modern London*: 187.

[158] LMA, LCC/MIN/574, Signed Minutes, February 1907–February 1908, 11 February 1908. LMA, LCC/MIN/575, Signed Minutes, March 1908–February 1909, 10 March 1908.

[159] LMA, LCC/MIN/575, Signed Minutes, March 1908–February 1909, 10 March 1908.

[160] LMA, LCC/MIN/575, Signed Minutes, March 1908–February 1909, 10 March 1908.

the London patients selected for these institutions were not visited, it would not entail any hardship on their part'.[161] Evidence from other sources suggested otherwise. When the Holborn Guardians asked that the patients chargeable to their board were returned to London asylums from the institutions in Birmingham and Hellingly in Sussex, the Committee responded that Out-County patients were 'specially selected, so that no hardship is occasioned to them or their friends because of the distance from London'.[162] This too was something that the Commissioners saw as intolerable, suggesting in 1908 that of the 2298 patients for whom no proper provision existed, 1880 were being boarded out at increased charges in other institutions.[163] For the Municipal Reformers, however, the maintenance costs involved in boarding out patients more than offset the capital costs involved in building and maintaining a new institution.

There were also implications for those who remained in LCC asylums too and when Goodrich announced the moratorium on the eleventh asylum, he stated that 'the Municipal Reform party hopes to be able by a judicious use of existing accommodation to avoid this enormous expenditure'.[164] On the plus side this led to almost immediate savings at the Horton Asylum, with the weekly cost of patients being reduced from 11s. 3 ¼d. in 1906–1907 to 10s. 1 ¾d. in 1907–1908. In addition, it was argued that the reformers saved '£10,417 in the administration of the asylum' and 'in no case has the general comfort and well-being either of the patients or the staff suffered, but the reverse is emphatically the case'.[165] In the same year, the Cane Hill sub-committee reported that, through a re-arrangement of beds in the wards, it had been possible to find accommodation for an additional 38 patients—without any additional expenses needed for equipment or staff.[166] While the Municipal Reformers may

[161] LMA, LCC/MIN/575, Signed Minutes, March 1908–February 1909, 14 April 1908.

[162] LMA, LCC/576, Signed Minutes, March 1909–July 1910, 22 June 1909.

[163] *Sixty-Second Report of the Commissioners in Lunacy*, 1908: 356.

[164] GL, LMS122. 1908. London Municipal Pamphlets and Leaflets, 'The Progress of Municipal Reform', Municipal Reform Pamphlet 26.

[165] GL, LMS72.1910, London Municipal Pamphlets and Leaflets, 'Municipal Reform and Model Management', Municipal Reform Leaflet A16.

[166] LMA, LCC/MIN/575, Signed Minutes, March 1908–February 1909, 13 October 1908.

have stressed the reorganisation of space, the Commissioners complained about overcrowding. By 1909, they complained that Cane Hill was overcrowded by 13 men and 24 women, while Hanwell in the following year was overcrowded by 50 men and 78 women.[167] By this time, the issue of overcrowding in both asylums generally, and individual wards specifically, had become a regular feature of the Commissioners reports. Hunter and Macalpine have described overcrowding as a perennial problem and, as was shown in Chapter 3, this was an issue that that pre- and post-dated the 1907 election.[168] In 1904, for example, the 'considerable' overcrowding of three of the male wards meant that the minimum space of 40 square feet per head had been reduced to 24.[169] At Claybury, one of the newest asylums and one that was often portrayed as a crowning achievement of LCC's Progressive administration, there was a considerable excess of 53 male and 133 female patients with beds made up in corridors and passages.[170] Nevertheless, while the Progressives were actively, if somewhat slowly, looking at options for additional accommodation, the Municipal Reformers were not.

Table 3.1 shows that when it came to the savings in the first few years after the 1907 election, the spending cuts on asylums were relatively low on the list but this tells only part of the story. Casting his eye over Asylum finances, Goodrich noted that the 'surplus' of £103,000 mentioned above might be used for other purposes. A new Municipal Reform dominated special committee concluded that only £55,000 was needed in working capital to avoid the need for overdrafts and potentially hefty banking charges. Rather than spend the money on improvements, the maintenance rate for patients was reduced by 1 ¾d. (to 10s 4 ¼d.) in January 1909 and at the same time negotiations were made so that each of the existing asylum's bank account accrued interest while in credit.[171] These examples are further evidence of the place of the management of London's asylums as part of the wider story of reform and,

[167] *Sixty-Fourth Report of the Commissioners in Lunacy*, 1910: 359, 365.

[168] Hunter and Macalpine, *Psychiatry for the Poor*: 57.

[169] *Sixty-First Report of the Commissioners in Lunacy*, 1907: 326.

[170] *Fifty-Ninth Report of the Commissioners in Lunacy*, 1905: 331, 340.

[171] LMA, LCC/MIN/575, Signed Minutes, March 1908–February 1909, 22 December 1908.

Table 3.1 Capital expenditure safeguarded[a]

	Amount voted (£s)	*Spent (£s)*	*Savings (£s)*	*Savings (%)*
Asylums	90,000	62,754	27,246	30
Education	500,000	383,525	116,475	23
Establishment	201,650	57,808	143,842	71
Fire Brigade	45,500	22,425	23,075	51
Tramways	1,300,000	1,046,235	253,765	20
Housing	130,000	81,447	48,553	37
Improvements	734,540	333,640	400,900	55
Main Drainage	500,000	363,918	136,082	27
Parks	43,500	31,732	11,768	27
Public control	3200	4	3196	100
Stores	20,000	Nothing	20,000	100
Contingency provisions	281,550	Nothing	281,550	100

aGL, LMS123. 1909. London Municipal Pamphlets and Leaflets, 'The Work of Municipal Reform in London, 1907–1909', Municipal Reform Pamphlet 37

as time progressed, the numbers increased with claims they reduced expenditures and cut back on Progressive commitments to the tune of £10 million.[172] Viscount Middleton speaking in 1909, put the figure at £7 million but this was a colossal figure nonetheless. 'I was appalled' he claimed, 'we were receiving an income of £10 million, and we were spending £15 million'. And this included the possible addition of £4 million or £5 million for Electric Lighting and another £3 million for asylums.[173] 'What was the result of all our efforts at economy?' he asked. 'The result has been that we have brought debt within moderate limits. I think in all we have knocked off about 7 millions of those 17 millions of commitments'.[174]

The Municipal Reformers continued to make political capital of the savings they had introduced, not just in their management of the asylums but in their management of the capital and, indeed, the capital's capital.

[172]GL, LMS116. 1912. Borough Council Elections 'Municipal Reform v Progressive Socialism'.

[173]GL, LMS108. 1910. *London County Council, Election 1910, Facts and Arguments Vol. 1.* London: London Municipal Society: 19.

[174]GL, LMS108. 1910. *London County Council, Election 1910, Facts and Arguments Vol. 1.* London: London Municipal Society: 20–1.

Somewhat ironically, the Municipal Reformers' plans to spend £175 on the opening of the asylums at Long Grove, was defeated by a Progressive Amendment.[175] The savings at Horton, along with savings to the ratepayers in other areas were used as both evidence of 'model managements' but also the mess, muddle and mismanagement of the progressive socialists.[176] In this respect, the management of asylums became useful evidence in wider ideological attacks. Significantly, the Municipal Reformers, had constituted a committee with a view to watching the progress of socialism in the capital and to advise on the best method of combatting it. The leaflets were part of that strategy and, as well as being circulated in London, were used to educate speakers who gave talks, mainly in London, but also in other parts of the country.[177] In the run up to the 1913 election, it was claimed that Municipal Reformers had reduced the average London rates by £750,000 since winning the election in 1907. When rates were hiked under the Municipal Reform administration, the blame was placed at the door of the 'Radical Progressive' national Government which, it was claimed, 'had added to the duties of the councils without giving any money to carry out those duties'.[178]

Conclusions

Although some contemporaries were apt to suggest that the financing of London's asylums rarely came before the Council or was untouched by its politics, this was far from the case. It is true that the privileging of the role of lunacy legislation and also of the role of the Commissioners in Lunacy can be seen in the latter's continuing pressure on the Council to build the institutions it had a statutory responsibility to provide, both before and after 1907. Such a straightforward overview, however,

[175] LSE, JS/57–60. Gilbert, J.D. 1909. *Two and a Half Years Record of the Moderate Party*. London: London Reform Union: 4.

[176] GL, LMS72. 1910. London Municipal Pamphlets and Leaflets, 'Municipal Reform and Model Management', Municipal Reform Leaflet A16.

[177] LMA, CLC/088/MS19528, London Municipal Society, Minutes Executive Committee Meetings: 19 September 1907, 20 November 1907.

[178] GL, LMS126. 1909. London Municipal Pamphlets and Leaflets, 'Rising Rates', Municipal Reform Leaflet 136. 'How the Radical-Progressive Government Raises Your Rates', Municipal Reform Leaflet 140.

dismisses the importance of political views on the provision of asylums and, crucially, on the economics of doing so. To be sure, both Progressives and Moderates (Municipal Reformers) made political capital of what they saw as the efficient management of the capital's institutions, but this was undoubtedly influenced by their wider visions for the governance of London. As a result, when it came to financial questions, spending on asylum stock became useful ammunition in critiques of spending, rather than the main issue in and of itself.

The internal wrangling of the Finance and the Asylums Committee was important, but it was also indicative of a political battle surrounding public spending and what represented value for money. This focussed on the employment of public labour on the one hand and the role of private enterprise on the other, and the part played by the Works Committee in both. At the very least this was indicative of contemporary political disagreement about the role of the Asylums Committee which became framed in terms of wider debates about 'intervention'. As a corollary, the Asylums Committee's ability to negotiate with the internal watchdog in the form of the Finance Committee and the external watchdog in the form of the Commissioners in Lunacy was governed to some degree by political majorities in the Council chamber. Here, the Council as a whole had a right to approve or veto the spending plans of individual committees, but the effectiveness of its Standing Orders was largely governed by the willingness and ability of the Council or, indeed, the Finance Committee to enforce them. Thus, in the case of London, the Finance Committee did not simply become stronger as its role became more clearly defined. Instead, it became stronger after 1907 when the Municipal Reformers swept to power. Their election victory allowed them to introduce new Standing Orders to govern the role of the Finance Committee, but it also meant that the majority of Councillors were more sympathetic to spending reform. Crucially, it allowed the new majority administration to pack the committees with their own men. In turn, this meant that the Council chamber and also the individual committees were more likely to act in concert, just as they had done under the previous Progressive regime. Whether the Asylums Committee was dominated by Progressives or Municipal Reformers, it was unable to meet the demand for accommodation and, as a corollary, the demands of its stakeholders in the form of the Poor Law Guardians and the Commissioners in Lunacy. Under the Progressives, issues of overcrowding had not gone away and questions have to be asked why they did not put any surpluses to good use in terms of improving their existing stock. Nevertheless, the attempts of the Municipal Reformers to place more people in the same accommodation, while at the same time reducing expenditure on extensions and repairs must have had an impact on the patients—whatever their election literature might have had to say about 'efficiency'. Here, there was the primacy of the lunacy legislation but even then the direction of travel from the parties was clearly defined. While the Progressives wanted smaller, newer, more local institutions, the Municipal Reformers wanted largely cheaper and more efficient ones—a theme that will be explored in more detail in the next chapter.

CHAPTER 4

The Politics of Innovation

With the passing of the LGA, LCC inherited a coterie of medical staff that was to grow with the opening of each of its additional asylums. By this time, the expansion of the asylum sector more generally had emphasised the role and influence of the medical professionals that worked within it. The Association of Medical Officers of Hospitals for the Insane was founded in 1841 and morphed into the Medico-Psychological Association 24 years later.[1] Those who worked in asylums were able to share ideas and update their professional knowledge in sector-specific, as well as broader medical journals, and at conferences and in research trips to other institutions at home and abroad.[2] Andrew Scull has argued that the status of doctors was, legally speaking, that of salaried employees of individual asylum committees but noted that most committees were content to leave medical matters in the hands of their medically trained subordinates.[3]

[1]The association became the Royal College of Psychiatrists in 1971. Fennell, Phil. 1996. *Treatment Without Consent: Law Psychiatry and the Treatment of Mentally Disordered People Since 1845*. London: Routledge: 4–5.

[2]The *Asylum Journal* was launched in 1853 and became the *Asylum Journal of Mental Science* three years later. Fennell, *Treatment Without Consent*: 5.

[3]Scull, *The Most Solitary of Afflictions*: 247. See also McCrae, Niall and Nolan, Peter. *The Story of Nursing in British Mental Hospitals: Echoes from the Corridors*. London: Routledge: Michael Finn describes the West Riding Asylum under James Crichton-Browne was a 'classic example' of a committee happy to leave the Medical Superintendent to work in a way that he saw fit. Finn, Michael. The West Riding Lunatic Asylum: 66.

R. Ellis, *London and its Asylums, 1888-1914*,
Mental Health in Historical Perspective,
https://doi.org/10.1007/978-3-030-44432-7_4

More recently, Louise Hide has written of some of the tensions between medical staff and management, particularly in the case of Robert Jones at LCC's Claybury Asylum.[4]

In terms of the shaping of a broader vision for the Council, however, the role of these staff is less clear. As has already been shown in earlier chapters, much of the party political rhetoric relating to the management of madness privileged the administrative reforms introduced by politicians, rather than the introduction of medical initiatives. Moreover, it has been argued that there is limited evidence to suggest that those outside of the medical profession were influenced by the dissemination of medical knowledge.[5] Indeed, the effect of wider medical discourses on LCC policy and practise appears to be contradictory. Cochrane describes the opening of the Maudsley Hospital as being 'out of step' with mainstream preoccupations of the Asylums Committee, but both he and others see medical practitioners as the driving force behind such successful innovations.[6] While Jones et al. do explain some of the administrative and legalistic issues in the Maudsley's development, the role of individual councillors, sub-committees and party politics is absent. Thus, the aim of this chapter is to consider the influence of governance and of party politics on medical discourses, discussions and initiatives, and vice versa.

To address these issues, this chapter will be framed around London's growing lunacy 'problem'. In particular, it will focus on the belief that more resources needed to be directed towards acute services, to stem the apparently never-ending tide of 'chronic' or incurable in-patients.[7] Chris Philo has challenged Foucault's notion that the social separation of the insane was a 'given', and to understand the 'historically

[4] Hide, *Gender and Class*: 48.

[5] Bartlett, *The Poor Law of Lunacy*: 18.

[6] Cochrane, The Asylum and Its Psychiatry: 265. See also Jones, Edgar, Rahman, Shahina and Woolven, Robin. 2007. The Maudsley Hospital: Design and Strategic Direction, 1923–1939. *Medical History* 51: 357–78. Allderidge, Patricia. 1991. The Foundation of the Maudsley Hospital. In *150 Years of British Psychiatry, 1841–1991*, eds. G.E. Berrios and H. Freeman, 79–88. London: Gaskell.

[7] From the earliest days of asylum medicine, it was felt that capturing insanity in its incipient form offered the best chance of recovery and the best chance to prevent individuals becoming long-stay chronic cases.

contingent' factors behind this, party politics will necessarily play a role in this analysis.[8] So too will an understanding of asylum governance and the potential for medical professionals from within and outwith LCC's asylum stock to influence broader policy on those terms. To achieve this there will be an examination of three key initiatives. The first will be the attempts in the early years of LCC to found a Hospital of the Insane for London, which, it was hoped, would work towards finding a cure for insanity. The second will explore an LCC proposal to develop Receiving Houses in the County of London which would act as triage services with a view to stemming the flow of people accessing asylum services. This section aims to extend the understanding of political and medical discussions taking place to include Poor Law officials who acted as key gatekeepers to London's asylums, as well as the Commissioners in Lunacy and Parliament. The relative successes and failures of these extra-institutional attempts to create new spaces and places for the management of London's madness will be extended with a third section which will consider the appointment of a pathologist for London whose aim was to conduct research into the causes and prevention of insanity. While these three activities might look like a concerted and organised effort to respond to the rising numbers of lunacy, this chapter will show how each activity was framed by political manoeuvring, and describe the limitations of what could be achieved in each case. In all cases there will be examination of the relationships and the discussions taking place between politicians and medical professionals. In doing so, it builds on the resurgent interest in the study of asylum medical staff but, in this case, it will argue that the success or failure of large-scale initiatives rested with an understanding of the politics and governance of LCC, rather than just medical opinion or innovation.[9]

[8] Chris Philo cited in Moran, J. and Topp, L. 2006. Introduction. In *Madness, Architecture and the Built Environment*, eds. Leslie Topp, James E. Moran and Jonathan Andrews, 1–16. London: Routledge: 7.

[9] Wallis, *Investigating the Body*. Finn, *The West Riding Lunatic Asylum*.

London and a Plan for a Hospital for the Insane

The impact of lay administrators on medical regimes already has a place in the historiography of madness. Suzuki, for example, saw the campaign to get rid of mechanical restraint at Hanwell 'as a political gesture on the part of the magistrates'.[10] It was, he concluded, indicative of changes that moved the Medical Superintendent from the asylum's 'autocratic guiding spirit' to 'a mere cog in a huge bureaucratic machine'.[11] His focus was on the first half of the nineteenth century but some sense of this bureaucracy in the period covered by this book has already been seen in Chapter 3. Pertinent here were the new politics of the post-1888, post-LGA landscape. Indeed, immediately after the first election in 1889, a resolution was put forward by Councillor Robert Brudenell Carter asking LCC to convene a committee to consider the building and operation of a Hospital for the Insane for the new county. Brudenell Carter's vision for the hospital was one that would 'complement' the existing asylum system but also focus on the 'curative treatment of insanity'.[12] In the debate that followed in the council chamber, there was a failed attempt to pass this matter to the Asylums Committee and, in the end, a new Committee was formed with its progenitor in the chair.

At the time, Brudenell Carter was Vice Chairman of LCC's Sanitary and General Purposes Committee and an Ophthalmic Surgeon at St George's hospital. In addition, he wrote articles for both *The Times* and the *Lancet* and served as the representative of the Apothecaries Society on the General Medical Council.[13] Here was a man with a long history of medical practice but no practical experience of asylums. As a young man he had treated 'a not inconsiderable number of cases of hysteria' but Alexander Walk argues that Brudenell Carter took his lead for the Hospital initiative from John Batty Tuke who had published an overview of Scottish open-door care in Scotland at the beginning of 1889.[14]

[10] Suzuki, The Politics and Ideology of Non-Restraint: 2.

[11] Ibid: 17.

[12] LMA, LCC/18.6, London County Council Minutes of Proceedings, January–December 1889, 11 April 1889.

[13] Anon. n.d. Robert Brudenell Carter, Royal College of Surgeons. http://livesonline.rcseng.ac.uk/biogs/E000859b.htm. Accessed 4 July 2019.

[14] Scull, Andrew. 2009. *Hysteria: The Disturbing History*. Oxford: Oxford University Press: 66. Walk, Alexander. 1976. Medico-Psychologists, Maudsley and the Maudsley Hospital. *British Journal of Psychiatry*: 128: 19–30.

Table 4.1 Meetings of LCC's Committee on a Hospital for the Insane

Date	*Witnesses examined*
13 May 1889	None
30 May 1889	Dr Batty Tuke, Sir J. T. Banks
20 June 1889	Sir J. Crichton Browne
4 July 1889	Dr C. Allbutt, Sir A. Clarke and Dr Ferrier
11 July 1889	Mr J. Marshall, Dr Quain, Dr Buzzard and Dr S. Mackenzie
18 July 1889	Prof V. Horsley, Dr Gowers and Mr T. Bryant
25 July 1889	Dr Charlton Bastian, Dr Whipham and Mr J. Hutchinson
3 October 1889	None
17 October 1889	None
30 June 1890	None

Source LCC/CL/PH/01/276, Report of the Committee on a Hospital for the Insane, LCC, 1890

As a council member of the then recently formed College of State Medicine, Brudenell Carter delivered its inaugural lecture at the Chemical Society's Burlington House. In the course of his lecture, he stated that 'the province of state medicine might be held to comprise of all the acts or precautions which were necessary for the prevention or cure of disease, and, which, for any reason, were beyond the power of isolated individuals and within the power of the organized community alone'.[15] The terms of reference for the Committee on a Hospital for the Insane reflected this emphasis on cure and was a move welcomed by the General Council of Medical Education and Registration.[16]

Appendix 4 shows the membership of what became known, informally, as Brudenell Carter's Committee. Unusually for LCC, the political affiliation of its membership was evenly split and while some had medical experience, and/or were serving members of the Asylums Committee, others were not. Brudenell Carter had a clear agenda but his aim was to draw on wider expertise and, at its first meeting, the Committee agreed a strategy whereby a list of 'eminent medical practitioners' was drawn up and who were then asked to attend a series of meetings. Table 4.1 shows the medical practitioners who attended these preliminary meetings, including the well-known experts on insanity and former asylum

[15] The College of State Medicine. *Times*, 4 May 1888: 3.

[16] Anon. 1889. General Council of Medical Education and Registration, Spring Session 1889. *BMJ*, 15 June.

superintendents, Batty Tuke and Sir James Crichton Browne. It is likely, that personal as well as professional contacts were utilised in those initial consultations. As the Committee members recognised, not all the people they interviewed were specialists in the field and their aim was to boost their understanding with a wider process of consultation.[17]

Following the first witness statements, a circular was drawn up along with a list of three key questions which was distributed to 'a wider circle of authorities', including every medical superintendent of a public asylum in England and Wales. The questions asked were:

> Is it your opinion that the organisation of public asylums for the insane, as at present conducted, makes sufficient provision, or allows sufficient opportunity, for the investigation of the pathology of insanity by the light of modern methods of research, or for the careful adaptation of medical or surgical treatment to the cases of individual patients?
>
> If you recognise deficiencies in the directions indicated above, is it your opinion that they might be supplied, at least to some extent, by a hospital in London in which the work of the resident medical officers would be supplemented by that of a sufficiently numerous medical and surgical visiting staff, and by that of a skilled pathologist?
>
> Would it be agreeable to you, if requested, to appear before the Committee as a witness?

The circular was prefaced with some leading information which spoke of the Committee's belief that there had been a failure to find workable solutions for the cure and prevention of diseases of the brain because of the administrative and disciplinary demands placed on the Medical Superintendents in large asylums.[18] The focus on cure and prevention bears Brudenell Carter's mark but this had been a recognisable issue for those working in the sector for some time. In 1854, a critic of the North Riding Asylum had complained that more time was spent on farming

[17] Sir John (J.T.) Banks, for example, was the Regius Professor of Physic at the University of Dublin, and other held positions relating to their roles as either physicians or surgeons. LCC/CL/PH/01/276. LCC. 1890. Report of the Committee on a Hospital for the Insane.

[18] LCC/CL/PH/01/276. 1889. R. Brudenell Carter, Committee on a Hospital for the Insane.

than it was on medical and curative arrangements.[19] The development of scientific and other initiatives into the causes and prevention of mental diseases in the decades that followed, did not prevent Montagu Lomax claiming, in 1921, that some superintendents still devoted more time and energy on drains than they did on brains.[20]

The Committee's preliminary findings were presented at the weekly meeting of LCC, presided over by its Chairman, Lord Rosebery, and included the recommendation that

> an adequately equipped hospital, containing one hundred beds for the study and curative treatment of insanity in pauper lunatics of both sexes, be established in the metropolis, and that it be under the direction and control of the Council.[21]

This was reiterated at the presentation of the final report in March 1890 and, given that Brudenell Carter had proposed the Committee on this basis in the first place, and given that the findings were based on its consultation with the medical profession, the conclusions were not, on the face of it, surprising. Indeed, Brudenell Carter, Walk argues, 'had his way and the Committee, over which of course he naturally presided, duly reported in accordance with his wishes'.[22]

Cochrane has described the hospital plan as a 'unique opportunity' and as a logical progression stemming from the asylum systems' 'low cure rates' but, at the time, not everyone saw it in those terms.[23] Indeed, the presentation of report's recommendations, and the plans to carry them forth at a meeting of LCC led to what *The Times* described as 'considerable argument'.[24] An important feature of this was the role

[19] Anonymous critic of the North Riding and Bedford asylums writing in 1854, cited in Philo, Chris. 1987. "Fit Localities for an Asylum": The Historical Geography of the Nineteenth-Century "Mad Business" in England as Viewed Through the Pages of the Asylum Journal. *Journal of Historical Geography* 13:4: 398–415: 407.

[20] Montagu Lomax cited in Hide, *Gender and Class*: 47. For an example of scientific initiatives in asylums see Wallis, J. 2015. *Investigating the Body in the Victorian Asylum*. London: Palgrave Macmillan.

[21] Anon. 1889. Proposed Hospital for the Insane of London, 9 November.

[22] Walk, Medico-Psychologists, Maudsley and the Maudsley Hospital: 26–7.

[23] Cochrane, Humane, Economical and Medically Wise: 263.

[24] Anon. 1889. The London County Council. *The Times*, 13 March.

and scope of medical expertise that featured in the report. The committee had 'received and analysed' 65 written responses but the fact that no more witness were called to give evidence to the Committee after 25 July 1889 would prove to be significant.[25] Dr George Cooper (Progressive, Southwark) raised concerns that only two of the 'eminent' gentlemen invited to present evidence (Crichton-Browne and Batty Tuke) had any real connection with asylums. Dr William Bott (Progressive, Newington West) 'contended that there was universal dissatisfaction by medical men at the manner in which the Committee had selected their witnesses'.[26] Reflecting on the report almost 25 years later, Robert Jones, the superintendent at the Claybury Asylum from its opening in 1893, asked why the 'great authorities' of Dr Hack Tuke, Dr George Savage and Dr Henry Maudsley had not been consulted.[27] Moreover he asked why 'no-one engaged at the time in the actual management of asylums for the insane was invited to give evidence'.[28]

The *BMJ* described the report as raising 'a whirlwind of indignant protest from medical officers of asylums throughout the country' and others too spoke of the apparently unexplained but keen opposition from alienists.[29] It is difficult to see just what was 'unexplained' as many, including Dr David Yellowlees, Physician Superintendent at the Glasgow Royal Asylum at Gartnavel, wrote at length about their concerns. Yellowlees was based in Scotland and not, therefore, included in the distribution of the circular that was sent to his peers in England and Wales. This explains, in part at least, why he complained in the 'strongest terms' at the 'absolute unfairness with which medical superintendents of the United Kingdom had been treated by men who seemed absolutely

[25] Proposed Hospital for the Insane of London. *BMJ*, 9 November 1889.

[26] Anon. 1890. The Proposed Hospital for the Study of Insanity. *BMJ*, 15 March.

[27] Robert Jones added Armstrong to his surname in 1913. I am grateful to Louise Hide for this biographical information. Armstrong Jones, Robert. 1914. The Rational Treatment of Incipient Insanity. *BMJ*, 7 February.

[28] Armstrong Jones, Robert. 1914. The Rational Treatment of Incipient Insanity. *BMJ*, 7 February.

[29] Alienist was term to describe those specialising in the treatment of lunatics, usually in asylums. Anon. 1891. The Second Annual Report of the County of London Lunatic Asylums. *BMJ*, 3 October. Horsley, V. 1891. The Student and the Practitioner. *BMJ*, 3 October.

ignorant of the subject they were dealing with'.[30] That ignorance included the 'absurd' way in which medical superintendents were canvassed by only being allowed to respond to three questions, but he also claimed that their responses were treated with 'contempt'.[31] Jones went further describing the report as casting a deliberate 'slur upon the whole body of medical men practising in the department of lunacy'.[32] To put this into context, another report suggested that Medical Superintendents would 'not feel flattered' by LCC's [*sic*] contention that the staff in its asylums were concerned with custody, when it seemed that madness was, in fact, curable.[33] At the West Riding Lunatic Asylum, William Bevan Lewis complained of the 'scant justice' done 'to many a conscientious Superintendent who ha[d] struggled against the odds to establish the treatment of lunacy upon a scientific basis', but he qualified this on the grounds that he believed the plan to be the correct one and he hoped it would eventually be realised.[34]

Certainly, the rising numbers of apparently incurable patients was an issue vexing many authorities. As Jeremy Taylor has suggested, 'As a result [of the Committee's work], the general level of debate promoted improvements in the detailed planning of new asylums from the 1890s onwards, and encouraged an increasing provision of separate "acute" hospital buildings on asylum sites'.[35] This included acute hospitals at Bevan Lewis's West Riding Asylum at Wakefield and the East Sussex Asylum at Hellingly, while G. T. Hine identified other counties following suit, including the Middlesex Asylum at Napsbury.[36] In reality,

[30]Proposed Hospitals for Lunatics in London. *BMJ*, 23 August 1890: 447. Richard Green, the Medical Superintendent of the Berry Wood Asylum in Northampton was another vocal critic. Greene, Richard. 1889. The Care and Cure of the Insane. *The Universal Review* 4: 493–508: 504–6.

[31]Proposed Hospitals for Lunatics in London. *BMJ*, 23 August 1890: 447.

[32]Armstrong Jones, Robert. 1914. The Rational Treatment of Incipient Insanity. *BMJ*, 7 February.

[33]E.M.L and C.B.L. 1890. Lunacy Law Reform. *The Westminster Review* 134: 128–42: 12.

[34]West Yorkshire Archive Service (hereafter, WYAS), C85/1/12/5. 1890. Report of the Sub-Committee and Medical Superintendent of the West Riding Asylum for the year 1889, West Yorkshire Printing Co, Wakefield: 10.

[35]Taylor, Jeremy. 1991. *Hospital and Asylum Architecture in England 1840–1914*. London, Mansell: 153.

[36]Ibid.

as the nineteenth century neared its end, a twin track system of care was developing in many institutions with acute cases being treated in smaller clinical facilities within asylum grounds.[37] As a result, the emphasis given to the prevention and cure of insanity in a hospital that was outside the existing model of care, was seen as an attack, not just on the system, but on the people who operated within it.

At the presentation of the report and its recommendations, Brudenell Carter attempted to address the issue directly. He 'entirely repudiated the idea of making any charge against the asylum superintendents, who had worked well under most difficult circumstances - circumstances which absolutely precluded them from attaining the object the Committee had in hand'.[38] Unfortunately for him, not everyone agreed with the report's recommendations. Cooper described the plans as 'at the best but an experiment', and called for proof that the medical authorities had 'no other means of educating medical students than by a hospital paid out of the rates'.[39] Similarly, Jones focussed on

> the inexperienced hands of a visiting staff who were to cure insanity with "stuff out of a bottle" and were to take the statical [*sic*] view of the dead-house rather than actual clinical experience of mental diseases as the guiding star in treatment.[40]

Richard Greene of the Berry Wood Asylum also failed to see how a visiting physician, assisted by newly qualified men and clinical clerks, could cure more cases than the present system. The suggestion that asylums did not have acute hospitals attached to them was flawed from the outset. It may have been true if 'hospital' meant a detached building, he argued, but there was not a single county lunatic asylum 'through the length and breadth of England' that did not have an infirmary or admission ward for acute cases.[41] For him, the hospital plan would be

[37] Hide, *Gender and Class*: 4.

[38] Anon. 1890. The Proposed Hospital for the Study of Insanity. *BMJ*, 15 March.

[39] Cooper pointed to the two large hospitals at St Luke's and Bethlem; both of which had visiting medical staffs. Anon. 1890. The Proposed Hospital for the Study of Insanity. *BMJ*, 15 March.

[40] Armstrong Jones, Robert. The Rational Treatment of Incipient Insanity. *BMJ*, 7 February 1914.

[41] Greene, The Care and Cure of the Insane: 504–6.

an expensive experiment, especially when it had been unsuccessful in 'German university towns' and the cures provided by the New South Wales acute hospital were lower than the cures in New Zealand which did 'not possess the boon'. The number of superintendents that saw the efficacy could be described as 'very few' and Greene concluded that he hoped LCC 'will think twice before expending a quarter of a million or even a quarter of that sum on these hospitals'.[42]

Significantly, more recent analysis has concluded that the decision to reject the Committee's recommendation was in deference to such widespread opposition of medical superintendents.[43] Certainly, the influence of medical opinion can be seen in the response of Cooper and Bott (above) but this was far from unequivocal. Martineau, the Asylums Committee's first Chairman, reminded the Council that the 65 asylum superintendents who had written to the Committee were largely in favour of the plan, and Hine argued that LCC overturned the 'very comprehensive report showing that the evidence adduced was greatly in favour of the scheme'.[44] Of the 65 'gentlemen' who responded, 24 approved of the proposed hospital 'without qualification'. A further 17 approved of it with 'some qualification' but this included one respondent who thought that equally good results would be achieved with an increase in asylum staff, and nine who thought that the hospital 'would "to some extent", or "to a limited extent", supply existing deficiencies'.[45] A minority of 15 respondents 'disapproved' of the plan and another nine responses were described as 'ambiguous'.

The report produced by the Committee on a Hospital for the Insane created much debate and disagreement within medical circles and both sides of the argument could draw on evidence to claim they held the majority opinion. The debate that took place focussed as much on the collection of witness statements, as it did about the efficacy or otherwise of the proposal, and its tone was influenced by its participants and the seven-man team that lead the investigation. As Brudenell Carter

[42] Ibid.

[43] Taylor, *Hospital and Asylum Architecture in England*: 153.

[44] Hine, George T. 1901. Asylums and Asylum Planning. *Journal of the Royal Institute of British Architects* February: 161–84: 171.

[45] LMA, LCC/CL/PH/01/276, Miscellaneous Papers. LCC. 1890. Report of the Committee on a Hospital for the Insane.

concluded, 'the non-medical members of the Committee have been compelled to lean, to some extent, upon the information supplied to them by their medical colleagues' when dealing with what were very technical questions.[46] This in itself appears to privilege the role of medical opinion but to understand the fate of the final report there has to be an understanding of the LGA, LCC, its committee structure and the devolution of decision-making.

LCC and the Politics of the Hospital Plan

Although Brudenell Carter had a longer-term interest in both the prevention and cure of disease, it was his election to LCC in 1889 that enabled him to first propose and then chair the Insane Hospital Committee. Beyond this, his success or otherwise in achieving his aims rested with the reading of the LGA. As Brudenell Carter's Committee discussed with medical practitioners the site and size of the proposed hospital, its potential location and the costs to LCC's ratepayers, it recognised the proposals were in no way reflective of the duty of LCC. Instead the Committee focussed on the 'public interest' of 'facilities for the conduct of medical education' and argued that the establishment of an Insane Hospital would be a 'legitimate exercise' of LCC's powers and 'a proper application of the funds of which it has control'.[47] Unfortunately for Brudenell Carter, this was to be an important first hurdle.

In the debate that followed the presentation of the report to LCC, calls were made to adjourn the matter so that it might be considered more fully by the Asylums Committee. Rosebery, as Chairman, concluded that such an adjournment would allow the Council to feel 'its legs a little more firmly', arguing that an 'experiment of that kind' would demand assistance from imperial funds as it would benefit the community and the 'Empire at large', and was not just for the good of London.[48] Once again, the mention of Empire emphasised London's

[46] LMA, LCC/CL/PH/01/276, Miscellaneous Papers. LCC. 1890. Report of the Committee on a Hospital for the Insane.

[47] LMA, LCC/CL/PH/01/276, Miscellaneous Papers. LCC. 1890. Report of the Committee on a Hospital for the Insane.

[48] London County Council. 1890. *A Review of the First Year's Work of the Council in a Series of Addresses Delivered by the Chairman, the Earl of Rosebery*. London: LCC: 30–1.

role as a potential exporter of ideas, as well as goods and people. If it was to be a question for LCC, however, then consideration would have to be given to the justification for such a project 'when the rates were acknowledged to be too high and they had vast and new responsibilities to discharge in adding this fresh burden upon the people (Hear, Hear).[49] The issue of the rates was a familiar refrain but, having been given licence to explore the possibility of a hospital in the first place, it was only on the publication of the report that consideration was to be given to the legislative power of the Council to build such an institution.

Brudenell Carter argued that if the plan could not be accepted, 'it would not be strengthened by being referred to the Asylums Committee' and *The Times* soon weighed in on his side.[50] The Asylums Committee, it stated, was 'perfectly competent to deal with questions connected with the management of asylums, and to discharge those functions', but it could not 'for a moment pretend to the authority of men like those' who gave their evidence to Brudenell Carter's Committee.[51] Instead, it described the supplementary consideration given to the power of building an insane hospital and its costs as 'merely the plausibilities which are employed to excuse a policy of delay'.[52] Indeed, the matter came to an end when the Council, following a recommendation from the Asylums Committee, concluded that this was an issue that affected 'national rather than metropolitan interests'.[53]

For Alexander Walk 'the decision to postpone was [probably] influenced by cost; the population of London was still rising and the Council was advised that new asylums would be needed before long; they were indeed built and were of the same inordinate size which the report had so severely condemned'.[54] Similarly, Cochrane argues that the proposed plans for a hospital were 'shelved' by the Asylums Committee as they became 'overwhelmed by the torrent of referrals' from [Poor Law] unions'.[55] Indeed, the Asylum Committee's second report revealed

[49] Anon. 1890. The London County Council. *The Times*, 13 March.

[50] Anon. 1890. The Proposed Hospital for the Study of Insanity. *BMJ*, 15 March.

[51] Anon. 1890. The Proceedings of the London County Council. *The Times*, 13 March.

[52] Ibid.

[53] LMA, LCC/MIN/565, Signed Minutes, 1889–1891, 1 July 1890.

[54] Walk, Medico-Psychologists, Maudsley and the Maudsley: 27.

[55] Cochrane, Humane, Economical and Medically Wise: 264.

that 381 potential admissions had been refused 'for want of accommodation' and this was in addition to the 2000 plus London's lunatics distributed across a range of English asylums for the same reason.[56] Undoubtedly, figures such as these were on the mind of the Committee but they were not included in the explanation for passing the report back to the Council. In this case, a straightforward reading of the Asylum Committee's fudging of Brudenell Carter's report show no direct references to either the medical debates taking place or the huge numbers of London's insane in the decision-making process. Instead, the 'shelving' of the report came to be seen as the result of the inter-related issues of LCC's politics, its committee structure, and its membership.

In part, at least, this sense of political manoeuvring stemmed from Brudenell Carter himself and the matter was behind his decision not to seek re-election in 1892. In a letter to *The Times* in that year, he complained that it was difficult for a busy professional man to promote reforms without being called upon to make 'unreasonable sacrifices'.[57] In particular, he was concerned with the size of committees, their membership, the number of meetings that were held and the attendance at them. In highlighting his concerns he singled out the Asylums Committee for being 'composed of the preposterous number of 60 members on the ground [*sic*] that it has been called upon to furnish a sub-committee for each asylum'.[58]

As was shown in Chapter 2, attendance at these Committees, and the commitment to them, became framed in political terms and Brudenell Carter's polemic against the Asylums Committee was coloured by his distaste for both it and LCC's majority membership. Two-thirds of Councillors, he complained, had radical or socialist opinions. They were 'mere politicians' and 'faddists' who had an 'undeveloped sense of duty' and they were not interested in the good government of London.[59] Both *The Times* and the *Spectator* magazine offered their support for this critique, with the former stating that Brudenell Carter had shone a

[56]LMA, LCC/ 26.21, Annual Reports for LCC Asylums Committee for 1889–1892, The Second Annual Report of the Asylums Committee of the London County Council, for the year ending 31 March 1891.

[57]Brudenell Carter, R. The London County Council. *The Times*, 6 January.

[58]Ibid.

[59]Brudenell Carter, R. 1892. The London County Council. *The Times*, 6 January.

light on the work of the faddists, whether in suspending 'metropolitan improvement' or in perpetrating 'all sorts of absurdities' that were 'going on in every committee room and over every detail of business'.[60] The *Spectator* used the letter as a rallying call to its readership, hoping it would 'startle even Londoners out of their apathy' so that the 'faddist' Progressives might be 'summarily dismissed' in the 1892 election.[61]

The main focus of these articles then, was in response to Carter's suggestions of faddism and a reminder to Londoners of their electoral duties to elect a government 'fit' for the capital in the forthcoming election. Given the readerships of both *The Times* and the *Spectator* this is hardly surprising but, in the immediate aftermath of the Brudenell Carter's failure, and in the years that followed, vocal critics focussed, not on the medical debates about the efficacy of the Insane Hospital plan, but on the political reasons for the postponement. The scheme 'was wrecked', according to the *BMJ*, 'by the political cross-currents in which so many useful proposals set afloat in the Council are submerged'.[62] Sir John Batty Tuke, who had given evidence at the original Committee could not understand why the 'modest scheme' was not carried into effect.[63] He stopped short of identifying the reason for, or the influences on the 'pigeon-holing' of the report but Brudenell Carter was clear. Writing to *The Times* in the context of a proposal to build a hospital villa at the Bexley Asylum, he concluded that his proposal for an Insane Hospital was shelved by the 'Radical caucus of the asylum determined that no action should be taken on this report'.[64]

In the fallout that followed, the Asylums Committee's 'preposterous' membership of 60 members came to represent a point of political debate in which the national media played an important role. This included the Liberal-supporting *Speaker* newspaper which argued that the Asylums Committee was 'perhaps, the most brilliantly successful of

[60] Anon. 1892. County Council and Organization. *The Times*, 6 January.

[61] Ibid.

[62] Anon. 1905. The London County Council and the Treatment of Insanity. *BMJ*, 5 November 1904.

[63] Anon. 1905. The Treatment of Incipient Insanity. *BMJ*, 4 March.

[64] Brudenell Carter, R. 1904. Insanity and the London County Council. *The Times*, 31 October 1904.

the chief administrative bodies on the Council'.[65] Moreover, it portrayed Brudenell Carter's letter, and the support for it offered by *The Times*, as 'the kind of tactics employed to ensure the return of the corrupt and effete system which the Council superseded'.[66] Philip Martineau and John Williams Benn attempted to use the press as a platform to defend the Asylums Committee and the Progressive majority on the Council, writing to the *Spectator* and *The Times*, respectively. Both reiterated the huge amount of work involved in the administration of London's asylums but Martineau's polemic was subject to severe editing and a rebuttal from the editor.[67] Benn had more success, noting Brudenell Carter's absence from any of the Asylum Committee's meetings, even though he was a member.[68] While some of these issues appeared to be procedural or administrative, they were also political and Benn concluded that Brudenell Carter's letter would not be a surprise to any of his colleagues who were 'quite used to his political animus and general inaccuracy'.[69]

It is pushing it to suggest that the failure of Brudenell Carter's proposal failed on political grounds alone. Indeed, some Progressives, including Martineau, spoke in favour of its report but it was the lack of support within the Council chamber that was crucial to its abandonment.[70] For the plan to have gained any traction it needed the support of the Asylums Committee and the Council itself. Brudenell Carter's attempt to circumvent the former while, at the same time, being in the minority opposition camp condemned the plan to oblivion. His failure only draws the attention back to LCC's ongoing asylum building programme and sequestration but to understand this more fully there has to be a wider consideration of initiatives that garnered much wider political support.

[65] Anon. 1892. Back to Vestrydom? *The Speaker*, 9 January.

[66] Ibid.

[67] Only part of Martineau's letter was published by the *Spectator* on the grounds that the magazine 'was compelled by reasons of space' to do so. 'Does he think', the editor asked, 'his committee manages more institutions than the Local Government Board does?' Martineau, P.M. 1892. London County Council. *The Spectator*, 16 January.

[68] Benn, J. Williams. 1892. The Internal Working of the London County Council. *The Times*, 7 January. Carter explained that once he realised the meetings were in the morning he withdrew from the Committee. Brudenell Carter, R. 1892. The London County Council. *The Times*, 9 January.

[69] Benn, J. Williams. 1892. The Internal Working of the London County Council. *The Times*, 7 January.

[70] Anon. 1890. The Proposed Hospital for the Study of Insanity. *BMJ*, 15 March.

LCC and the Politics of Receiving Houses

One of the issues that LCC had in governing London was the negotiation it had to undertake with the other bodies that had responsibility in the capital. 'London governance in the early 1900s was a bewildering tapestry' and included the MAB, 28 Borough Councils, and 31 Boards of Guardians.[71] This was responsible for a lack of joined-up thinking when it came to the cross-boundary running of trams and wider initiatives around slum clearance, but it was an issue that can also be applied to the management of madness.[72] In the discussions leading up to the introduction of the LGA, radicals and others had called for 'Home Rule for London'. Young has shown that of the 73 Progressive Councillors elected in 1889, 66 of them were associated with London Municipal Reform League and another four were sympathetic to its aims of an area-wide municipal authority for London.[73] Influenced by demands for Irish Home Rule, reformers lobbied for self-government and what the Fabian Society called the 'Unification of London', with a centralised authority responsible for all municipal powers and duties.[74] London, wrote Webb, 'was far too important to be made the shuttlecock of the Imperial parties' and would later complain that the 'half and half' council of 1895 was a disappointing one for those interested in social reform because of the imposition of Imperial politics into County Council affairs.[75]

Unification was to include the abolition of the Poor Law Boards of Guardians and the MAB, and these were to be replaced by executive councils 'subordinate in all matters' to the County Council.[76] Alex Windscheffel describes Home Rule for London as eclipsing Irish Home Rule as the key issue in the 1892 election and, for voters, this

[71] Ball and Sunderland. *An Economic History of London, 1800–1914*: 410.

[72] Ibid: 377.

[73] Young, *Local Politics and the Rise of Party*: 35–7.

[74] BI 228/10. 1898. Fabian Society, Questions for London County Councillors. Pennybacker, The Millennium by Return of Post: 140.

[75] LSE, JS203–211. Webb, Sidney. 1895. Six Years' Work on the London County Council: 7.

[76] During this period the Fabians lobbied for 'municipal reform'. This should not be confused by the same phrase adopted by the Moderates later in the period as their party name. BI P3008, Fabian Society. 1890. Questions for Reform Candidates. BI 229/12. Davies, A. Emil. 1937. The LCC 1889–1937, a Historical Sketch: 6.

was recognisably a party political issue.[77] 'When I choose a man to look after my streets and sewers, it never occurs to me to ask what his views are on Home Rule', wrote one critic, '... [but] as politics have been imported into the business by the Radicals, I shall vote next time for a Conservative streets and sweepers man, not because I am a Tory, but because Conservatives appear to recognise that there is some difference between the parish and the empire'.[78]

It was not until 1892 that the first members of the Fabian Society were elected to the Council. As part of the election campaign of that year, John McDougall and Will Crooks had put forward a joint Progressive and Labour programme in Poplar, where they were both duly elected. With McDougall standing as a Progressive and Crooks representing the trade union and labour movements, they put forward a programme that drew on both radical tradition and *The Fabian Municipal Programme* that included a call for the self-government for London.[79] It is no coincidence that shortly after that date John McDougall suggested the formation of a joint committee consisting of members drawn from the Asylums, Industrial Schools, and Public Health Committees.[80] Other Progressives would later argue that LCC asylums should be passed to the MAB but with W. J. Collins in the Chair, this new joint committee made a series of recommendations that included an aspiration that all lunatics and imbeciles in the capital would be under the control of one authority, and that authority would be LCC.[81]

[77] Windscheffel, 72.

[78] BI 230/4. Baumann, Arthur A.C. 1890. The London County Council. *The Universal Review*: 493–502: 493.

[79] Tyler, Paul. 2007. *Labour's Lost Leader: The Life and Politics of Will Crook*. London: Tauris Academic Studies: 44–5. Gillespie has shown that the revival of interest Progressive municipalisation, after the 1907 election defeat came in 1915 with the formation of the London Labour Party and its post-war revival of the old Progressive slogan of 'Home Rule for London'. Gillespie, James. 1989. Municipalism, Monopoly and Management: The Demise of Socialism in one County, 1918–1933. In *Politics and the People of London, The London County Council 1889–1965*, ed. Andrew Saint, 103–26. London: Hambledon Press: 103, 108.

[80] LMA, LCC/18.6, London County Council Minutes of Proceedings, January–December 1893, 20 June 1893.

[81] Anon. 1898. London Awake. *Reynold's Newspaper*, 27 February. LMA, LCC/18.6, London County Council Minutes of Proceedings, January–June 1894, 5 June 1894, 19 June 1894.

The opposition to this wider policy of unification became known as 'Tenification' and, according to Young, took its name from early plans to create ten corporations that would ensure that there was no centralisation of power in the capital. The London Reform Union produced evidence to show that the combined expenditure of London's 43 Vestries was more than that of the Council. Additionally, it argued that while a Royal Commission on Unification had stated that there should be one Central Municipal Authority to co-ordinate the work common to London as a whole, it had concluded that no powers ought to be exercised by it which could be equally well discharged by existing local bodies.[82] This party political debate about a centralised and interventionist Council versus a disparate and devolved system for delivering London's services was settled to some degree by the passing of the 1899 Local Government Act. Introduced by a Conservative national government, the Act created 28 Boroughs to act as a counterweight to the power of the Progressive LCC.[83] In the interim, the Progressives argued that 'Unification is the cause of public government. Tenification is the Game of Private Interests', and the management of the capital's asylums was intimately connected to these diverse political views.[84]

Collins was a House Surgeon at London's St Bartholomew's Hospital, specialising in ophthalmics, but his place within this new subcommittee did not rest on his medical experience alone. Elected in 1892 as a Councillor for the West St Pancras ward, Collins soon became a Progressive party 'whip' and in 1897–1898 became Chairman of LCC itself.[85] Even when McKinnon Wood assumed leadership of the party, Collins along with Dickinson was described as qualified for leadership due to his 'judgement and experience'.[86] Described by the *BMJ* as a 'prominent member of the Asylums Committee', like others in the party, he was an advocate of teetotalism (see Chapter 2).[87] The committee

[82] LSE, Coll Misc 904. London Reform Union. 1896. *The County Council and the Vestries: The Two Partners in London Government.*

[83] Young, *Local Politics and the Rise of Party*: 54–9. Smellie, *A History of Local Government* London: 178. See also Davies, Local Government 1850–1920: 51.

[84] LSE, Coll Misc 904. n.d. How to Reform London Government, Progressive Leaflet 20.

[85] LMA, ACC/1632/001, Minutes of the Progressive Party of the London County Council, 1890–1895.

[86] LSE, F35/41. c. 1905. Radford, G.H. The Story of London County Council 1901–4: 1.

[87] Anon. 1897. Young Men in Public Life. *BMJ*, 4 September.

which he chaired, drew on a report entitled 'Initial Procedures in Lunacy' written by Partridge, the Asylums Clerk. Partridge had recommended the creation of a Receiving House to act as a triage centre for the reception and classification of all new cases of insanity and this, it was hoped, would effectively replace workhouses as the gateways into LCC asylums.

Alexander Walk has suggested that it was Frederick Mott who 'possibly stimulated' the idea of Receiving Houses but the discussions on this matter pre-dated his appointment.[88] Moreover, the initial work of McDougall and Collins soon found other allies in the Accommodation Sub-Committee, chaired by another Progressive, Dr George Cooper. Cooper, that most 'active and useful' member of the Asylums Committee, was influential and his Committee had a grand vision and called for the establishment of four Receiving Houses in 'convenient districts' of the county of London. The proposed inclusion of facilities for the 'treatment of acute cases of a recoverable nature' here seemed to recall the issues raised by Brudenell Carter but, as Cooper pointed out, the scope of the considerations were beyond the remit of that earlier sub committee.[89] Besides, here was a broader political aim that foresaw the abolition of workhouse lunatic wards, which reflected the wider concerns of some Progressives in terms of Poor Law reform.

In presenting its findings, Cooper's committee predicted a reduction in the number of certified lunatics, economies in the costs of reception and treatment, and the removal of the 'hardship of going through the workhouse'.[90] As a corollary, the Committee spoke to a number of concerns that also recognised a need for early treatment and the equitable treatment of private, as well as pauper patients. Nevertheless,

[88] Walk, Medico-Psychologists, Maudsley and the Maudsley: 19–30.

[89] Later discussions included the expectation that Receiving Houses would include an Out-Patients' Clinic. Some already existed in other parts of the country but their growth followed the introduction of the Mental Treatment Act in 1930. LMA, LCC/MIN/710, Accommodation Sub-Committee Minute Book, 1896–1905, 25 January 1897, 20 October 1897. LMA, LCC/18.6, London County Council Minutes of Proceedings, September–December 1902, 21 October 1902.

[90] It was envisaged that magistrates and medical offices would be on hand to sign any certificates required under the lunacy legislation and that an ambulance service would be provided to ferry people from their homes to the Receiving House and on to an asylum where necessary. LMA, LCC/MIN/568, Signed Minutes, 1897–1899, 14 December 1897.

it was probably the potential for a 'considerable pecuniary saving to the ratepayers' that explains why the Council, as whole, supported the scheme so readily.[91] Beyond this, the political aspiration to take control of all lunacy procedures in the capital demanded negotiations with the Commissioners in Lunacy, the LGB, the MAB, and to a lesser degree London's Poor Law Unions.

The 'Consultation' with the Poor Law

In his initial report, Partridge had recommended the establishment of a 'special representative body' to manage and deal with London's lunatics, and cited a parliamentary act relating to the County of Lancashire as a legislative precedent.[92] The political aspiration to extend LCC's management of madness meant that there would be less cross-administrative co-operation in this case, with the Council seeking to impose its vision on London via parliamentary legislation. Nevertheless, after the matter was passed to the Housing and Accommodation Sub-committee, and a resolution from one of its members, Partridge was tasked with consulting with the Boards of Guardians in London in a bid to gauge their views.[93]

Cochrane has argued that the Asylums Committee approved 'a series of expensive capital projects, the suitability of which it profoundly doubted' because of demand placed for spaces from the Poor Law Unions.[94] For him this was influenced by changing views about the workhouse and its suitability for the detention of lunatics, which in turn meant that the workhouse 'was purely a place of reception for lunatics prior to automatic transfer to an asylum'.[95] It is clear, however, that the workhouses were already acting as triage centres and figures collected

[91] LMA, LCC/18.6, London County Council Minutes of Proceedings, September–December 1899, 10 October 1899, 11 July 1899. LMA, LCC/18.6, London County Council Minutes of Proceedings, September–December 1902, 21 October 1902.

[92] The Lancashire County (Lunatic Asylums and Other Powers) Act, 1891 enabled the convening of a Board consisting of Councillors and also representatives of the various boroughs. LCC/CL/PH/01/276, Partridge, R.W. 1893. Report of the Clerk. London: LCC. See Also Hayes, Lancashire Public Asylums Provision: 84.

[93] LMA, LCC/MIN/710, Accommodation Sub-Committee Minute Book, 1896–1905, 11 May 1898.

[94] Cochrane, Humane, Economical and Medically Wise: 253.

[95] Ibid.

during the consultation period revealed that 46% of those deemed to be lunatics were not, in fact, transferred from the workhouse to the asylum. Significant numbers were, instead, discharged by Poor Law medical officers as 'not certifiable'.[96]

In reality, removal to the asylum was not automatic but the fact that London's asylums were already bursting at the seams meant that there was a knock-on effect of demand on Poor Law Services. In January 1892, the Medical Officer of the St Olave's workhouse at Tanner Street reported that 'the sick wards are all full and sick cases keep coming in' to such an extent that within a few days there was no room for any more cases.[97] This was also the case in the Fulham Union where the Medical Officer of the Workhouse explained that

> In many acute cases almost irreparable damage is done to the patient by his [*sic*] enforced stay in the workhouse, where the accommodation is frequently severely over-taxed and the nursing rarely the best. And this is an important fact, viz:- That when the wards are over-crowded the extra attendants engaged are wither paupers or person who have rarely had any experience of nursing – usually ex-policemen.[98]

There is some recognition of the additional problems that arose from the relatively slow speed of an asylum building programme that did not keep pace with demand. It was this ongoing pressure that helped to explain the focus on Receiving Houses and, at various times, the Asylums Committee used the investigations into their development as a reason for further delaying the building of new asylums.[99] As a

[96] In the year ending 31 March 1898, 6599 individuals were alleged to be insane in the County of London. 6280 of them were removed to a Parish Workhouse or Infirmary. Of those, 3573 (54%) were certified for removal to an asylum with the remainder being discharged from the workhouse as not certifiable. Of the 3573 certified, only 26 were taken to an asylum from their home and in every other case, each patient, unless they were already an inmate was taken to the asylum via the workhouse. LMA, LCC/MIN/568, Signed Minutes, 1897–1899, 11 July 1899.

[97] LMA, BBG/423, St Olave's Union Committee Reports, 1892–1893, 2 January 1893, 4 June 1893.

[98] LMA, LCC/CL/PH/01/276, Marsh, T.A. 1898. Scheme of London Asylums Committee for Providing Receiving Houses &c., Fulham Union.

[99] LCC/MIN/710, Accommodation Sub-Committee Minute Book, 1896–1905, 2 July 1902.

corollary, such delays meant further stresses on supply and demand but a narrow majority of Poor Law officials in London supported the moves to build Receiving Houses, rather than simply press for more asylum accommodation.[100]

Of the records that survive, it was the Fulham Union that provided the most detail in support of the plans with Mr Marsh, the Clerk to the Guardians, alive to the issue of where their charges might find themselves. As he pointed out, patients were frequently removed to Licenced Houses, and the out-county asylums at a considerable distance from London, 'and in many such cases, great hardship arises owing to the wife or other relatives being in poor circumstances and unable to bear the expenses of a visit'.[101] For those who were better off, the proposed Receiving Houses offered a way of separating or classifying the different classes, and a chance to remove 'the stigma of pauperism'.[102] As Marsh noted, 'many of the better class people on their recovery appear greatly concerned that they have been brought to a workhouse, and until their discharge by a justice compelled to mix with some of the very lowest of their sex'.[103]

Moreover, Unions such as Lambeth that offered context to their opposition to the scheme, did not simply press for more asylum accommodation and, instead, argued that it would not obviate the need for workhouse accommodation for certain cases.[104] As Peter Bartlett has shown, workhouse care could have many advantages, not least its locality to the people it served, and the St Olave's Union was just one example of a Poor Law authority that had already looked to improve the conditions for staff in a bid to encourage them to stay longer in service.[105] The fact

[100] Of the 29 Unions in London, 15 supported the scheme, 10 did not and 4 did not reply to the Clerk's letter. LCC/MIN/710, Accommodation Sub-Committee Minute Book, 1896–1905, 18 July 1898.

[101] LCC/CL/PH/01/276, Marsh, T.A. 1898. Scheme of London Asylums Committee for Providing Receiving Houses &c., Fulham Union.

[102] LMA, LCC/MIN/568, Signed Minutes, 1897–1899, 11 July 1899.

[103] LCC/CL/PH/01/276, Marsh, T.A. 1898. Scheme of London Asylums Committee for Providing Receiving Houses &c., Fulham Union.

[104] Of the 29 Unions in London, 15 supported the scheme, 10 did not and 4 did not reply to the Clerk's letter. LCC/MIN/710, Accommodation Sub-Committee Minute Book, 1896–1905, 18 July 1898.

[105] This included improvements to salaries and accommodation for nursing staff. LMA, BBG/514/001 Letters from Government Departments 1890–1892, Letter from LGB to the Guardians of St Olave's Union, 10 April 1890. See also Bartlett, *Poor Law of Lunacy*.

that these Unions were in the minority, and that the fact that LCC was looking to impose changes on them anyway, meant that their opposition would prove to be moot. After a discussion of all the responses, the process of finding sites for the new Receiving Houses was set in train. After this time, the Asylums Committee was to receive regular missives from the Poor Law Unions, including those who has opposed the scheme in the first instance, asking for updates on progress and others who continued to express strong opposition.[106]

Commissioners in Lunacy and Parliamentary Assistance

More important than the support from the Poor Law Unions was the 'cordial approval' received from the Commissioners in Lunacy who promised to co-operate by affording any assistance in their power.[107] The first step was to meet and negotiate with the Lord Chancellor, the Earl of Halsbury, and by 1900, it was suggested that clauses were added to a proposed Lunacy Bill so that the institutions administered by the MAB would come under the control of LCC.[108] The Lunacy Bill of that year failed but Halsbury remained open to discussions with members of the Asylums Committee and, after further negotiations, he reiterated his support for the endeavour, recommending that the Council introduce its own Bill in parliament, and promising to assist in the process.[109]

[106]For example, the Hammersmith Board of Guardians explained that if the Receiving Houses plan was dropped, they would be 'at once compelled to provide Lunatic Wards for their parish'. LMA, LCC/MIN/572, Signed Minutes, June 1904–November 1905, 14 November 1905. See also LMA, LCC/MIN/568, Signed Minutes, 1897–1899, 11 July 1899. Holborn Guardian expressed strong opposition as did the Guardians of Bloomsbury, Wandsworth, Fulham, Islington, Westminster, St George's and Hackney. LMA, LCC/576, Signed Minutes, March 1909–July 1910, 12 July 1910.

[107]LMA, LCC/18.6, London County Council Minutes of Proceedings, May–August 1899, 18 July 1899.

[108]The Lord Chancellor was a member of the Cabinet and mainly responsible for judicial matters. Halsbury (Conservative) was well known for the appointment of judges on party political grounds, rather than on merit. Woodhouse, Diana. 2001. *The Office of Lord Chancellor*. Oxford: Hart Publishing: 139. LCC/MIN/569, Signed Minutes, 1899–1901, 13 March 1900.

[109]The 1900 bill was one of six attempted reforms of the Lunacy Laws that failed in the period between 1890 and 1914. Takabayashi, Akinobu. 2017. Surviving the Lunacy Act of 1890: English Psychiatrists and Professional Development During the Early Twentieth

To move this forward, the Asylums Committee needed and received the support of both the Commissioners in Lunacy and the LGB, but it also needed support from within the Council. On reading the Standing Orders, the Council's Solicitor agreed that LCC had the power to spend money to permute legislation, and its Parliamentary Committee recommended that proceedings were taken with a view to introducing a Bill in Parliament.[110]

The motion to introduce a bill for London was carried but only after support was received from the Finance Committee.[111] As was explained in Chapter 3, the Finance Committee had a role to play in overseeing and agreeing any costs incurred and it was the same here. Although the Clerk had originally recommended one Receiving House, the Asylums Committee pushed for four to be built and suggested two sites on the north of the River Thames and two on the south of it.[112] The Finance Committee noted that the costs for such sites could vary wildly, and would later suggest that the Council should proceed 'experimentally' by building only one Receiving House in the first instance.[113] Moreover, it reported that any immediate savings would 'belong' to the Poor Law authorities as the cost of conveyance to the Receiving Houses and asylums, and some of the operational costs covered by the weekly maintenance charge, would be shifted from them to the County. It was hoped that the new system would impact on the growth of lunacy and, as a corollary, reduce the demand for additional large asylums. Any savings here, the Finance Committee concluded, were 'only speculative', while the

Century. *Medical History* 61:2: 246–269. LCC/MIN/569, Signed Minutes, 1899–1901, 13 March 1900. LCC/MIN/570, Signed Minutes, 1901–1902, 26 March 1901, 6 May 1902. LMA, LCC/18.6, London County Council Minutes of Proceedings, September–December 1902, 21 October 1902.

[110] LMA, LCC/18.6, London County Council Minutes of Proceedings, September–December 1902, 21 October 1902.

[111] LMA, LCC/18.6, London County Council Minutes of Proceedings, September–December 1902, 4 November 1902.

[112] LMA, LCC/18.6, London County Council Minutes of Proceedings, September–December 1902, 21 October 1902.

[113] It noted that land in south-eastern and south-western districts would cost £2000–£3000, while land in northern and eastern districts would cost £8000–£10,000 per acre. LMA, LCC/18.6, London County Council Minutes of Proceedings, September–December 1902, 4 November 1902.

BMJ described the estimates of costs to LCC as 'somewhat alarming'.[114] Nevertheless, the report of the Finance Committee concluded that the 'time has arrived when London, which has to deal with one-fifth of the lunatics of England and Wales, should make better and more humane provision for the early treatment of its insane population'.[115] In this respect, the Progressives were playing a potentially expensive and interventionist long-game. The Finance Committee's conclusion is entirely consistent with the themes explored in Chapter 3 with it acting in concert with both a Progressive Asylums Committee and the wider Progressive Council.

With the support from every relevant committee, plans were set in place for a London County Asylums (Receiving Houses for Patients) Bill to be introduced in parliament at the earliest opportunity.[116] This was to be a private bill, pertaining specifically to London, and its exact wording demanded negotiation between Asylums Committee, the Parliamentary Committee and the Council's Solicitor, as well as with the LGB, and the Commissioners in Lunacy.[117] Halsbury, the Lord Chancellor, was also involved in the negotiations and he pressed the Council to re-draft the proposed legislation as a public bill; one which would effectively amend and sit alongside the existing acts that governed the whole country.[118]

It had, thus far, taken nine years to move from the initial recommendation to provide Receiving Houses to the introduction of a public bill but the tortuous process was not to end there. On its first reading, it was passed by the House of Lords without amendments but 'time did not permit it making progress in the House of Commons'.[119] In 1905, it was introduced by Sir John Batty Tuke, the man who had been one of Brudenell Carter's expert witnesses, but it was found 'impossible

[114] LMA, LCC/18.6, London County Council Minutes of Proceedings, September–December 1902, 4 November 1902. Anon. 1902. Receiving House for the Insane. *BMJ*, 8 November.

[115] LMA, LCC/18.6, London County Council Minutes of Proceedings, September–December 1902, 4 November 1902.

[116] LMA, LCC/18.6, London County Council Minutes of Proceedings, September–December 1902, 9 December 1902. LMA, LCC/18.6, London County Council Minutes of Proceedings, January–June 1903, 3 March 1903.

[117] LMA, LCC/MIN/572, Signed Minutes, June 1904–November 1905, 11 July 1905.

[118] LMA, LCC/18.6, London County Council Minutes of Proceedings, January–June 1903, 10 March 1903.

[119] LMA, LCC/18.6, London County Council Minutes of Proceedings, July–December 1903, 3 November 1903.

to make any progress with the Bill and it was dropped before the second reading'.[120] It was this failure that was to prove to be fatal to the Receiving Houses scheme. Plans to reintroduce the Bill in 1906 prompted a discussion within the Council. To re-submit the Bill meant a suspension of a key standing order, for which the Council, as a whole, had to vote on and approve.[121] Standing Order 161 stated that any schemes had to be put before the Council in June and, as the meeting was taking place in December, this meant that the Council had to first agreed to suspend it before they could agree the re-submission. A majority of 66-32 voted for the suspension but this was eight short of the number demanded by Standing Order 89.[122] As a result, it was the procedures of the Council condemned the Receiving Houses plan into political limbo but this was undoubtedly informed by the Finance Committee's 'approval' of the scheme. Prior to the discussion around the suspension of Standing Orders, its 1902 report was circulated to every member of the Council. Rather than focussing on the benefits of 'humane provision', Councillors were reminded that the capital commitments of the Council were more pressing in 1905, than they were when the report was made.[123]

There were a few more attempts to press ahead with the Receiving Houses plan but by this time the Municipal Reformers had seized control of the Council. In May 1907, the Parliamentary Committee of LCC decided that 'in regard to the extension of the reference to the Royal Commission of the Feeble-minded, they had decided to advise the Council not to proceed with the Lunacy Acts Amendment (London) Bill in the present session' but this was undoubtedly informed by the Council's moratorium on all capital projects (see Chapter 3).[124] Similarly, it was suggested in 1909, that the proposed (Maudsley) Mental Hospital

[120]LMA, LCC/18.6, London County Council Minutes of Proceedings, September–November 1905, 28 November 1905.

[121]LMA, LCC/18.6, London County Council Minutes of Proceedings, December 1905, 12 December 1905.

[122]Standing Order 89 stated that any suspension of the Councils Standing Orders had to be approved by three quarters of the Councillors present. LMA, GLC/DG/AE/ROL/82/001, LCC Standing Orders, 1906–1907: 89, 161.

[123]LMA, LCC/18.6, London County Council Minutes of Proceedings, September–November 1905, 28 November 1905.

[124]LMA, LCC/MIN/574, Signed Minutes, February 1907–February 1908, 14 May 1907.

might operate as a Receiving House, probably because the conditions of Henry Maudsley's £30,000 gift for its establishment stipulated that it should deal exclusively with recent and acute cases and include provision for out-patients.[125] The Finance Committee rejected this because it felt that the establishment of more than one was unnecessary but they were opposed to the plan on financial grounds anyway. Unless the matter was withdrawn, they reported, they would have little option than to report their strong adversity to the plan to the Council.[126] Nevertheless, in February 1910, the Clerk once again submitted a draft Bill for consideration but with one important revision; there was to be only one Receiving House.[127] This was still subject to opposition from the Parliamentary Committee and the Finance Committee, and in 1910, the Asylums Committee finally admitted defeat.[128] So far then, the failure of two attempts to introduce new extra-institutional innovations had failed, even if they had failed for different reasons. The Asylums Committee and LCC was to have more success with the appointments of a Pathologist, even if a central London laboratory would prove to be a step too far.

LCC and the Politics of Pathology

Just as Brudenell Carter had tried to claim some credit for the idea of Receiving Houses, he also wrote to *The Times* stating that the appointment of a pathologist for LCC stemmed from recommendations made by his committee.[129] In response, Robert Jones, with the permission of the Chairman of the Claybury Committee, wrote, instead, to honour the work of William Collins. Jones pointed to Brudenell Carter's association with at least one failure, while Collins himself explained that the two things were unconnected.[130] Nothing, Collins remarked, was

[125] Jones, *Mental Health and Social Policy, 1845–1959*: 103–4.

[126] LMA, LCC/576, Signed Minutes, March 1909–July 1910: 10 May 1909.

[127] Ibid: 8 February 1910.

[128] Ibid: March 1909–July 1910, 12 April 1910, 12 July 1910, 26 July 1910, 13 December 1910.

[129] Brudenell Carter, R. 1904. Insanity and the London County Council. *The Times*, 31 October.

[130] Jones, Robert. 1904. Insanity and the London County Council. *The Times*, 8 November. Collins, William J. 1904. Insanity and the London County Council. *The Times*, 22 November.

Table 4.2 Special sub-committee (appointment of pathologist)

Committee member	*Party*	*Attendance (first year)*
Dr William Collins (Chairman)	Progressive	3/3
Dr William Blake	Progressive	3/3
Dr William Bott	Progressive	0/3
Dr George Cooper	Progressive	1/3
Dr Elijah Baxter	Moderate	3/3

Source LMA/LCC 26.21. The Fourth Annual Report of the Asylums Committee of the London County Council, for the year ending 31 March 1893

heard of Carter's report after it had been passed back to the Council by the Asylums Committee. It was only after the election of 1892 that an 'entirely new enquiry was set on foot', and, as Collins pointed out, Brudenell Carter was not a member of LCC after that date.[131] 1892 was the date that Collins was elected, as well as the election of the second Progressive Administration and it is these factors that help to explain the development and direction of London's pathological services in this period.

In line with what was becoming the usual practice, the Asylums Committee appointed a Pathology sub-committee to deal with the issue but, for the first time, it was made up entirely of its medical members. Doyle has explored the levels to which medical staff could influence decision-making but, just as was the case with Brudenell Carter's committee, their relative power stemmed from their election as councillors and not from their expertise in the treatment of lunacy.[132] As the names in Table 4.2 show, this committee was dominated by Progressive members and it was Collins, one of only two of its members that attended all three of its meetings who was appointed its Chairman. It is little wonder that he was described as the Committee's 'moving and guiding spirit'.[133] With Collins in the Chair, the first task of the appointment sub-committee was to read a report by 'Dr Alexander of Hanwell Asylum to the

[131] Collins, William J. 1904. Insanity and the London County Council. *The Times*, 22 November.

[132] Doyle, *The Politics of Hospital Provision*: 143.

[133] Anon. 1899. The Pathology of Insanity. *BMJ*, 18 February.

Hanwell sub-committee upon the question of a appointing a pathologist'.[134] Following this, a list of questions were formulated for each of the medical superintendents of London's Four County Asylums and also to the members of the sub-committee.[135] Just as had been the case with Brudenell Carter's Committee, the Pathology sub-committee engaged in a consultation exercise. Crucially, however, that consultation included LCC medical staff from the outset but, more significantly still, it had drawn its authority from the Asylums Committee itself. In this respect, it made it much more likely that any of its recommendations would be approved as they made their way through the Committee structure.

The Pathology Committee also engaged in an international consultation exercise and utilised their status within the Council to good effect. Lord Rosebery, the first Chairman of LCC and an *ex-officio* member of the Asylums Committee, enabled the Pathology Committee to make important connections with the Foreign Office. In turn, it was agreed that written questions concerning the efficacy of pathological investigations could be distributed via embassies in European capitals and in Washington.[136] The response rate was impressive with details of the *post-mortems* carried out in almost eighty asylums in Europe and the United States.[137] Jennifer Wallis has shown how pathological studies enabled alienists and others to be 'cautiously' optimistic about the potential to relieve, or even cure mental diseases and we can see evidence of that here too.[138] The consensus reached from the consultation was that any benefit arising from pathological investigations could not be guaranteed but, as the *BMJ* pointed out, there was a general feeling within the medical profession that investigations should be made.[139] The proposed appointment of a pathologist was a 'wise and useful step ... of

[134] LMA, LCC/MIN/747, Pathologist Sub-Committee Minute Book, 1892–1901, 8 November 1892.

[135] Ibid.

[136] LMA, LCC/MIN/747, Pathologist Sub-Committee Minute Book, 1892–1901, 3 March 1893.

[137] LCC/CL/PH/01/276, Report of the Special Sub-Committee appointed to consider the appointment of a Pathologist, LCC, 1894.

[138] Wallis, *Investigating the Body*: 144.

[139] Anon. 1894. Pathology of Insanity. *BMJ*, 8 September.

great value in the advancement of this important branch of the healing art'.[140] This was a view shared by the Commissioners in Lunacy, who regularly pressed LCC to appoint individual pathologists and to provide equipment for the scientific and pathological investigation into the causes of insanity at several of its institutions.[141] On a visit to Hanwell, they reminded the Committee that 'The provisions of the Lunacy Act, 1890, point to the necessity for the employment of a stronger medical staff than heretofore, and there can be no advance in the care and treatment of the patients without scientific enquiry'.[142]

The concerns of the medical profession and the Commissioners in particular, seemed to chime with the will of Collins's committee to appoint a pathologist. Even by 1908, however, the Commissioners were complaining that, while the majority of staffs in the majority of asylums was adequate to carry out the everyday tasks of keeping case notes and encouraging their charges to engage in pursuits that were conducive to good mental health, it left them little, if any time to study their cases scientifically.[143] Such comments reflected the findings of LCC's pathological consultation exercise which showed that some medical staff in asylums had made 'several valuable communications' to medical periodicals on the pathology of insanity', but the pressure of administrative duties precluded others from conducting such research.[144]

There were limits, however, as to how far the politicians were willing to go and the Pathology sub-committee remained wedded to the idea of one pathologist for the whole service. As *post-mortems* were already taking place in individual asylums, it concluded that a pathologist at each asylum would not be needed. Instead the appointment of a man 'of standing and position who should have access to pathological material in all the asylums and who would, no doubt, direct and encourage research

[140] Anon. 1893. The London County Council and the County Lunatic Asylum. *BMJ*, 22 July 1893.

[141] *Forty-fifth Report of the Commissioners in Lunacy*, 1891: 199. *Forty-sixth Report of the Commissioners in Lunacy*, 1892: 213. *Forty-seventh Report of the Commissioners in Lunacy*, 1893: 212. *Sixty-second Report of the Commissioners in Lunacy*, 1908: 17–18.

[142] *Forty-fifth Report of the Commissioners in Lunacy*, 1891: 199.

[143] *Sixty-second Report of the Commissioners in Lunacy*, 1908: 17–18.

[144] LMA, LCC/MIN/747, Pathologist Sub-Committee Minute Book, 1892–1901, 3 March 1893.

by younger men who are resident at each asylum'.[145] After consultation with both the Claybury sub-committee and the Asylums Committee, Claybury, then in the course of being furnished, was chosen as the site for the new Pathology laboratory.[146]

The choice of one pathologist in one asylum who would be responsible for surveying the work of all of LCC's asylums emphasised an apparent level of medical independence previously unseen in asylum administration. The sub-committee ordered that the Pathologist

> should be required to devote himself exclusively to the work, to report from time to time, to publish the various researches in which he has been engaged and also those which other medical officers have carried on under his guidance; he should not have charge of or interfere with, the clinical treatment of the patients; and his work need in no way conflict with that of the medical superintendents.[147]

This independence was reiterated in the interview process and when Jones, the Medical Superintendent at Claybury, asked if his presence was required on the 'selecting committee', his offer was politely declined.[148] After two rounds of interviews, Frederick Mott was appointed and the *BMJ* congratulated LCC on securing the services of such a man of distinction.[149] Not everyone was quite so gushing and nor did everyone see the appointment of a Pathologist in quite such positive terms. The Victoria Street Society, an anti-vivisection organisation, had been lobbying against the use of animals in research from 1875 and, after the passing of the Cruelty to Animals Act in the following year, only those with dispensation from the Home Office were allowed to do so.[150] Following the decision to appoint a Pathologist, the Asylums Committee received letters from a range of individuals and organisations concerned at the use

145 Ibid.

146 Ibid.

147 Ibid.

148 LMA, LCC/MIN/747, Pathologist Sub-Committee Minute Book, 1892–1901, 18 January 1895.

149 Anon. The Pathology of Insanity. *BMJ*, 18 February 1899.

150 Wallis, *Investigating the Body*: 169.

of vivisection.[151] More recently, Andrew Scull has argued that, in reality, clinicians had little interest in treating and curing patients, which, in turn meant that the living were abandoned to their fate.[152] Some sense of this will be explored in the following chapter but in medical circles these attempts were seen as progressive and much of the praise for them was directed towards LCC.

Pathology, LCC and Civic Pride

To be clear, it is important to reiterate that the attempts to stem the never-ending tide of lunatics was as much a political one as it was a medical one. 'The reports of the asylums generally were of an encouraging character as regards their administration and efficiency' concluded the *BMJ* in 1894,

> but the dull shadow of the fearful increase of lunacy hung over the work of the committee, and it was devoutly to be hoped that science would be enable by research to judge more accurately of the active causes of these diseases that the necessity of erecting a new lunatic asylum every two of three years might be obviated.[153]

Such a rolling programme of building took significant sums of money and this was always a feature of discussion in any attempts to innovate or, indeed maintain the *status quo*. Nevertheless, praise for LCC's pathological initiatives from the medical press focussed on two overlapping areas. The first of these was LCC's place as a world leader in the field. Indeed, in its annual report for 1892–1893, the Asylums Committee reported that the lessons learned from the practice of pathology in foreign asylums would allow 'London to take a leading place in this scientific branch of

[151] Concerned groups included the Electoral and Church Anti-Vivisection Leagues, and the International Anti-Vivisection Council. Mr. W.L. Humfrey wrote to the Asylums Committee 'protesting against such a wicked appointment' and Mrs Annie Goff raised concerns about the potential use of vivisection. LMA, LCC/MIN/747, Pathologist Sub-Committee Minute Book, 1892–1901, 1 May 1895, 7 May 1897. LMA, LCC/MIN/748, Pathologist Sub-Committee Minute Book, 1901–1908, 22 April 1902.

[152] Scull, *Madness and Civilisation*: 262–3.

[153] Anon. 1894. Lunacy in the Metropolis. *BMJ*, 28 July.

medical work'.[154] For the *BMJ* it was the appointment of a person of 'standing and position' that would place 'London in the front rank in regard to research into the pathology of lunacy', but Collins saw this as part of a wider strategy.[155]

As the negotiations for the building of the Pathological Laboratory and the appointment of a Pathologist continued, Collins drafted a letter asking the London's medical superintendents for suggestions on how London's County Asylums could be used for clinical instruction.[156] This was informed by new regulations of the conjoint board of the Royal Colleges of Physicians and Surgeons which, from January 1892, required all medical students to produce certificates of having attended clinical demonstrations at a recognised lunatic asylum before they could sit their examination. With other licensing bodies, including the University of London, requiring similar certificates, a special sub-committee consisting of medical officers of the Committee was convened to consider how best to utilise the asylums for clinical instruction'.[157]

Having obtained recognition from the conjoint board for London's asylums, it was recommended that those medical superintendents who were also lecturers at a medical school, should conduct their clinical demonstrations in that asylum. Those who were not lecturers, should demonstrate clinically 'at his asylum to students attending the course of lectures in Psychological Medicine at London Medical schools'.[158] Although not all superintendents wanted to 'demonstrate', Collins vision was that all of London's asylums, rather than just the laboratory at Claybury, would play a part in medical education. These new arrangements were circulated to the Deans and Wardens of medical schools in the capital. Shortly afterwards, students from the London School of Medicine for Women attended sessions at Colney Hatch, students of the Westminster School attended Cane Hill and students at St

[154]LMA, LCC 26.21. The Fourth Annual Report of the Asylums Committee of the London County Council, for the year ending 31 March 1893.

[155]Anon. Pathological Laboratory at Claybury. *BMJ*, November 1893.

[156]LMA, LCC/MIN/747, Pathologist Sub-Committee Minute Book, 1892–1901, 9 March 1894.

[157]LMA, LCC 26.21. The Fifth Annual Report of the Asylums Committee of the London County Council, for the year ending 31 March 1894.

[158]LMA, LCC/MIN/747, Pathologist Sub-Committee Minute Book, 1892–1901, 9 March 1894.

Bartholomew's attended sessions at Banstead.[159] Collins's own links with St Bartholomew's must have been important here and, while placing London's asylums at the centre of medical training must have enhanced LCC's civic reputation as an innovative administrator of lunacy, there were still some practical limitations to consider.

From the outset, the Commissioners in Lunacy had been concerned that the establishment of the laboratory at Claybury would lead to the diminishing or abolishing of any pathological work taking place in the individual asylums.[160] Even by this time, the number of *post-mortems* carried out in London's asylums differed across the various institutions. At Bexley the figure was 98% of all deaths, while at Colney Hatch it was nearer 80% and, a few years later at Banstead, the figure was as low as 67%.[161] At other places, such as Hanwell, they noted the 'careful and intelligent attention … devoted to the keeping of *post-mortem* records and of the case books', but regretted that 'no pathological work of the finer kind appears to be done in this asylum' and it was the same at Cane Hill.[162]

The uneven nature of scientific endeavour across London's asylums was also reflected in the research that was taking place within them, and both LCC and Mott were playing catch up with other, more well-known asylums and individuals. In his first report for LCC, Mott wrote of his aspirations to emulate the longer-term pathological initiatives that had taken place at the West Riding Asylum at Wakefield.[163] Indeed, the Commissioners in Lunacy would later praise Mott for the publication of three volumes of the *Archives of Neurology* as a 're-vindication' of work carried out by James Crichton-Browne at the West Riding Asylum in the 1870s.[164] The *BMJ* also wrote of the longer-term lineage of pathological

[159] LMA, LCC/MIN/747, Pathologist Sub-Committee Minute Book, 1892–1901, 18 December 1894.

[160] *Fiftieth Report of the Commissioners in Lunacy*, 1896: 293.

[161] Ibid.

[162] *Fifty-seventh Report of the Commissioners in Lunacy*, 1903: 327.

[163] LMA, LCC 26.21. Report of the Pathologist, April 1896. The Lancashire County Asylum at Whittingham also appointed a pathologist in 1890, with the then superintendent at the West Riding Asylum, William Bevan-Lewis, claiming they had followed 'our' example. WYAS, C85/1/13/5, Medical Director's Journal 1888–1894, 20 June 1890.

[164] Crichton-Browne had published or influenced the publication of six volumes of the 'West Riding Medical Reports'. *Sixty-second Report of the Commissioners in Lunacy*, 1908: 16.

pioneers but, nevertheless, claimed that the appointment of Mott and the new facilities at the Claybury Asylum marked the dawn of a new era while the Commissioners claimed Mott's work marked 'an epoch in this kind of asylum research'.[165] There can be little doubt that this praise was welcomed by LCC and the first edition of the *London County Council Staff Gazette* recorded its congratulations to Mott on the reaction in medical circles to his work at the Claybury Asylum. 'It is not often', it was noted, 'that the professional and scientific journals award such enthusiastic praise as they have given in reviewing what the *Lancet* calls "this magnificent record of research"'[166]

In the third volume of the *Archives*, Mott contributed 12 of the 24 papers. Robert Jones, the Medical Superintendent at Claybury included a paper on injuries to the frontal region of the brain, while Dr Candler, Mott's assistant pathologist, looked at the impact of dysentery with a study of the bacteria present in the excreta of patients.[167] These contributions reflect the mixed picture of scientific research taking place in London's asylums and further afield. The edited collections drew on contributions from other institutions and, in 1907, the Commissioners in Lunacy undertook a review of the scientific work in England and Wales that demonstrated its breadth.[168] Along with their contributions to Mott's *Archives*, the staff working in these institutions published in journals including the *British Medical Journal*, the *Journal of Mental Science*, the *Review of Neurology and Psychiatry* and *Brain*. In the years that followed, the number of asylums undertaking research was to grow but Mott was seen as the driving force and the Claybury Asylum continued to maintain its prominence.[169] As the Commissioners in Lunacy would later report, while the ongoing work in places like Lancashire and Yorkshire was to be commended, the laboratory at London was

[165]The pioneers cited were 'Bevan Lewis, Batty Tuke and others in this country; and Gressinger, Westphal, von Gudden and others abroad.' Anon. 1899. The Pathology of Insanity. *BMJ*, 18 February. *Fifty-fourth Report of the Commissioners in Lunacy*, 1900: 317.

[166]BL, *London County Council Staff Gazette* (1900), 1:1: 3.

[167]*Sixty-second Report of the Commissioners in Lunacy*, 1908: 68.

[168]Along with the work undertaken by Mott at Claybury, the research taking place include that at the Lancashire Asylums at Lancaster and Prestwich, the Essex County Asylum at Brentwood and the Sunderland Borough Asylum. *Sixty-second Report of the Commissioners in Lunacy*, 1908: 69.

[169]*Sixty-third Report of the Commissioners in Lunacy*, 1909: 80–95.

the 'ideal plan' as it was attached to several asylums under a 'conjoined authority'.[170]

These examples shed light on a second area of praise for LCC's pathological initiative and that was on Mott himself. Significantly, just as commentators had suggested a level of independence of the Asylums Committee from the Council, so too the *BMJ* claimed that 'this was the first pathology laboratory founded by a public body on a basis of complete independence from the administrative authorities of the asylum'.[171] It praised LCC's 'enlightened policy in leaving him a free hand in the organisation of the laboratory, and on their liberality in the supply of whatever he thinks necessary for the successful carrying on of the work with which they have entrusted him'.[172] Once again there was a privileging of the medical story behind the work of Mott but this does not adequately explain either his place within the Council hierarchy or the continuing importance of the politically-constituted Pathology and Asylums Committees.

Mott the LCC Employee

It seems clear that, for the medical profession at least, Mott became the public face of LCC's operations. It was to him that the Anatomical Department of St Thomas's Hospital wrote, asking for his permission to receive the bodies of the inmates of LCC asylums who died without relatives or friends.[173] The existing agreement with Boards of Guardians was, according the hospital, 'inadequate' and, as a result the capital lagged behind both the continent and the provinces.[174] There was nothing particularly unusual about the Guardians unwillingness to hand over bodies, which St Thomas's put down to 'sentimental considerations'.[175] While Mott's views may have been influential, the decision to accede to

[170] *Sixty-second Report of the Commissioners in Lunacy to the Lord Chancellor*, 1908: 16. *Sixty-third Report of the Commissioners in Lunacy*, 1909: 65.

[171] Anon. 1899. The Pathology of Insanity. *BMJ*, 18 February.

[172] Ibid.

[173] LMA, LCC/MIN/748, Pathologist Sub-Committee Minute Book, 1901–1908, 7 November 1905.

[174] Ibid.

[175] Strange, Julie-Marie. 2005. *Death, Grief and Poverty in Britain 1870–1914*. Cambridge: Cambridge University Press: 8.

this request rested with first the Pathology sub-committee and then the Asylums Committee itself.[176]

Moreover, Mott did not have quite the 'free hand' that was suggested by the medical press and, just like others working in LCC, Mott's aspirations were limited by agreed budgets. When he presented his wish list for 'the furnishing and fitting of the pathological buildings', he was asked to revise the estimate down to the £820 already agreed by the Council for the purpose.[177] Similarly, when he was approached by London University to be their examiner in Pathology, the Committee recommended he accept the position on the understanding that his fees were paid into the county fund.[178] These examples emphasise Mott's role as an employee and the relatively limited number of papers submitted to medical journals by LCC staff, and the disparate nature of scientific research taking place in London's asylums, call into question just how far Mott was able to 'direct and encourage research' within them. Indeed, even the sharing of knowledge within London's asylums was limited by budgets and, after it was suggested to send copies of the *Archives* to each of London's Medical Superintendents, it was, instead, agreed that they would only be sent to those who applied for one.[179]

Often, Mott was involved in other duties that took him away from the study of the pathology of insanity and he became involved in some aspects of scientific work that spoke to the general management of asylums. This included time invested in the physical well-being of the patients, such as his attempts to discover the roots of asylum dysentery. It was, according to the *BMJ*, Cooper who pressed for such a study, which was no doubt linked to his other interests, including his work on the Public Health Committee.[180] In 1902, Mott was involved in an investigation into the cases of tuberculosis at London's asylums using comparative data from the 'new' Claybury asylum and the older Hanwell

[176]LMA, LCC/MIN/748, Pathologist Sub-Committee Minute Book, 1901–1908, 20 November 1905.

[177]LMA, LCC/MIN/747, Pathologist Sub-Committee Minute Book, 1892–1901, 1 October 1895.

[178]LMA, LCC/MIN/748, Pathologist Sub-Committee Minute Book, 1901--1908, 5 April 1906.

[179]LCC/MIN/569, Signed Minutes, 1899–1901, 14 November 1899.

[180]LMA, LCC/MIN/748, Pathologist Sub-Committee Minute Book, 1901–1908, 16 October. Anon. 1909. George Joseph Cooper, MRCS, LAS. *BMJ*, 16 October.

asylum.[181] Similarly, in 1903, he worked with LCC's Medical Officer of Health to identify the causes of enteric fever at the Colney Hatch Asylum which involved him carrying out *post-mortems* at Colney Hatch.[182] These examples followed a study on an outbreak of 'the itch', which arose from the reception of some patients at Horton from a private asylum, and Mott was drafted into investigate. Significantly, the nature of these investigations occasionally brought a level of tension between the Pathology Laboratory and existing staff in Asylums. Commenting on the study of 'the itch', Dr Bryan of the Horton Asylum, who had been studying its prevalence for three years, concluded that Mott's work had not produced any 'fresh information'.[183] At the Banstead Asylum, one of the Assistant Medical Officers refused to follow instructions given by Mott during a *post-mortem* but it was a Claybury where tensions were most apparent.[184]

Whereas the *BMJ* saw the advantages of a 'free hand', there were those who saw Mott as an imposition and complained of his overstepping professional boundaries. Shortly after his appointment, Mott reported that the officers at Claybury could open the laboratory with their pass keys and he reported that 'under these circumstances he would not be responsible for the care and custody of the place'.[185] Some years later, when carrying out work into dysentery, Mott had reported that he 'came across' Dr Jones who said it was not right for him to go around the wards at Claybury without a Medical Officer.[186] In each of these cases, Mott appealed to the Pathology Sub-committee, which then liaised with the relevant asylum sub-committees on his behalf. Cooper, who sat on both the Pathology sub-committee and acted as Chairman of the Claybury sub-committee, as well as being a member of the Asylums Committee,

[181] LMA, LCC/MIN/748, Pathologist Sub-Committee Minute Book, 1901–1908, 3 December 1902.

[182] LMA, LCC/MIN/748, Pathologist Sub-Committee Minute Book, 1901–1908, 4 March 1903, 6 May 1903, 24 June 1903.

[183] LMA, LCC/PH/01/276, Bryan, F. 1905. Report of the Medical Superintendent on Dr Mott's Report on the Itch, LCC.

[184] LCC/MIN/569, Signed Minutes, 1899–1901, 13 November 1900, 11 December 1900.

[185] LMA, LCC/MIN/747, Pathologist Sub-Committee Minute Book, 1892–1901, 1 October 1895.

[186] LMA, LCC/MIN/748, Pathologist Sub-Committee Minute Book, 1901–1908, 24 April 1904.

was key. It had already been agreed that the person appointed would have access to asylum wards but he would not have 'charge of, or interfere with the treatment of the patients at any of the asylums, and he shall conduct his work so that it shall in no way conflict with that of the medical superintendents'.[187] However, subject to the Asylums Committee's directions, Mott was to 'have supreme and sole charge and control of the Pathological laboratory and museum at Claybury for the care and custody of which he shall be held responsible and no other person whatsoever shall be entitled to the possession of the keys of this building without his express sanction and permission'.[188] Similarly, while Mott acted as the main gatekeeper to the new facilities, applications to work at the new Claybury Laboratory had to be agreed by the Committee and while some were readily acceded to, others were not.[189]

This is not to suggest that Mott's tenure was beset only by tensions. Mott explained that he and Jones were 'very good friends' and the latter had an ally in Collins who was the best man at his wedding on 1894.[190] In other cases, Mott worked in concert with LCC's Medical Superintendents, including but not limited to, the negotiations needed for the development of a standard form to be used by all those conducting *post-mortems* in London's asylums.[191] Nevertheless, Cooper and Mott were firm allies and even co-authored reports together. This included a report on medical statistics in 1904, the introduction to which stated.[192]

[187] LMA, LCC/MIN/747, Pathologist Sub-Committee Minute Book, 1892–1901, 1 May 1895.

[188] LMA, LCC/MIN/747, Pathologist Sub-Committee Minute Book, 1892–1901, 1 October 1895.

[189] When Mott asked if his niece could work in the laboratory to help with the preparation and drawing of microscopic specimens, the sub-committee agreed to it 'readily'. LMA, LCC/MIN/747, Pathologist Sub-Committee Minute Book, 1892–1901, 27 January 1899. LMA, LCC/MIN/748, Pathologist Sub-Committee Minute Book, 1901–1908, 2 December 1903.

[190] I am grateful to Louise Hide for the details of Jones's wedding. LMA, LCC/MIN/748, Pathologist Sub-Committee Minute Book, 1901–1908, 2 December 1903.

[191] LMA, LCC/MIN/748, Pathologist Sub-Committee Minute Book, 1901–1908, 24 April 1904.

[192] LMA, LCC/PH/01/276, Cooper, G.J. and Mott, F.W. 1904. Interim Report on Medical Statistics, LCC.

> We are of the opinion that these statistical tables should be to afford clear and accurate information to the public concerning insanity and its causes, and thereby stimulate the feeling that ratepayers' money is expended to the best advantage in promoting and introducing remedial legislative measures for the prevention of insanity, failing that its cure and, failing that, the placing under suitable conditions the vast number of incurable cases, so that they may be relived of the responsibility of taking care of themselves and especially of reproducing their species'.[193]

Key here, of course, was the recurring issue of ratepayers' money but so too was the order in which they hoped to address London's growing lunatic populations. As with other initiatives, the priority was to somehow address the need for more expensive in-patient accommodation. This is entirely consistent with the other attempts already seen in this chapter but here we can see evidence of eugenical ideas relating to the limits that might be placed on reproduction more generally. In the north of England, Mary Dendy had been hugely influential in advocating colonies designed for the permanent sequestration of the feeble-minded, while Wallis has shown that the 'drive to gather information about heredity and illness grew with the success of the British Eugenics Society in the 1930s'.[194] The point she made here is that 'the social aspects of diseases were not erased by *post mortem* or laboratory investigation, and that asylum doctors were not operating in a vacuum without reference to wider social or political ideas'.[195] Sequestration was expensive and, in this case, what may appear to be a straightforward medical story is also a political one. Eugenical ideas were key 'features of the ethos of Progressivism' and 'mainstays of Fabian rhetoric' and fears about the degeneration of the imperial population seeped into the *fin de siècle* social and political consciousness.[196]

[193] Ibid.

[194] Wallis, *Investigating the Body*: 207. See also Jackson, *The Borderland of Imbecility*: Chapter 3.

[195] Wallis, *Investigating the Body*: 207.

[196] Pennybacker, *A Vision for London*: 4, 78. Pennybacker also describes the educational work of the Council as 'eugenic work'. Pennybacker, The Millennium by Return of Post: 146. Fee, Elizabeth and Porter, R. 1992. Public Health, Preventive Medicine and Professionalization: England and America in the Nineteenth Century. In *Medicine in Society*, ed. Andrew Wear, 249–76. Cambridge: Cambridge University Press: 271. See also Pick, Daniel. 1989. *Faces of Degeneration: A European Disorder, c. 1848–1918*. Cambridge: Cambridge University Press.

Mott and Cooper's views on long-term sequestration were mediated by the ongoing pressures on LCC's institutional stock. A study of discharges in LCC asylums by Louise Hide suggests that some Medical Superintendents actively blocked the discharge of some patients. This included Thomas Stansfield who, in 1911, claimed that insanity was still on the increase and that the 'only remedy' was to sterilise the insane because while 'feeble-mindedness ... appears in all ranks of life' the poorer classes 'tend to gravitate to the lowest ranks, where they mate with their kind without let or hindrance, and reproduce a further crop of feeble-minded'.[197] Stansfield was just one member of LCC's medical staff who was influenced by and published work on eugenical ideas but not everyone arrived at the same conclusions.[198] Robert Jones, for example, advocated some eugenical practices but argued, in 1911, that 'suggestions in regard to sterilisation ... have no moral support and ... no legal justification' and this was reflected in the Asylums Committee minutes.[199] As such, this was not a debate that was limited to the medical profession and the Bexley sub-committee, which rubber-stamped the discharge of patients, was not always prepared to maintain patients for eugenically based reasons. Stansfield, explains Hide, expressed his frustration when trying to persuade a committee of laymen 'as to the necessity for the detention of the feeble-minded hooligan or erotic imbecile after they have been converted into quiet, industrious members of an asylum community by treatment'.[200]

Thomson has recently concluded that responses to the 1934 Brock Report, and support or otherwise for sterilisation, was not bound by party affiliations. Rather it was personal, constituency and even administrative factors that mediated responses to it.[201] Similarly, while the Asylums Committee was prepared to canvas the opinion of medical men more

[197] Hide, *Gender and Class in English Asylums*: 129–30.

[198] LMA, LCC/MIN/759, Stansfield, T.E.K. Hereditary and Insanity. See also Faulks, E. 1911. The Sterilisation of the Insane. *JMS*, 57. January. Clarke, Geoffrey. 1912. Sterilisation from the Eugenical Standpoint. *JMS*, 58. Daniel, A.W. 1912. Some Statistics About the Sterilisation of the Insane. *JMS*, 58.

[199] Hide, *Gender and Class in English Asylums*: 132. LMA, LCC/MIN/575, Signed Minutes, March 1908–February 1909, 16 June 1908, 14 July 1908.

[200] Hide, *Gender and Class in English Asylums*: 130.

[201] Thomson, Social Policy and the Management of the Problem of Mental Deficiency: 137.

widely on sterilisation, they had their own views on it and there were political points to be made here. The relief of Mafeking in May 1900 and the celebrations in the streets of London had followed the Jubilee celebrations of 1897, and represents a highpoint of the popularity of Empire.[202] Among Liberals and Socialists there were concerns that any moves towards social reform might be deflected by what Harrison describes as 'hysterical, flag-waving jingoism.[203] It is no coincidence that, after 1907, the Municipal Reformers sought to celebrate Empire day and purchased flagstaffs so that London's schools could proudly display the Union flag.[204] As Pennybacker argues, however, Mafeking 'shook the Progressives' while they were in power' and, as a result, 'LCC parties attempted to outdo each other in constructing a rhetorical link between the municipality and the fate of empire and race, often sharing the national perspectives of the parliamentary parties in the proximate general elections'.[205]

Schneer argues that while some radicals might have claimed to be anti-imperialist, they were in fact 'anti-jingo' and even John Burns' messages were 'rife' with the link between reform and the country's world status.[206] 'The elimination of the poorest conditions and the poorest sections of the working class could only make London and the nation more fit'.[207] As a Progressive member, Cooper could not have been immune from this rhetoric or unmoved by events in the capital.

The Politics of a Central Laboratory

For all the praise in medical circles, and all the civic pride in the new Claybury asylum, both Mott and Cooper recognised its limitations. Part of this was its physical distance from London and, time and again, Mott reiterated that 'many eminent men' had visited the laboratory

[202] Harrison, J.F.C. 1990. *Late Victorian Britain 1875–1901*. London: Fontana Press: 211.

[203] Ibid.

[204] LSE, J2/210. Anon. 1909. *London Under the Moderates*. London: Alexander and Shepherd Ltd.

[205] Pennybacker, The Millennium by Return of Post: 140.

[206] Schneer, *London 1900: The Imperial Metropolis*. New Haven: Yale University Press: 166.

[207] Pennybacker, The Millennium by Return of Post: 140.

and commented on the difficulties involved in reaching its otherwise world-leading facilities. This included Sir Arthur Arnold, a former Chairman of the Council, but he also drew on the support of medical practitioners from abroad. By this time, the transnational sharing of medical and psychiatric ideas already had a long-term history and this will be explored more fully in the next chapter. In this case, Mott used the laboratory's situation at Claybury to press for new facilities. Professor Wilson of the University of Chicago had written to Mott to thank him for his time at Claybury but bemoaned the relative inaccessibility of the laboratory which precluded him from spending more time on his research.[208] Similarly, a party of distinguished French physicians visited Claybury and expressed surprise that such an institute of scientific research should be in so inaccessible a place.[209] 'If the Asylums Committee is in earnest in its endeavour after a better condition of things', the *BMJ* concluded 'its next step should be to recommend the removal of the laboratory to London'.[210]

The *BMJ* was taking its lead from Mott who had already argued that a more central institution would easily accessible for London's asylums which, in turn, would allow their medical officers to work there.[211] He also thought that the medical profession, more generally, would be more inclined to take advantage of its research facilities, while the University of London would be more likely to recognise it as a place of teaching and learning.[212] Mott also argued that the costs of moving to London would be relatively small. 'The expenses of upkeep would not be greater than at present', explained

[208] LMA, LCC/MIN/748, Pathologist Sub-Committee Minute Book, 1901–1908, 9 June 1904.

[209] Anon. 1904. The London County Council and the Treatment of Insanity. *BMJ*, 5 November.

[210] Ibid.

[211] LMA, LCC/MIN/748, Pathologist Sub-Committee Minute Book, 1901–1908, 9 June 1904.

[212] Ibid: 25 March 1903.

> and the only outlay would be in the fitting up of the laboratory. I do not expect at present that so handsome a building as that at Claybury could be obtained but the co-operation of intelligent workers is the most important furniture of a laboratory, and the prospects of many additional workers would far outweigh any defects of the building.[213]

In each of these cases, Mott was speaking directly to the issues that were of interest to LCC and its Asylums Committee but it was Cooper who played an important role in progressing the issue. Cooper had already been the driving force in the setting up and development of key services and, along with the Pathology laboratory, he was feted with within LCC and the medical press as the driving force behind the Epileptic Colony.[214] In 1903, the Pathology Sub- Committee sought clarification from LCC's Solicitor, W. A. Blaxland, on the issue of a new pathology laboratory. Blaxland argued that, under the regulation of the 1890 Lunacy Act, the Committee had no power to establish separate pathology facilities in central London. The laboratory at Claybury was an annexe of the asylum and linked to the statutory responsibility for the reception and treatment of lunatics. This appeared to mirror the issues raised in Brudenell Carter's Hospital plan, but Blaxland read the provision of a separate laboratory as an 'entirely different matter' and saw no reason why the Asylums Committee should not find a clause in the General Powers Bill authorising them to incur the necessary expenditure.[215]

As a result of these discussions and this evidence, the Pathology Sub-Committee recommended in 1904 that the Asylums Committee insert a clause in the next general powers bill for the authorisation of a new laboratory in London. Time and again, the Asylums Committee adjourned any discussion of the report until the issue was dropped for good after the Municipal Reformers came to power in 1907.[216] By this time Cooper has already resigned from the Council to take up his role in the House of Commons but the offer of £30,000 from Henry Maudsley

[213] Ibid: 9 June 1904.

[214] Anon. 1909. George Joseph Cooper. *BMJ*, 16 October.

[215] LMA, LCC/MIN/748, Pathologist Sub-Committee Minute Book, 1901–1908, 25 March 1903.

[216] LMA, LCC/MIN/748, Pathologist Sub-Committee Minute Book, 1901–1908, 11 July 1905, 5 April 1906, 8 July 1907.

to build a hospital meant that the issues had shifted. As with the earlier examples in this chapter, there were limits to how far the Council as a whole was prepared to go, especially when it meant building new facilities away from existing institutional structures.

Conclusions

The initiatives presented in this chapter appear to be very different, but they share two important characteristics. On the one hand, the proposed Hospital for the Insane, the plans for Receiving Houses, and attempts to gain traction for a pathology laboratory in central London, all sought to move some aspect of the management of madness away from the large institutions that had come to dominate the landscape of care and treatment in the nineteenth century. On the other hand, their relative successes and ultimate failures, depended on the politics of the Council and the procedures in place to manage madness in the capital. On the face of it Brudenell Carter's failure rested with his vocal critics in the medical profession, but this is to misunderstand the importance of the council chamber. By trying to circumvent the Asylums Committee, he was already pushing his luck in terms of what he could hope to achieve. While his claims that it was the radicals within the Council that scuppered his plans for an Insane Hospital may seem fanciful, there is a hint of truth in it. It was the Progressives who dominated the Council and any plans that sought to push the boundaries of the Council's terms of reference in relation to its management of madness, needed widespread support.

Just as Brudenell Carter had limited experience of the treatment of insanity, so too had Cooper and Collins. The difference was that they worked within the Committee framework to push through their ideas. While the Receiving Houses plan never made it past the drawing board, the ongoing time and energy spent on the plan rested with its place within an ideology that foresaw a unified London, but also the allies within the Asylums Committee and within the Council who were prepared to support the initiative and to vote in support of it at Committee level. The same can be said for the appointment of Mott as the Pathologist. The sub-committee involved in that were also medical members of the Council, but they drew their authority from their membership of the Asylums Committee and also their membership of the Progressive majority. Once appointed, some of Mott's activities became subservient to the needs to present the existing institutions as bastions of good practice but this emphasises just how important those institutions were. It is easy to conclude, as Cochrane has done, that the 'overriding policy objective' of the Asylums Committee was one of sequestration and link this to Foucault's focus on the segregation and isolation of the mad.[217] These examples disrupt that narrative, and point instead to the importance of key individuals and their ability to garner wider political support for their visions and aspirations. Ultimately, there were more failures than successes but we can see the antecedents and longer-term political story behind what Thomson has described as LCC's 'surprisingly well developed and integrated community care service' in the early twentieth century.[218] To understand this further, the next chapter will explore how LCC looked abroad to further develop its institutional provision.

[217] Cochrane, Humane, Economical and Medically Wise: 265.

[218] Thomson, Social Policy and the Management of the Problem of Mental Deficiency: 138–9.

CHAPTER 5

The Politics of Architecture

Introduction

When it came to the administration of mental health policies, LCC was a relative newcomer. Despite the fact that the 1890s saw renewed energies in asylum construction throughout the country, it did not prevent some commentators from boasting about the almost immediate impact that the new Council had in that field too.[1] 'An annual expenditure exceeding £300,000 passes through [the Asylums Committee's] hands', wrote Sidney Webb,

> and it is not too much to say that under their zealous care the London lunatic asylums have become models for the world. The new asylum at Claybury, which was opened in 1893, with its magnificent pathological laboratory, now nearing completion, will take rank, indeed, amongst the greatest of many advances in the provision for the insane which this generation has witnessed.[2]

Within earlier chapters, it has already been shown that there were challenges to such hubristic declarations, with claims of innovation in administration and care as part of a wider strategy of talking up the new

[1] Taylor, *Hospital and Asylum Architecture in England*: 151.

[2] Webb, *The Work of the London County Council*: 6.

R. Ellis, *London and its Asylums, 1888-1914*,
Mental Health in Historical Perspective,
https://doi.org/10.1007/978-3-030-44432-7_5

political landscape in the face of domestic criticism. Moreover, shortly after Webb's comments, a working party was briefed to study asylum design abroad as LCC looked for inspiration in foreign paradigms of care.[3] As was shown in the previous chapter, this kind of consultation exercise was not that unusual, and neither was it one that was limited to an understanding of the care and control of lunatics. By this time, innovations in transportation and communication meant international travel had never been easier, and professionals, politicians and lay practitioners took the opportunity to travel abroad to share ideas and learn from others across a range of contexts. Significantly, this period saw the development of a range of new networks and a transnational exchange of ideas were part of an 'Atlantic economy' and evidence of 'public knowledge at a world scale'.[4]

Initial sorties into the transnational histories of psychiatry have sought to tease out the various actors in this process and tended to focus the medical motives and connections in the sharing of ideas.[5] Some of this reflects the key issues identified by Steven V. Ward in his overview of the transnational diffusion of ideas in relation to urban planning, which included the mechanisms for diffusion of knowledge and the extent to which ideas and attitudes were changed as a result.[6]

[3] Cochrane, Humane, Economical and Medically Wise: 259.

[4] Ball and Sunderland, *An Economic History of London*: 83–6.

[5] Roelcke et al. *International Relations in Psychiatry*. Rochester: University of Rochester Press. Previous studies have focussed on international examples of psychiatric care but are not necessarily comparative in their analysis. See, for example, Porter, R. and Wright, D. 2003. *The Confinement of the Insane: International Perspectives 1800–1965*. Cambridge: Cambridge University Press. Gijswijt-Hofstra, M. Oosterhuis, H. Vijselaar, J. and Freeman, H., eds. 2005. *Psychiatric Cultures Compared: Psychiatric and Mental Health Care in the Twentieth Century Comparison and Approaches*. Amsterdam: Amsterdam University Press. Ernst, Waltraud. 2010. Practising "Colonial" or "Modern" Psychiatry in British India? Treatments at the Indian Mental Hospital at Ranchi, 1925–1940. In *Transnational Psychiatries, Social and Cultural Histories of Psychiatry in Comparative Perspective, c.1800–2000*, eds. Waltraud Ernst and Thomas Mueller, 80–115. Newcastle: Cambridge Scholars Publishing.

[6] Ward notes that 'great men' were able to assert key ideas in some parts of the world, such as India, because of colonial power. Ward, Stephen V. 2000. Re-examining the International Diffusion of Planning. In *Urban Planning in a Changing World: The Twentieth Century Experience*, ed. Robert Freestone, 40–60. London: E. & F.N. Spon.

Despite this, it is only relatively recently that historians of mental illness have sought to explore, substantively, transnational psychiatric networks. Waltraud Ernst and Thomas Mueller, for example, have charted the moves in the histories of psychiatry from edited collections that feature regional and national contexts, to ones that have provided international overviews in countries across the world.[7] They point to the volumes where 'comparative and network-focussed methodology has begun to feature' but note that their volume on *Transnational Psychiatries* is the first one where all the contributors offer comparative methodologies.[8] What remains less clear, however, is the role of politics and politicians in those processes. In this case, Cochrane notes that an 1897 working party was briefed by LCC to study asylums abroad and reported its findings in 1902. However, there has been no attempt to explain how the politics and governance of LCC mediated the working party's terms of reference or the role they played in the hiatus between its conception and the publication of its findings.[9]

To address this, this chapter will explore the lineage of transnational networks in relation to the history of psychiatry, and place them within the orbit of the municipal networks that developed from the end of the nineteenth century. This will necessarily mean consideration of LCC's committee structure and its role in the sharing of medical and other ideas in relation to the treatment of madness. In the section that follows, there will be an overview of the role that the wider council chamber had in instigating an international fact-finding tour but also how concerns about the costs involved in such consultations stymied progress. To consider the matter further, there will be an analysis of those who were able to make consultative trips abroad and how their findings, and the impact of them, were mediated by the demands on London's already stretched services, the civic pride in the new administration and as a corollary, its politics. Cochrane cites John McDougall, the one-time chairman of the Asylums Committee, who stated that that

[7] Ernst, Waltraud and Mueller, Thomas. 2010. Introduction. In *Transnational Psychiatries, Social and Cultural Histories of Psychiatry in Comparative Perspective c.1800–2000*, eds. Waltraud Ernst and Thomas Mueller, ix–xxiii. Newcastle: Cambridge Scholars.

[8] Ibid.

[9] Cochrane, Humane, Economical and Medically Wise: 259.

> We have always been pressed with much asylum work. I have never known the day when we were not building an asylum ... we have repeated and repeated, mainly from stress of time and going along the path of least resistance.[10]

Cochrane argues that the Asylums Committee had little option but to buckle under the pressure from the Commissioners in Lunacy to build barrack style asylums. This chapter challenges that straightforward assumption and contributes to the relatively recent interdisciplinary interest in the place and space of madness.[11] It places key individuals and the Asylums Committee at the centre of what it was prepared to accept and, crucially, reject from international consultation.

The Lineage of Psychiatric Transnational Dialogue and the Development of Municipal Networks

From the outset, it must be made clear that there was a long-standing tradition of dialogue when it came to the management of madness. In the nineteenth century, this usually meant visits to, and tours of the specialist institutions designed and built to deal with the mentally ill. Staff at hospitals welcomed visitors and it was a crucial way for the latter to 'acquire information about new or alternative treatments, as well as the general organisation of institutions'.[12] Opening up asylums to both medical and lay visitors also allowed institutional managements to challenge what they saw as negative stereotypes of inhumane care, and the West Riding Pauper Lunatic Asylum at Wakefield in the north of England, is just one example of visitors 'much gratified' by the work being carried out there.[13]

[10] Ibid.

[11] Topp, Leslie, Moran, James E. and Andrews, Jonathan, eds. 2007. *Madness, Architecture and the Built Environment*. London: Routledge.

[12] Mooney, Graham and Reinarz, Jonathan. 2009. Hospital and Asylum Visiting in Historical Perspective: Themes and Issues. In *Permeable Walls: Historical Perspectives on Hospital and Asylum Visiting*, eds. G. Mooney and J. Reinarz, 7–30. Amsterdam: Rodopi: 18.

[13] Yanni, Carla. 2007. *The Architecture of Madness: Insane Asylums in the United States*. Minneapolis: University of Minnesota Press: 45. Ellis, R. 2001. A Field of Practise or Mere House of Detention. Unpublished PhD thesis, University of Huddersfield: 85.

On an international scale, different countries could seem to offer paradigms of best practice but, in reality, this was dependent on a number of factors, including the individuals involved and the chronology of their travels. Pliny Earle, who would go on to be the superintendent at the Bloomingdale Asylum in New York, and co-founder of the Association of Medical Superintendents of American Institutions for the Insane, for example, visited asylums in England, Scotland, Ireland and continental Europe.[14] 'Our country has caught the spirit', he wrote in 1841, 'and is imitating the good example of her transatlantic sisters'.[15] As Carla Yanni points out, however, John Charles Bucknill would later visit Uttica and other institutions in the United States to see what improvements he could make to his own practise as a result of his 'natural devotion to the field of medicine'.[16] Similarly, whereas Heinz-Peter Schemeideback has shown that German psychiatrists in the second half on the nineteenth century tended to see British asylums as superior to their own, Rhodri Haywood has described Frederick Mott, LCC's Pathologist as being 'infatuated' with the German psychiatric system.[17]

[14] Frosch, William and Richardson, Diane. 2004. Pliny Earle MD, 1809–1892. *American Journal of Psychiatry* 161:11: 1989. Barton, Walter E. 1987. *The History and Influence of the American Psychiatric Association*. Washington, DC: American Psychiatric Association: 38–9.

[15] Earle, *A Visit to Thirteen Asylums in Europe*: 135.

[16] Bucknill was the co-editor of the *Manual of Psychological Medicine*. Tomes, Nancy. 1988. The Great Restraint Controversy: A Comparative Perspective on Anglo-American Psychiatry in the Nineteenth Century. In *The Anatomy of Madness, Vol. III, The Asylum and Its Psychiatry*, eds. W.F. Bynum, Roy Porter and Michael Shepherd, 191–225 London: Routledge: 191–2.

[17] Schemeideback, Heinz-Peter. 2010. Inspecting Great Britain. German Psychiatrists' Views of British Asylums in the Second Half of the Nineteenth Century. In *International Relations in Psychiatry*, eds. Volker Roelcke, Paul J. Weindling and Louise Westwood, 12–29. Rochester: University of Rochester Press. Hayward, Rhodri. 2010. Germany and the Making of 'English' Psychiatry: The Maudsley Hospital, 1908–1939. In *International Relations in Psychiatry*, eds. Volker Roelcke, Paul J. Weindling and Louise Westwood, 67–90. Rochester: University of Rochester Press. See also Allmond, Gillian. 2017. Liberty and the Individual: The Colony Asylum in Scotland and England. *History of Psychiatry* 28:1: 29–43, 31. For a range of international examples see Ernst and Mueller, *Transnational Psychiatries, Social and Cultural Histories of Psychiatry*. Novella, E.J. 2016. Travel and Professional Networks in the Origins of Spanish Psychiatry, História, Ciências, Saúde-Manguinhos, 23:4: 1023–40.

This complex web of knowledge exchange was not limited to visits to institutions and the broader sharing of ideas was reflected in other parts of the world. As result, we should not be fooled into thinking that this was a straightforward process.[18] Not all ideas were shared in quite the collegiate way that is sometimes represented here. In the 1870s an 'often acrimonious' debate was contested between English and American alienists over the uses and abuses of non-restraint, and the abolition of anything that might be used to restrain patients.[19] Although Tomes has identified dissenting voices on both sides, those in England were largely in favour of its introduction, while those in the United States were broadly against. Matters came to a head when an editorial written by J. Mortimer Granville appeared in the *Lancet* in 1875 'excoriating' the work of American superintendents.[20] In a bid to offer a more constructive criticism of the American system, Bucknill wrote to the *Lancet* and a subsequent series of articles were published as *Notes on Asylums for the Insane in America*. Although Bucknill reiterated Granville's claim that the latter had 'neither said, nor implied that there were no good and well managed asylums in the United States nor has he stigmatised the alienists of America as mad-doctors', his stipulation that the controversy was 'happily ended' proved to be premature.[21] In part this rested with Bucknill's own assertion that the resistance to the abolition of restraint was the 'great stumbling block of the American superintendents' and, as the debate rumbled on, lines were being drawn on national grounds.[22]

The fact that LCC was to include the United States on its list of places to visit is indicative of some *rapprochement* but these examples privilege

[18] D.E. Dhunjibhoy of the Ranchi Indian Mental Hospital, for example, kept a well-stocked library of medical texts and journals, engaged in correspondence with other practitioners and attended conferences and congresses abroad. Ernst, Practising "Colonial" or "Modern" Psychiatry in British India? See also Jackson, Mark. 2010. Permeating National Boundaries. European Influences on the Emergence of 'Medico-Pedagogy' in Late Victorian and Edwardian Britain. In *International Relations in Psychiatry*, eds. Volker Roelcke, Paul J. Weindling and Louise Westwood, 30–47. Rochester: University of Rochester Press.

[19] Tomes, The Great Restraint Controversy: 191–2.

[20] Ibid: 210–11.

[21] Bucknill, J.C. 1876. *Notes on Asylums for the Insane in America*. London: J&A Churchill: 67.

[22] Bucknill, *Notes on Asylums for the Insane*: 67. See also Tomes, The Great Restraint Controversy: 191–2.

the role of medicine and medical staff. One critique of Foucault has been, that for all his focus on the asylum as a microcosm of social and political tendencies, he ignored the geographical specifics of particular social and political networks.[23] Urban historians, turning their attention to the concept of networks, such as Marjatta Hietala, have shown that there were four key ways in which ideas were shared—the employment of foreign experts; study abroad and personal contacts; research papers and journals; and international congresses and exhibitions.[24] Some of this reflects the sharing of medical ideas, but politicians and municipalities were also important here too.[25] John Griffiths, for example, has argued that a close reading of *the Municipal Journal* reveals 'a prodigious global circulation of ideas' and this is particularly relevant as it was originally titled *London* when it first appeared in 1893 and was closely linked to LCC and Progressive ideas.[26] Furthermore, he argues the Progressivism inherent in the *Municipal Journal* found support as far afield as Cape Town in South Africa, and Auckland and Christchurch in New Zealand.[27] This, however, was a slippery concept and even though Progressivism found a constituency in number of international contexts, its finer details were not necessarily transferable or even palatable and were dependent on local factors. As Ewen and Hebbert point out, the interventionist examples that Albert Shaw, a pioneering US journalist, advocated would have been seen as a 'creeping collectivism or an infringement of personal liberty' by some in his own country.[28]

[23]Topp, L. 2007. The Modern Mental Hospital in Late Nineteenth-Century Germany and Austria: Psychiatric Space and Images of Freedom and Control. In *Madness, Architecture and the Built Environment*, eds. Leslie Topp, James E. Moran and Jonathan Andrews, 241–62. London: Routledge: 245.

[24]Despite the evidence above, there was a sense in some circles that transnational interconnections had their roots in the 1960s but this was 'debunked' by the end of the twentieth century. Saunier, Introduction: Global City, Take 2: A View from Urban History: 2–3. Cited in Griffiths, Were there Municipal Networks in the British World: 576–7.

[25]See, for example, Kirk. Neville. 2017. *Transnational Radicalism and the Connected Lives of Tom Mann and Robert Samuel Ross*. Liverpool: Liverpool University Press.

[26]Griffiths, Were there Municipal Networks in the British World: 577.

[27]Ibid.

[28]Ewen and Hebbert, European Cities in a Networked World: 329–30. See also Sutton, John, R. 1991. The Political Economy of Madness: The Expansion of the Asylum in Progressive America. *American Sociological Review* 56:5: 665–78.

Nevertheless, the transnational readership of the journal and its political and administrative focus was significant, and the stories of LCC's asylums were of interest to these non-medical networks and the administrators responsible for their management. Key examples of this include the opening of the Ewell Epileptic Colony which made the front cover of the *Municipal Journal* in July 1903, along with overviews of the new Croydon Mental Hospital and the MAB's Tooting Bec Asylum. The opening of the tenth asylum at Long Grove was the sole story of one front cover in 1907.[29] Long Grove was also covered by the *Local Government Journal* and the editor of *Public Works* magazine wrote to the Asylums Committee asking for permission to include a descriptive account of the Horton Asylum in another, later edition.[30] Even LCC's *Staff Gazette* ran a series of short articles titled 'How other Cities are Governed', which focussed on cities around the world and often included a paragraph on the treatment of the insane.[31] These examples place the administration of asylums firmly within what Ewen and Hebbert have described as a burst of municipal activity that began in the late nineteenth century and peaked in 1913 with the foundation of the International Union of Local Authorities'.[32]

Included within this were the visits of politicians and representatives of municipal authorities, such as those from the Municipal Council of Paris during an event LCC branded the *Entente Municipale*. During that visit, the President and members of the Municipal Council of Paris travelled to London for a six-day tour of London and the work of LCC. A visit to London's asylums was not included, no doubt because of the logistics involved in moving the party out of London and back again, but the illustrated programme of activities include an overview of the work of the Asylums Committee, along with photographs of the Claybury Asylum and a new ward at the Bexley Asylum.[33]

[29] Anon. 1907. A New London Asylum. *Municipal Journal*, 14 June.

[30] LMA, PH/Ment/3/5, Newspaper Cuttings. *Municipal Journal*, 14 June 1907. *Local Government Journal*, 15 June 1907. LMA LCC/MIN/572, Signed Minutes, June 1904–November 1905, 11 October 1904.

[31] See, for example, Anon. 1901. How Other Cities Are Governed. *London County Council Staff Gazette* 2:22: 112.

[32] Ewen and Hebbert. European Cities in a Networked World: 327.

[33] BI 229/14. 1905. Entente Municipale, Visit of the Municipal Council of Paris, to London.

A review of London's Victorian architecture has shown that large-scale building projects were at a relatively low level in this period.[34] Within this context, the huge asylums built by LCC became statements of power, dominance and prestige. Claybury was brand new, and although its antecedents pre-dated the passing of the LGA it was, from the outset, recognisable as an LCC institution. This, along with an updating of the facilities at Bexley Asylum, allowed LCC to showcase its impact on the care and treatment of the insane to an international municipal audience. Indeed, the French visitors from the *Conseil Général de la Seine* and officials connected with the Seine Asylums were allowed to visit Cane Hill, Bexley, Ewell, Long Grove and Horton but not the older Middlesex asylums. 'They have in previous years visited most asylums', the Clerk reported, 'but they think the London County Council have provided the last word – *le dernier cri* – in asylum buildings'.[35]

Such international recognition for this 'last word' was also reflected at conferences. After receiving requests from the International Congress on the Care of the Insane, held in Milan in September 1906, and again when the congress was held in Amsterdam in 1907, the Asylums Committee agreed to lend plans of some of Council's most recent asylums for inclusion in an exhibition.[36] There had been medical conferences before 1888 but the important point here was the emphasis being placed on the management of London by the new Council.[37] 'The work of the Council in the provision of asylums cannot fail to be of great use', recorded the Asylum Committee minutes, and this was confirmed when Great Britain was awarded the *Grand Prix d'honeur* for the plans of the Ayr Asylum, Hellingly Asylum and the London Asylums that had been exhibited in Milan.[38] Other medical visits too, were represented as civic success stories with the Annual Report of the Asylums

[34] Summerson, J. 1973. The Artifact. *The Victorian City: Images and Realities, Vol. 1*, eds. H.J. Dyos and M. Wolff, 311–32. London: Routledge and Kegan Paul.

[35] LMA, LCC/MIN/574, Signed Minutes, February 1907–February 1908, 8 October 1907.

[36] Ibid: 26 March 1907.

[37] Burdett, Henry. 1891. *Hospitals and Asylums of the World. Vol. I, History and Administration*. London: J&A Churchill: 164.

[38] LMA, LCC/18.6, London County Council Minutes of Proceedings, April–June 1906, 15 May 1906. LMA, LCC/MIN/575, Signed Minutes, March 1908–February 1909, 22 December 1908.

Committee for 1908–1909 revealing that LCC asylums received visitors from Sao Paulo and Tokyo, as well as from other parts of Europe and the United States.[39] Professor Wilson and Dr Waldemar Koch, both of the University of Chicago, wrote to the Pathology Sub-Committee independently to express their appreciation of the access and privileges they enjoyed at the Claybury laboratory. There was nowhere in America, or on the continent, they concluded, that could match LCC's facilities.[40]

At the International Congress of Medicine in 1913, the Committee agreed to loan old methods of restraint from the Hanwell Asylum to Henry S. Wellcome who curated an exhibition of rare and curious objects. Wellcome assured the Committee that the exhibition would be held in a fireproof building that would be guarded day and night. He also agreed to pay for the insurance on the objects and for their transportation to and from the site. Keen to ensure that the delegates were aware of the strides being made by LCC in the care of the insane, a party from the congress was invited to visit and tour the much more modern asylum at Claybury.[41] Similarly, when the Congress of Alienists and Neurologists met at Amiens in France, the Asylums Committee invited a group of them to Claybury, where they were met by Councillor John McDougall. This hosting of medical staff by municipal authorities was also matched by medical staff reaching out to lay administrators. It was hoped, for example, that the Fourth International Congress for the Care of the Insane in Berlin in 1910 would attract municipal officials, lawyers and school masters (*sic*) as well as physicians.[42]

In other cases, however, it may have been that LCC's reputation as an asylums administrator was less important than its status as a world city and this seems to have been the case when the Asylums Committee received a letter from the Acting Agent General for Victoria in Australia

[39]LMA, LCC 26.21. The Twentieth Annual Report of the Asylums Committee of the London County Council, for the year ending 31 March 1908.

[40]Wilson also mentioned Claybury's relative inaccessibility—see Chapter 4. LMA, LCC/MIN/748, Pathologist Sub-Committee Minute Book, 1901–1908, 9 June 1904. LMA, LCC/MIN/748, Pathologist Sub-Committee Minute Book, 1901–1908, 20 November 1905.

[41]LMA, LCC/578, Signed Minutes, March 1912–October 1913, 25 February 1913.

[42]Anon. 1910. International Congress for the Care of the Insane. *Journal of Mental Science* 56:234: 583–4. The Third International Congress was held in Vienna. See Percy Smith, R. 1908. Third International Congress on the Care of the Insane, Vienna, October 1908. *Journal of Mental Science* 55:28: 172–9.

in 1902. The purpose of that letter was to ask whether a Medical Superintendent of one of London's Asylums 'would be permitted to visit that colony for the purpose of reporting to the government on the best mode of ameliorating the existing conditions of lunacy there, should the government decide to avail itself of such expert assistance'.[43] The Asylums Committee agreed to this 'very exceptional request' on the understanding that all costs, including any salaries would be covered by the state of Victoria.[44] That administrators in Australia should look to London was not a given and, by this time, there were other authorities and other institutions with a longer track record in the management of madness, and there were other municipalities with reputations for innovation in other areas too. The US journalist, Julian Ralph, proclaimed Birmingham to be the 'best governed city in the world' and, from at least 1892, Bernard Aspinwall has argued that it was Glasgow that represented the beacon of effective and efficient municipal government to Progressive Americans.[45] At the height of Empire, the letter from Victoria can be explained, perhaps, by colonial ties but Waltraud Ernst, has recently challenged any suggestions that psychiatry and institutions in places such as India were simply 'offshoots of colonial medicine' and that knowledge travelled in one direction.[46] Nevertheless, the examples above allowed LCC to promote its administration of lunacy as an exemplar of innovation and modernity in the UK and further afield.

London and the Politics of International Fact Finding

Despite LCC's confidence in its own administration, it was not averse to learning from others. Indeed, its Housing of the Working Classes Committee visited Glasgow, the second city in the Empire, and 'made a very careful inspection of the municipal lodging houses' there. Similarly,

[43] LMA, LCC/MIN/570, Signed Minutes, 1901–1902, 10 June 1902.

[44] LMA, LCC/18.6, London County Council Minutes of Proceedings, May–August 1902, 24 June 1902. LMA, LCC/MIN/570, Signed Minutes, 1901–1902, 8 July 1902.

[45] Briggs, *Victorian Cities:* 55. Aspinwall, Bernard. 1984. *Portable Utopia, Glasgow and the United States, 1820–1920*. Aberdeen: Aberdeen University Press: 157.

[46] Ernst, Practising "Colonial" or "Modern" Psychiatry in British India?: 80–115.

the Education Committee sent its Medical Officer and the Assistant Educational Advisor to Holland and Germany to report on the school systems in place in continental Europe.[47] Within this context, the decision to task a party to visit asylums abroad is understandable but given that the Council as a whole, the committee structure and individuals on committees affected other parts of asylums administration it seems obvious that they would have a role here too.

A reading of LCC minutes reveals, once again, the vital role of the administrative structure of LCC. The working party was, in fact, a sub-committee appointed by the Asylums Committee following an Instruction from the Council. At the weekly meeting of LCC, held at Spring Gardens in October 1896, Lieutenant Colonel Charles Ford moved

> That, having regard to the growing demands upon the ratepayers of the County of London in connection with the care of pauper lunatics, it be referred to the Asylums Committee to consider and report as to the expediency of adopting a better and less expensive method of housing and treating such persons, and that in dealing with the question the Committee do consider the system adopted in principal and European cities.[48]

Ford was also a member of the Asylums Committee but raising the motion in the Council chamber improved the chances of it being adopted. Although not a member of the Progressive Party Committee, the driving force behind the organisation of Progressives on LCC, Ford was active in party affairs and often in dispute with it. In the 1890s, he audited the Party's accounts, but he was also of the opinion that more party meetings should be held than the monthly meetings taking place at that time. Moreover, he was at odds with the party in 1897, when he moved that the 'Chairman of the Council for the ensuing year be left in the hands of the Moderate Party'. Ford lost this proposal by 17 votes

[47] London County Council. 1890. *A Review of the First Year's Work of the Council in a Series of Addresses Delivered by the Chairman, the Earl of Rosebery*. London: LCC: 9. John Rylands Library [Hereafter JRL], LCC, 1907. *Report of the Education Committee of the London County Council Submitting a Report of the Council's Officers on the bathing arrangements in Schools in Germany and Holland*. London: P.S. King and Son: 5.

[48] Anon. 1896. The London County Council. *Morning Post*, 28 October.

to 5, which revealed a modicum of sympathy for his suggestion, but in the following year he expressed his concern that the Party Committee was usurping the rank and file of the party in deciding which proposals it would support.[49] In this respect, it is easy to see why he ignored the Asylums Committee, which was dominated by the Progressives, and raised the motion in the larger Council chamber.

For Ford, the 'less expensive' element of his motion was the key, and this was not the first time that he had moved to impact on the rates. In June 1893, he had failed to convince the Council 'that any alteration to the present county rate ought to be in the direction of a decrease and not an increase'.[50] More specifically, he had already suggested an increase in the employment of asylum patients with a view to bringing costs down and complained bitterly that 'this committee never considered the pockets of the ratepayer' when plans were passed to make improvements at the Hanwell Asylum.[51] The latter plans included the abolition of basement dormitories in recognition of Hanwell's age which meant it was sorely in need of an update. In these cases, Ford was seen as out of touch with the aspirations of the wider Committee and his motions were rarely seconded. While his call to find a better and less expensive system was seconded by George Cooper, also a Progressive member of LCC, his motivations were somewhat different to Ford's. Cooper was to suffer an untimely death after being elected Liberal Member of Parliament [MP] for Bermondsey in 1906 with his demise being attributed 'to the severe strain which the prolonged discussion on the Budget' had imposed on MPs.[52] Prior to that he had served as an LCC councillor from 1889 and, as a member of the Asylums Committee, he had played a prominent role in the failure of Brudenell Carter's plans for the proposed Hospital for the Insane but also in the more successful development of the Pathological Laboratory at Claybury (Chapter 4). Thus Cooper was

[49] LMA, ACC/1632/002, Minutes of the Progressive Party of the London County Council, 1895–1900.

[50] LMA, LCC/18.6, London County Council Minutes of Proceedings, January–December 1893, 27 June 1893.

[51] LCC/MIN/566, Signed Minutes, 1891–1894, 21 August 1893. Anon. 1894. Hanwell Asylum Improvements. *The Times*, 2 May.

[52] Anon. 1909. George Joseph Cooper. *BMJ*, 16 October. Pennybacker describes the LCC as a 'nursery' for parliament because so many councillors were later elected to the House of Commons. Pennybacker, The Millennium by Return of Post: 133.

active in those discussions that sought to somehow arrest the apparently continuous growth of London's lunatic population, via innovative and extra-institutional medical means.

Beyond this, the prospect of a better and less expensive system was one that had broad appeal and the motion was easily passed in the Council Chamber. Once approved, Ford moved that that a special sub-committee should be formed to consider the issue and a new Accommodation sub-committee was constituted shortly afterwards. As with other sub-committees, this new one reported to, and was part of the management of asylums and, as such, reported to the main Asylum Committee, from which it drew its membership. Key members of the new committee included Ford and Cooper, and also William Collins, another medical man (see Chapter 4) who was voted the new sub-committee's Chairman.[53] In the meantime, the immediate impact of Ford's motion was to halt the building of a second asylum on the Horton estate and an eighth for London, when the Asylums Committee voted 11:10 to hold plans in abeyance until the new accommodation sub-committee had an opportunity to present its findings. This left the immediate issue of how to consider the substantive issues in Ford's motion and, meeting for the first time a month later, the sub-committee identified four ways to gather evidence.[54]

First, the Clerk was instructed to forward a copy of Brudenell Carter's report on the Hospital for the Insane (see Chapter 4) to every member of the new Accommodation sub-committee. At the same meeting, and second, Frederick Mott, the Pathologist, was invited to make any suggestions in writing.[55] Third, using Lord Rosebery's connections at the Foreign Office, an information gathering exercise was set in train when the Clerk prepared a list of questions which were approved by Collins and sent to the Medical Superintendents in the United States and Canada.[56] Fourth, and most important, were the plans to gather information

[53]LMA, LCC/MIN/710, Accommodation Sub-Committee Minute Book, 1896–1905, 17 November 1896.

[54]LMA, LCC/MIN/00567, Signed Minutes, 1894–1897, 3 November 1896.

[55]LMA, LCC/MIN/710, Accommodation Sub-Committee Minute Book, 1896–1905, 17 November 1896.

[56]LMA, LCC/MIN/710, Accommodation Sub-Committee Minute Book, 1896–1905, 7 May 1897, 20 October 1897.

first-hand and Collins and the Clerk agreed to compile 'a list of the asylums, which in their opinion, it would be advantageous to visit'.[57]

At the outset, the consultation was framed around institutions and this was undoubtedly linked to the fact that the Council was already exploring extra-institutional options (see Chapter 4). Having provided a list of asylums in France, Germany, Belgium, Canada and the United States, the sub-committee proceeded to elect members of a visiting party so they could approach the Council for funds for travel and 'out-of-pocket' expenses.[58] It was 'impossible', the Asylums Committee reported, 'to proceed further in forming a definite or practical opinion as to the merits of the modern Continental system' without a personal examination of some of the asylums.[59]

Already then, there is further evidence of the sometime glacial movement of the County Council's business in relation to its committee structure. Ford had proposed the amendment in October, but it took four months to constitute a sub-committee and then organise its terms of reference. Part of the delay resulted from the committee structure which meant that the Accommodation sub-committee had to report back up the hierarchy to the Asylums Committee which, in turn, then had to report to the full Council. Further delays were incurred in 1898, when plans to go abroad were temporarily put into abeyance while the Asylums Committee considered the development of Receiving Houses (see Chapter 4).[60] In other cases, the sheer weight of asylums' business meant that some discussions were adjourned as time ran out, such as in the case of longer discussions relating to the boarding out of epileptic patients.[61] Going forward, an ongoing stumbling block was to be the personnel likely to be involved in any international consultations and the differing views on the roles of finance and 'expertise'.

[57] Ibid: 17 November 1896.

[58] Ibid: 7 May 1897.

[59] Anon. 1897. London County Council, *Morning Post*, 10 February.

[60] LCC/MIN/710, Accommodation Sub-Committee Minute Book, 1896–1905, 18 Jul 1898.

[61] Ibid: 11 May 1898.

Politics and the Financing on International Fact Finding

When the Lancashire Asylums Board visited continental Europe in 1900, the party consisted of its Vice Chairman and two of its Medical Superintendents.[62] Similarly, in 1902, a deputation of those involved in the proposals for an Epileptic Colony at Warford near Alderley Edge visited the United States. The party was to consist of Dr J. Milson Rhodes, who was a councillor, GP and Poor Law Reformer and Secretary Edwin W. Marshall. It would also have included Councillor John Royle had he not been debarred on his doctor's advice.[63] Predating both these, the initial plan of LCC was to send a six-man 'commission' abroad with three members of the Accommodation sub-committee and three of its officers.[64] The officers were Dr Claye Shaw of the Banstead Asylum, Mott, the Pathologist and Partridge, the Clerk. Claye Shaw was chosen, no doubt, because of his knowledge of asylums in France, Switzerland and Germany, as was Mott.[65]

The proposed inclusion of politicians on the party was entirely consistent with a Council that had been eager to stress its pioneering impact on the management of madness. Those Councillors and members of the sub-committee nominated for the party included Mr McDougall, Dr Forman and Mr White, who all declined to accept the invitation and this was to become an important sticking point.[66] Without volunteers from the body of Councillors, Ford moved that the matter be left to three officers who would be requested to visit the asylums and report back to the sub-committee for consideration. This resolution was lost by six votes to four and, instead, the matter was referred back to the Asylums Committee for further discussion.[67] The Asylums Committee had similar

[62] Lancashire Asylums Board. 1900. *Report of a Deputation Appointed Visit Asylums on the Continent*. Salford: W.F. Jackson and Sons.

[63] BL, Rhodes, J. Milson and Marshall, Edwin W. 1902. *Report on a Visit of Inspection to Colonies and Hospitals*. London: P.S. King and Son. See also Allmond, Liberty and the Individual: 36.

[64] LMA, LCC/MIN/710, Accommodation Sub-Committee Minute Book, 1896–1905, 7 May 1897.

[65] BL, *London County Council Staff Gazette* (1901), Vol. 2, No. 16: 42.

[66] LMA, LCC/MIN/710, Accommodation Sub-Committee Minute Book, 1896–1905, 7 May 1897, 17 May 1897.

[67] Ibid: 17 May 1897.

difficulty in moving the matter forward. An amendment that proposed sending only the officers led to 'considerable discussion' and, with little sign of agreement on whether Councillors should be involved in international trips or not, the matter was dropped.[68]

Eventually, the Asylums Committee took the issue to the Council and requested £150 to cover 'travel and out of pocket expenses' that would allow 'three members of the sub-committee and two [sic] expert medical officers to visit the various asylums at Paris, Berlin, Leipsic [*sic*], and other continental cities'.[69] Before the request went to a show of hands in the Council chamber, Thomas Corbett (Moderate) requested an amendment to remove the Asylum Committee members from the visiting party. 'He objected', reported the *Morning Post*, 'to members of the Council being allowed to make Continental trips at the expense of the ratepayers' and this was met with 'cheers' from those who supported his amendment and cries of 'oh, oh' from those who did not.[70] Significantly, those who supported Corbett's amendment (John Fletcher and Lionel Holland) were also Moderates and they too were concerned at such apparent profligacy. In response, Collins spoke of the value for money to be gained from the plan but it was Sir John Lubbock, (a former Chairman) who spoke of the balance between expenditure and results. As a rule, he stated, 'expenditure of this sort was undesirable (hear, hear) but … it was unwise to treat such matters under one fixed rule'.[71] This would not be a journey of pleasure, he argued, and would save the ratepayers much more than the initial outlay of £150.

Thus a political debate on the issue of expenses became too big for the Accommodation sub-committee, the main Asylums Committee and the Council itself and the matter was referred 'to the General Purposes Committee to consider and report upon the whole question of the system to be adopted by the Council for investigating questions of importance in relation to the Council's work'.[72] The Committee scrutinised two of the Council's standing orders (no. 147 and no. 148), which stated that Councillors could reclaim from the County Fund,

[68] LCC/MIN/00567, Signed Minutes, 1894–1897, 18 May 1897.

[69] Anon. London County Council. *Morning Post*, 10 February 1897.

[70] Ibid.

[71] Anon. London County Council. *Morning Post*, 10 February 1897.

[72] LMA, LCC/18.6, London County Council Minutes of Proceedings, January–June 1897, 9 February 1897.

travelling costs, 'not exceeding the cost of locomotion' and that those visiting LCC's asylums and industrial schools could 'avail themselves of the stores…on payment of their value'.[73] In presenting evidence from a Water Committee trip to Wales, where Councillors recouped travelling expenses, and a Housing Committee trip to Glasgow, where they did not, the General Purposes Committee fudged the issue. Rather than recommending a definite system, they concluded that each case was considered on its merits and this meant that a similar 'heated and painful debate' took place in 1901 when the issue of expenses was raised to pay three delegates to attend a housing conference in Glasgow.[74]

In the interim, the awarding of expenses, or otherwise, for visiting asylums abroad was debated again. Corbett tried and failed to pass the issue back to the Asylums Committee so that it might consider the request for funds and reconsider who it might send abroad.[75] As a result the issue became dependent on a missive from the Finance Committee which offered 'no observations' on whether or not it was appropriate to send Councillors abroad but did note that in line with Standing Order 212, any expenses for such should be subject to inclusion in the vote, and subsequent passing of the annual maintenance bill. It resolved that the Council would authorise the travelling and out of pocket expenses of three members of committee and three officers 'subject to the passing of the annual maintenance vote' and then the matter was dropped again.[76]

Finally, in 1899, the Asylums Committee was awarded £1000 by the Council for the drawing up of preliminary plans for a new asylum but also to cover the costs of visiting foreign asylums.[77] This followed a warning from the Committee to the Council that 'active steps' needed to be taken by the Council, given that the numbers of patients was rising by 600 per annum and that existing accommodation, including that currently being contemplated, would be filled

[73] Ibid: 9 March 1897.

[74] Ibid: 9 March 1897. BL, *Municipal Journal*, 19 July 1901: 549.

[75] LMA, LCC/18.6, London County Council Minutes of Proceedings, January–June 1897, 23 March 1897.

[76] Ibid.

[77] LMA, LCC/18.6, London County Council Minutes of Proceedings, September–December 1899, 10 October 1899. Anon. 1899. London County Council. *The Times*, 11 October.

by the end of January 1901.[78] In the following year, the Asylums Committee reported its plans for another international fact-finding mission, this time to the United States and Canada. Those chosen for this trip were the Committee's Assistant Clerk, the Asylums Engineer, one of the asylum superintendents and, once again, after three meetings of nominations and votes, three County Councillors in the form of committee members.[79] The cost of the deputation was estimated to be between £400 and £600 and, referencing the Council's desire for a better but less expensive system, Nathaniel Hubbard, the Chairman of the Committee, reported once again that it was impossible to report 'in the manner desired without the information to be acquired from such a visit'.[80] This, of course, was a similar refrain but Hubbard argued that the 'matter had been in hand for so many years that he hoped the Council would now come to some definite conclusion on the subject'.[81]

As was shown in Chapter 2, the role of 'experts' was and is important in the histories of local authorities and in the ensuing debate, the focus was, again, not so much on the value of the trip but the *costs* involved in sending 'non-specialist' members of the Asylums Committee.[82] Richard Beachcroft (Moderate) represented a common strand of opinion when he stated that the Asylums Committee 'should certainly not build another large block asylum without inquiry abroad'.[83] It was, however, 'highly desirable that the Council should stay clear of committing itself to the principle of sending out its members on roaming exhibitions at the cost of the ratepayers'.[84] On this occasion, however, Progressive members also spoke against the awarding of expenses and Benn moved to pass the recommendation back to the Asylums Committee, on the grounds that the 'important principle' that information should be

[78] LMA, LCC/18.6, London County Council Minutes of Proceedings, September–December 1899, 10 October 1899. Anon. 1899. London County Council, *The Times*, 11 October 1899.

[79] LCC/MIN/569, Signed Minutes, 1899–1901, 29 May 1900, 19 June 1900, 26 June 1900.

[80] Anon. 1900. London County Council. *The Times*, 4 July.

[81] Ibid.

[82] Doyle, The Changing Functions of Urban Government: 296–7.

[83] Anon. 1900. London County Council. *The Times*, 4 July.

[84] Ibid.

collected at Councillors own expense was in danger. Hubbard pointed out that that this would lead to only rich members of the Council being involved in such inquiries but, by this time, Benn's proposed amendment had been seconded by another Progressive Councillor, Sir Arthur Arnold. The latter stated that while 'he felt under deep obligation to the Asylums Committee for all the good work it had done for London … it had not', in his opinion, 'pursued in the past the path of economy so strictly as it might have done'.[85]

At the end of what the *Standard* described as a 'long discussion', the Chairman concluded that because the Council had refused to accept the recommendations of the Asylums Committee, and because they had also voted against sending the initial report back to it, they had in fact 'done nothing at all in the matter'.[86] The *Daily News* satirised this inaction under a subheading of 'Something about nothing' and described the two and half industrious hours as 'doing nothing in a manner at once elaborate, complete and artistic'.[87] So much for Hubbard's wish for a definite conclusion and an exasperated Ford complained that 'he almost despaired of getting any report from the Committee on this all-important issue'.[88] Finally, he got his wish when the Asylums Committee reported that it would send the Asylums Engineer, William Charles Clifford Smith, to inspect asylums in Scotland and the continent, and draw on the £1000 that had been granted in 1899. However, it would not be until 1901 that Smith would report on his findings.[89]

International Findings and Medical Opinion

Without the approval of the main Council for an international trip, the Accommodation sub-committee sought to review foreign asylums through existing means. In addition to the initial reports that were circulated at the outset, Dr Thomas (T.E.K.) Stansfield was asked to report

[85] Ibid.

[86] Anon. 1900. London. *The Standard*, 4 July 1900. Anon. 1900. London County Council. *The Times*, 4 July.

[87] Anon. 1900. London County Council. *Daily News*, 4 July.

[88] Anon. 1900. London County Council. *The Times*, 4 July.

[89] LMA, LCC/CL/PH/01/276, Smith, W.C.C. 1901. *Notes of a Visit to Continental and British Asylums*. LCC: London.

on his trip to American Asylums. Stansfield, who was described as an excellent junior medical officer when offered the opportunity to move from the Banstead Asylum to the new Claybury Asylum as First Assistant Medical Officer, often used his leave entitlement visiting other institutions designed for the care of lunatics.[90] The *BMJ*

> Doubted if any other example can be found of a mental hospital physician of his juniority [*sic*] so systematically devoting so large a share of annual leave to professional self-improvement by the visiting of other mental hospitals at home and abroad.[91]

Along with reports on a similar trip to Germany and, and the circulation of a paper on 'The Treatment of the Insane' which he delivered at the British Medical Association, the report on his US trip were all used as evidence by the sub-committee.[92] Stansfield's report pre-dated Ford's call for international consultation by two years and, in this case, municipal networks were less important than the longer-term tradition of medical staff visiting different institutions. His conclusions in this case were drawn from the descriptions of four of the eight asylums he visited during his vacation.[93] These were the St Lawrence State Hospital, the Uttica State Hospital (both New York), the McLean Hospital in Massachusetts and the Toledo Hospital in Ohio. Somewhat ironically, the governors of the McLean Asylum had sent their own architect, Mr Folson, to England to explore information that would lead to the building of a block or pavilion asylum at a time when, according to Bucknill, the only examples were the MAB asylums at Caterham and Leavesden and the new Lancashire County Asylum.[94]

Stansfield, like other medical men before him, focussed on the role of medical staff and their treatment regimes. He noted that the inmates

[90] LMA, LCC 26.21. The Report of the Claybury Asylum Sub-Committee for the year ending 31 March 1893.

[91] Anon. 1939. Obituary: T.E. Knowles Stansfield. *BMJ*, 15 April.

[92] LMA, LCC/MIN/710, Accommodation Sub-Committee Minute Book, 1896–1905, 17 November 1896.

[93] Hine, Asylums and Asylum Planning: 173.

[94] Bucknill referred to the new Lancashire Asylum at Wigan but he was more likely referring to Whittingham. Bucknill, *Notes on Asylums for the Insane in America*: 19.

in the United States had more freedom, that the open-door system was 'extensively in vogue', that upwards of 20% of patients enjoyed the privilege of parole and, significantly, that 'the hospital line of treatment is advancing'.[95] Stenographers, he continued, were employed to do a great part of the administrative work leaving the medical staff to concentrate on medical and scientific work. 'Palatial buildings and luxuries', Stansfield concluded, were wasted on the organically insane who were 'hopeless', and if the 'whole battery of medical sciences' could be brought to bear on the functionally insane, then recent cases had a real prospect of recovery. What was needed, Stansfield argued, was a 'hospital with all the most modern appliances and contrivances for the recent and recoverable cases, and homes for convalescents and chronic insane grouped according to their requirements'.[96] Given the large number of insane in the capital, focussing on those deemed to be curable would mean that LCC 'would naturally take the lead in its system of treatment and management'.[97]

These themes were reiterated in another report authored by Stansfield which detailed an earlier trip to Germany. Stansfield admitted that he had had no intention of writing on the subject when he visited German Asylums in the summer of 1896 and the content of the report was reliant on memory rather than any copious notes. Again, the trip had taken place during his absence from Claybury on annual leave and the purpose had been to 'amplify' his personal knowledge. He had been to Germany before and, while he visited the asylums at Alt-Scherbitz and Herzeberge for the first time, he also 'refreshed' his knowledge of those institutions he had previously explored.[98] Stansfield reported that there were two important issues 'in the modes of dealing with the insane in Germany'. The first was the clinics that dealt with recent and acute insanity and allowed a separation of these patients from 'the noisy and dirty chronic cases'. The second was the method of housing patients in detached pavilions and cottages.[99] 'Why the English architects should adhere so tenaciously to their present formulae for asylums', he wrote, 'I cannot quite

[95] LMA, LCC/CL/PH/01/276, Stansfield, T.E.K. 1894. Report on a Visit to some American Asylums. London: LCC: 7.

[96] Ibid.

[97] Ibid.

[98] Ibid: 1.

[99] Ibid: 8.

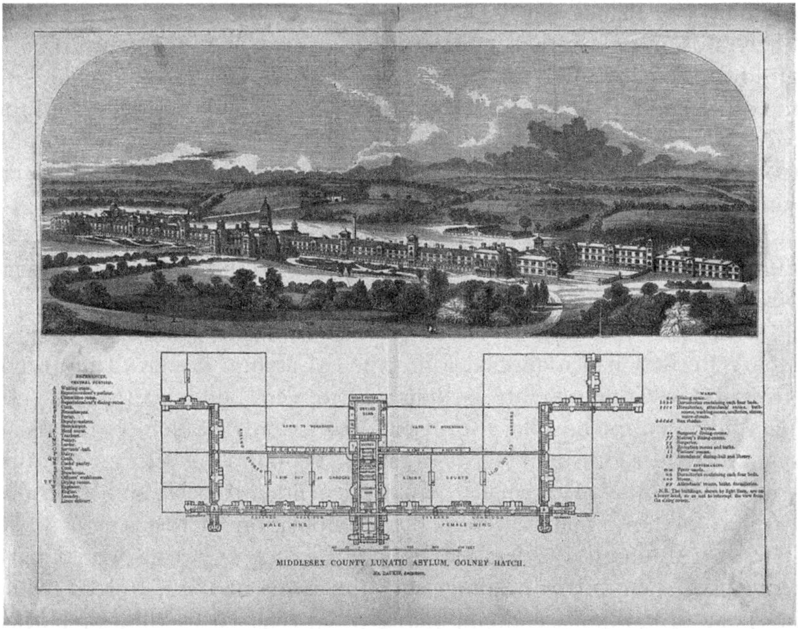

Fig. 5.1 Middlesex County Lunatic Asylum, Colney Hatch, Southgate, Middlesex: bird's eye view with detailed floor plan and key. Wood engraving by Laing after Daukes (Reproduced with permission. Wellcome Collection. CC BY)

understand'.[100] Systems of corridors, Stansfield concluded, were expensive and unnecessary and had a deleterious effect on the patients. Given that Burdett had already described Colney Hatch as a 'typical corridor asylum' with no special feature 'beyond its great size', Stansfield's comments emphasised the archaic nature of LCC's older institutions (see Fig. 5.1).[101]

Stansfield's findings echoed those of Mott who had already visited asylums in Germany, France and Switzerland. On the one hand, the latter had concluded, LCC's 'two modern asylums' were greatly superior to

[100] Ibid: 9.

[101] Burdett, Henry C. 1891. *Hospitals and Asylums of the World. Vol. II, Asylum Construction*. London: J&A Churchill: 74–5.

anything else that he saw. 'The buildings are more costly', he reported, 'the wards more cheerful and better furnished in every way, and the grounds are pleasanter and more extensive'.[102] On the continent, 'on the other hand, [he] was struck with the superiority of knowledge of the Medical Staff as a whole, and the larger number of such in proportion to the number of patients'.[103] The themes of investment in acute services here are redolent of those in the previous chapter but, while Mott's in particular, and Stansfield's accounts looks very much like the kind of thing that Brudenell Carter was canvassing for, the latter was, in fact, pushing for a move towards a cottage-style of asylum.

In his now well-known *Hospitals and Asylums of the World* (1891), Henry Burdett had identified four types of asylum design. These were 'Irregular or Conglomerate asylums' which were buildings that had not been intended for hospital use; 'Corridor Asylums', which, as the name suggests, had rooms and wards organised around connecting corridors; 'Pavilion Asylums' with smaller, semi-independent blocks; and 'Corridor Pavilion' asylums that represented a combination of the previous two styles.[104] Although Burdett was influential, not everyone would have recognised these broad headings, nor the terms he used. Indeed, while he spoke of pavilions, contemporaries often referred to villas or blocks. Design played a part in these definitions but so too did size and the smaller cottages that Stansfield referred to could also be described as semi-independent blocks.[105]

By this time, as was shown in the previous chapter, the development of institutional and extra-institutional responses was subject to debate and the architect of several of London's asylums, G.T. Hine, presented a paper in 1901 that laid out his vision for asylums in the early twentieth century.[106] This was a coalescing of familiar themes and included

[102] LMA, LCC/CL/PH/01/276 Mott, F.W. 1896. Housing of Lunatics. London: LCC.

[103] Ibid.

[104] Burdett, Henry C. 1891. *Hospitals and Asylums of the World. Vol. II, Asylum Construction*. London: J&A Churchill: 59–109.

[105] Topp, The Modern Mental Hospital in Nineteenth-Century Germany and Austria: 244.

[106] Taylor, Jeremy. 2007. The Architect and the Pauper Asylum in Late Nineteenth-Century England. G.T. Hine's Review of Asylum Space and Planning. In *Madness, Architecture and the Built Environment*, eds. Leslie Topp, James. E. Moran and Andrews Jonathan, 263–81. London: Routledge: 275–6.

two key developments in the form of an acute hospital on the one hand and smaller detached villas which would house the remaining patient population, on the other. Following his trips to the USA, Stansfield had shared the plans of American asylums with Hine and it is easy to see their shared viewpoint on the future of asylum accommodation.[107] As Louise Hide points out, the two collaborated on the plans for the Bexley Asylum, which was the first English pauper asylum to incorporate the villa system into its design.[108] This was not an issue limited to London and following a visit to Germany and France, the Lancashire Asylums Board also recommended that their next asylum should be in the villa style.[109]

Just like Stansfield, Hine was influenced by asylum design in America and also in Germany and by the end of the nineteenth century, asylum planners in both Germany and the Austrian Empire had 'universally embraced' the villa system.[110] The transferability of these models to the UK was far from straightforward, however, and referencing plans for a villa-style asylum near Edinburgh, Hine wondered how the central administration and food supply for 33 individual units would successfully work in a climate like Scotland's, and this was a wider issue of concern. Stansfield had also questioned how the wide-open spaces of villa-style accommodation would suit the English climate but he provided tables of metrological data, supplied by the Secretary of the Royal Meteorological Society which identified the similarities in 'climatic difficulties' in London (Greenwich), Leipsic [*sic*] and Berlin.[111] The message here was that if they could work in other places, why not in London?

Such views were not representative of the medical profession as a whole and this included Edward Marriott Cooke, one of the Commissioners in Lunacy, who argued that villa-style asylums would

[107] Hine, Asylums and Asylum Planning: 173.

[108] Hide, From Asylum to Mental Hospital: 61.

[109] Lancashire Asylums Board, *Report of a Deputation Appointed Visit Asylums on the Continent*: 68.

[110] Topp, The Modern Mental Hospital in Nineteenth-Century Germany and Austria: 244.

[111] LMA, LCC/CL/PH/01/276, Stansfield, T.E.K. 1896. Report to the Special Sub-Committee (Housing of the Insane) of the Asylums Committee: 9.

not work in England. Marriott had visited Germany too and for him the villa system there worked for mild cases who, in England, would be dealt with by the Poor Law, either in the workhouse or in their own homes.[112] To critics, even a change to the design of large-scale institutions left the main issues unresolved. The *BMJ* argued that

> villas conducted on strictly hospital lines are all very well, but what is wanted is the establishment of real hospitals for the insane in which the sufferers shall be under the care of a specially skilled visiting staff with all the necessary equipment for the clinical and pathological study of mental disease and facilities for the fullest therapeutic research.[113]

Whereas, many saw villa-style hospitals as the innovative response, the *BMJ* saw only a 'herding together of patients in all stages of disease, with the result that cases in which recovery might confidently be looked for become, incurable'.[114] This dissonance can be explained, in part at least, by the roles of Mott and Stansfield as LCC employees, and that of Hine as a contractor for several county authorities but, for both medical insiders and outsiders alike, Claybury was not quite '*le dernier cri*' that LCC was apt to proclaim.

In the period from Ford's resolution in 1896 until the end of their dominance of LCC in 1907, the Progressive Asylums Committee built and opened five large-scale institutions. Despite the discussions that were taking place, only one of them could be described as approximating anything like a villa-style asylum, and that was the Ewell Epileptic Colony which opened in 1903 at the Epsom site. Cochrane argues that that the Colony was based on the Asylums Engineer's trip to Europe and on the Galkhausen Asylum, near Cologne, but that trip post-dated the decision to build and the discussions already taking place about its design.[115] Indeed the issue was first raised in May 1898, when LCC's Medical Superintendents were invited by the Asylums Committee to contribute ideas but it was Dr George Cooper who was the driving force behind the

[112] Taylor, The Architect and the Pauper Asylum in Late Nineteenth-Century England: 276.

[113] Anon. 1904. The London County Council and the Treatment of Insanity. *BMJ*, 5 November.

[114] Ibid.

[115] Cochrane, Humane, Economical and Medically Wise: 256.

project.[116] As the name suggests, the 300-bed Colony was designed for epileptic patients drawn from LCC's other asylums and it was founded on three key principles. First, it was designed for the care and, if possible, beneficial treatment of the patients. Second, it was expected that it would be self-supporting with patients conducting all the work necessary on the Colony itself, and also manufacturing goods for sale to boost incomes. Third, any patient unwilling to work would be returned to their original asylum.[117] These three principles fitted neatly with the will to provide something better and cheaper, at least from an administrative point of view, but it did not address the calls from the medical profession to impact on the rates of cure more generally. Nevertheless, the Asylums Committee reported, in 1898, that the Colony afforded 'an opportunity for thoroughly testing the advantage or otherwise of the less institutional character of asylum construction which is much more vogue in Europe and the United States of America' and, on its opening, proudly reported that it was 'the first of its kind in the country'.[118]

Beyond this, the impact of medical and architectural views about acute hospitals and villas was to represent only relatively small steps in influencing the shape of London's institutional stock. A convalescent home was built at Colney Hatch and a cottage hospital at Banstead but the real chance to innovate was at the asylums that were still on the drawing board. Hine did include villas in his plans for the Bexley (1898) and Horton (1902) Asylums. These were for 35 patients in each case and a new hospital on the Bexley site in 1907 was furnished with 'appliances for electrical and other modes of treatment' for new patients. Those who showed early signs of recovery stayed there until their discharge while other, less hopeful cases were transferred to the main building.[119] Again, these changes were reflected elsewhere and the smaller and *Grand Prix d'honeur* award-winning Hellingly Asylum at East Sussex included an

[116]LCC/MIN/710, Accommodation Sub-Committee Minute Book, 1896–1905: 11 May 1898. Anon. 1909. George Joseph Cooper. *BMJ*, 16 October.

[117]Ibid: 25 October 1898.

[118]LMA, LCC/18.6, London County Council Minutes of Proceedings, July–December 1898, 20 December, 1898. LMA, LCC/CL/PH/01/276, LCC. c.1904. The Epileptic Colony, Ewell. London: LCC.

[119]*Sixty-First Report of the Commissioners in Lunacy*, 1907: 328.

acute hospital for 80 patients, a main building for patients of all classes, four detached villas, and a block for idiots and imbeciles.[120]

In London, the blame for this apparently slow pace of change was placed firmly at the door of the Commissioners in Lunacy. Commenting in 1907, Keene, the Clerk reported that,

> except in the case of the epileptic colony we have never been able to build an asylum entirely upon the villa principle. Bexley (The first asylum provided by the County of London) was designed on the continuous principle, in combination with villas to a certain extent, and when another large asylum at Horton was contemplated the need for the speedy provision of accommodation forced the Committee to reproduce the Bexley plans. The same thing happened with the plans of the Long Grove Asylum where the Lunacy Commissioners put pressure on the Committee to erect buildings of the old type and thus avoid the delay of preparing fresh designs.[121]

It seems odd that Keene would, in 1907, reflect upon the Asylums Committee's inability to innovate on asylum design, when it had consistently and regularly presented its administration of lunacy, and their institutional provision as world leading. Certainly, when the Long Grove Asylum opened in the same year, its footprint was similar to Bexley, and to a lesser degree, Claybury (see Fig. 5.2 and plans in Chapter 3). To understand this apparent contradiction there needs to be an understanding of how medical and architectural ambitions were mediated by politicians and administrators.

[120]Hine, Asylums and Asylum Planning: 175–6. Taylor, The Architect and the Pauper Asylum in Late Nineteenth-Century England: 276–7. LMA, LCC/CL/PH/01/276, Smith, *Notes of a Visit to Continental and British Asylums*: 101–2. Allmond, Liberty and the Individual: 31–2.

[121]LMA LCC/CL/PH/01/276, Keene, H.F. 1907. Report of the Clerk in Connection with Question of the Need for Additional Accommodation. London: LCC.

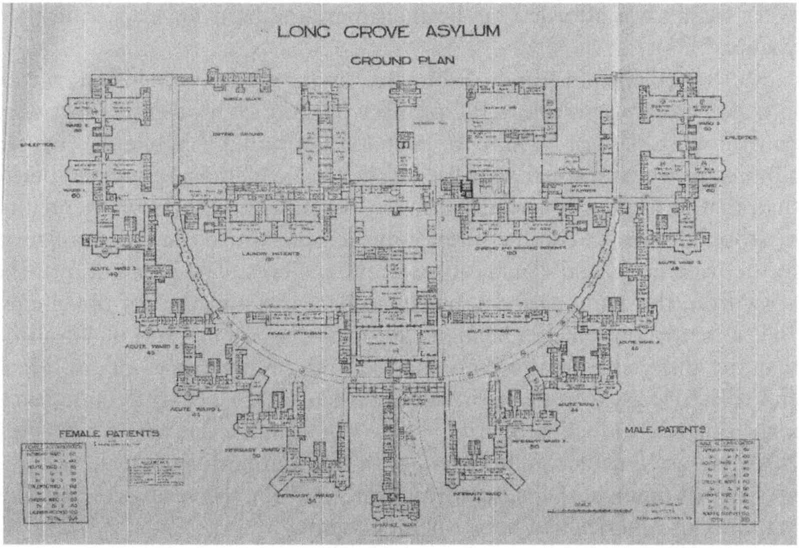

Fig. 5.2 Ground Floor Plan of the Long Grove Asylum. c.1906. LMA, LCC: 26.21. Asylums Committee Report, 1905–1906 (Reproduced with permission of London Metropolitan Archives, City of London)

Transnational Networks, the Maryland Asylum and the Limitations of Expert Opinion

As the discussions about expenses showed, it was not only medical staff who were visiting asylums in this period and included here was John McDougall, the Chairman of the main Asylums Committee, 1895–1898. In 1897, he visited Canada and the United States, sailing from Liverpool in the company of another Councillor who was making his way to America for information on the working of tramway systems. Before setting off, McDougall had arranged, via Partridge, the Asylums Clerk, to have letters of introduction provided by the Foreign and Commonwealth Office. These were 'unnecessary', McDougall wrote, 'as without exception on mentioning that I was from London, every facility was afforded me by the superintendents for inspecting their asylums'.[122]

McDougall visited some of the same asylums as Stansfield but, travelling after Ford's resolution, the primary purpose of his trip was to 'ascertain the best class of asylum to erect for London'.[123] While he covered administrative issues such as patients' dietary, which was generally better than that in London's asylums, and the pay and conditions of attendants, he stopped short of commenting on more substantive changes in relation to the treatments and classification of the patients. The separation of the noisy from the acute patients, he concluded, was a matter for the alienist and 'a matter on which a layman can give no opinion,' and he admitted that the difference in the construction and circumstances of the block and villa-style asylums he saw made it difficult to make any definite statement on their individual merits.[124] He noted, however, that while some villa-style asylums accommodated both chronic and acute patients, the majority of them were for the former only and the 'chief object' of building them in America had been one of economy.[125]

While the cost of treatment was always an issue for all Councillors, straightforward economy for the sake of it was not. By this time, there had been a number of failed attempts by individual councillors to press the Asylums Committee to economise by exploring options for boarding out old and infirm patients. The aim in these cases was to somehow manage the demand on existing resources in the hope it would preclude the need for additional, expensive institutions. Some Councillors argued that if new in-patient facilities were needed, then it would be better to build separate, cheaper, institutions for elderly and/or chronic patients but these were limited to individual, unsupported motions, either in the Asylums Committee or the Council chamber.[126] Similarly, when calls

[122] LMA, LCC/CL/PH/01/276, McDougall, John. 1901. *Notes of a Visit Made in 1897 to Canadian and American Asylums.* London: P.S. King and Son.

[123] Ibid: 23–4.

[124] Ibid.

[125] Ibid: 23.

[126] LMA, LCC/18.6, London County Council Minutes of Proceedings, January–December 1893, 28 July 1893. May–August 1900, 8 May 1900. LCC/MIN/568, Signed Minutes, 1897–1899, 8 November 1898. LCC/MIN/570, Signed Minutes, 1901–1902, 14 October 1902. LCC/MIN/571, Signed Minutes, November 1902–May 1904, 14 July 1903. In 1903, the MAB opened the Tooting Bec Asylum for the aged, epileptic and infirm imbeciles. BL, *Municipal Journal*, 3 July 1903.

were made to achieve economies of scale by moving almost 100 blind patients to one asylum it was rejected on the grounds that it would not benefit the patients already accustomed to their surroundings. As the Asylum Committee explained in their planning of the Epileptic Colony, 'on the question of housing and treatment we have always had at heart the best interests of the unfortunate patients entrusted to our care, and at the same time have exercised every economy'.[127] The working patients at the Colony might not have agreed with this assessment but it reflected LCC's and, to a lesser degree, the Commissioners' views about the nature of asylum accommodation in this period. As Patricia Clavin points out, transnational encounters did not or do not necessarily break down frontiers and can even reinforce barriers.[128] Extrapolating this in this context, it can be seen that the rhetoric concerning LCC's place as a world leader in the treatment of the insane, in part, explains McDougall's conclusions but then too were the demands on its institutional spaces.

This is not to say that LCC and the Commissioners in Lunacy were in complete agreement. The Asylums Committee resisted specific requests from the latter to provide accommodation for the quiet class of patients who were boarded out around the country.[129] Similarly, when LCC purchased the Horton Estate at Epsom, the initial plan was to convert the existing manor house there for administrative purposes and use temporary buildings to house chronic patients who had been sent to out-county institutions. After reaching agreement with the Commissioners of Lunacy and the Secretary of State for the Home Office to allow this, the Committee was asked by the former to

> consider, with a view to immediate action, the provision of an eighth asylum of a less expensive character for the accommodation of patients of a quiet and inoffensive character to be drafted in from their other asylums.[130]

[127] LMA, LCC/18.6, London County Council Minutes of Proceedings, January–April 1901, 30 April 1901.

[128] Clavin, Patricia. 2011. Introduction: Conceptualising Internationalism Between the World Wars. In *Internationalism Reconfigured, Transnational Ideas and Movements Between the Wars*, ed. Daniel Laqua, 1–15. London: I.B. Tauris: 2–3.

[129] LMA, LCC/MIN/710, Accommodation Sub-Committee Minute Book, 1896–1905, 25 January 1897.

[130] LMA, LCC/MIN/567, 1894–1897, 26 January 1897. LMA, LCC/MIN/710, Accommodation Sub-Committee Minute Book, 1896–1905, 25 January 1897.

For the Asylums Committee, this condition effectively 'pre-judged the character' of a new asylum, and was one that 'did not meet the pressing demands of London'.[131] Collins took the lead on the response and, after initially calling for a rejection of the Commissioners' demands on the grounds that the Committee were considering a better and less extensive system, replied that they would endeavour, as far as possible, to have regard to the wishes of the Lunacy Commissioners.[132] Once built, however, the filling up the temporary asylum with the kind of patients stipulated by the Home Secretary was open to interpretation.

At the time, LCC had 432 individuals boarded out and the Asylums Committee prioritised those who were being charged a weekly rate of 19s 6d, but who also met the stipulation laid down by the Home Secretary of being of the quiet class. The first 228 admissions to Horton Manor in 1899 were women transferred, in the main, from the relatively expensive licensed houses, in and around London but, as the Clerk pointed out, this meant that at least 362 beds at the institution remained unfilled.[133] The vacant accommodation, along with the conditions laid down by the Home Secretary, placed the London's ratepayers at a 'disadvantage' and the Clerk suggested that Committee write to Commissioners and, 'failing action by that body to memorialise the Home Secretary to relax his conditions'.[134] 'The Medical Superintendent', it was reported 'sees no reason why a proportionate number of present and acute cases should not be received at this asylum'.[135] After discussion, the Asylums Committee authorised the movement 'in' of recent cases and resolved only to inform the Secretary of State once this had been done.

This understanding of the political and economic landscape of care is crucial and, whatever those in the medical profession may have felt about

[131] LMA, LCC/MIN/710, Accommodation Sub-Committee Minute Book, 1896–1905, 25 January 1897. LMA, LCC/MIN/567, 1894–1897, 26 January 1897.

[132] LMA, LCC/MIN/567, 1894–1897, 26 January 1897.

[133] LCC/MIN/568, Signed Minutes, 1897–1899, 20 June 1899. The places listed were Fisherton (96 patients), Bethnall House (44), Camberwell House (37) Grove hall (29), Dorset County Asylum (12), Hoxton House (5) and Peckham House (3). The total number here is 226 which was two less than the figure cited by the Asylum Clerk. *Fifty-Fourth Report of the Commissioners in Lunacy*, 1900: 323.

[134] LCC/MIN/568, Signed Minutes, 1897–1899, 20 June 1899.

[135] Ibid.

foreign asylums, McDougall could not conceive 'that they would find in America any improvement on the system adopted in this country'.[136] In particular, he was referring to the small-scale changes that had taken place at the Bexley Asylum and he argued that the plans for the eighth asylum at Horton, should follow the same plan 'extending the villa system by degrees for the accommodation of convalescents, quiet chronics, and patients working on the farm'.[137]

These findings explain why the Asylums Committee was so keen to send Councillors abroad. McDougall was apt to talk up the Asylums Committee's strategy because, as was shown in previous chapters, it was one that was couched very much in political terms. Hennock described the Progressive movement, more generally, as 'an attempt to find a municipal expression for civic pride' and this goes a long way to contextualising McDougall's findings.[138] Moreover, in the same year that Keene was complaining about the pressure from the Commissioners, the Asylums Committee was presenting the piecemeal changes favoured by McDougall as particularly innovative. This included the detached villas (Fig. 5.3) but also the open corridors that were presented as 'special features' of the asylum that can be seen in Figs. 5.4 and 5.5. These were attempts to somehow open up the architecture of the asylum and, while they drew on the findings of Stansfield who had complained about the 'systems of corridors', his views were mediated by the Asylums Committee.

Within this context, it is no surprise that when Smith, the Asylums Engineer, reported on his trip to 28 asylums in England, Scotland, Belgium, France, Germany and Holland, he focussed on a 'most careful comparison of the French, German and Scottish systems of asylums arrangement with those of the Committee's asylums'.[139] Arguing that the next asylum for London should be arranged in three sections, he concluded that the first should be for recent and acute cases, with admission pavilions, acute and infirmary pavilions and pavilions or villas for

[136] Anon. 1900. London County Council. *The Times*, 4 July.

[137] LMA, LCC/CL/PH/01/276, McDougall, John. 1901. *Notes of a Visit Made in 1897 to Canadian and American Asylums*. London: P.S. King and Son: 24.

[138] Hennock, *Fit and Proper Persons*: 290.

[139] LMA, LCC/CL/PH/01/276, Smith, *Notes of a Visit to Continental and British Asylums*: 101.

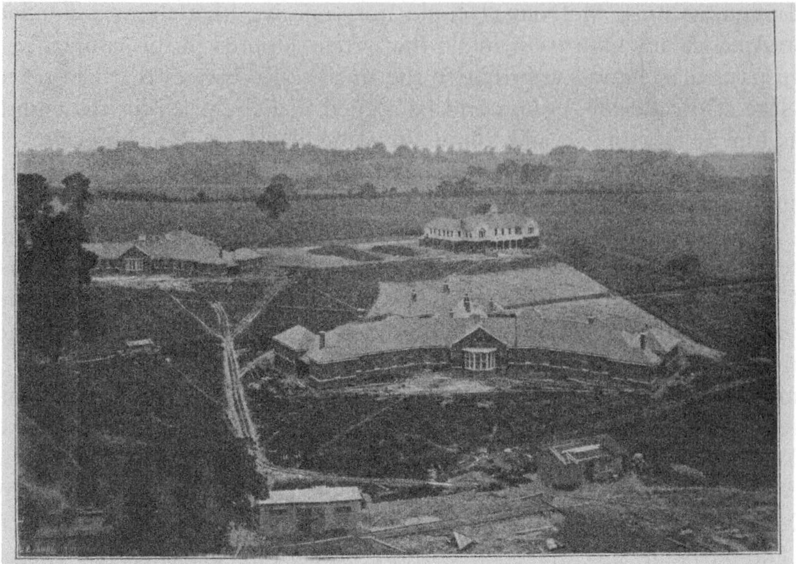
LONG GROVE ASYLUM.
VIEW FROM TOWER, SHOWING DETACHED VILLAS. (1) AND (3) VILLAS FOR CHRONIC PATIENTS. (2) VILLA FOR WORKING PATIENTS.

Fig. 5.3 Detached Villas at the Long Grove Asylum. c.1906. LMA, LCC: 26.21. Asylums Committee Report, 1905–1906 (Reproduced with permission of London Metropolitan Archives, City of London)

convalescing patients; the second section should be for refractory chronics and infirm chronics, while the third should be for quiet and harmless patients.[140] At this point, neither Smith, nor Stansfield or McDougall had managed to identify a specific model that LCC might follow and this helps to explain why the Long Grove Asylum followed much the same plan as its predecessor at Bexley.

In April 1902, the Accommodation sub-committee resolved to circulate Smith's report to its membership 'together with plans, descriptions and any information that Mr E. White can supply with regard to the

[140] Ibid: 101–2.

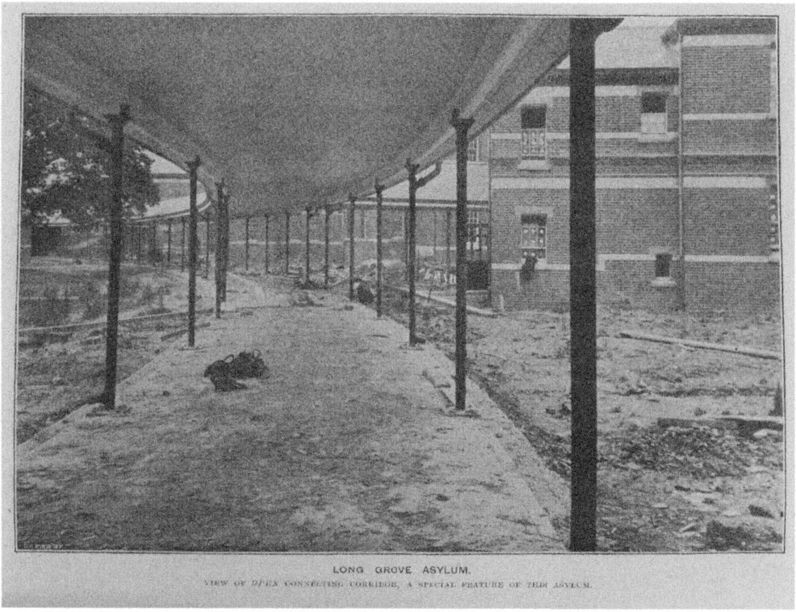

Fig. 5.4 Open Connecting Corridor at the Long Grove Asylum. c.1906. LMA, LCC: 26.21. Asylums Committee Report, 1905–1906 (Reproduced with permission of London Metropolitan Archives, City of London)

Springfield Asylum, Maryland, United States of America'.[141] Despite the fact that none of the three previous reports by Stansfield, McDougall and Smith had covered Maryland, it was this institution that was chosen as the potential model for the next asylum in London.

Like McDougall and Stansfield, Edward White had toured the United States and visited several asylums. He had also been asked to write a report on his trips there but if this was ever published, it is not preserved in the archives and it is not clear from the records that do remain why Maryland was pushed to the fore. By 1903, the Accommodation sub-committee finally settled on a villa-style asylum based on its design

[141] LCC/MIN/710, Accommodation Sub-Committee Minute Book, 1896–1905, 7 April 1903.

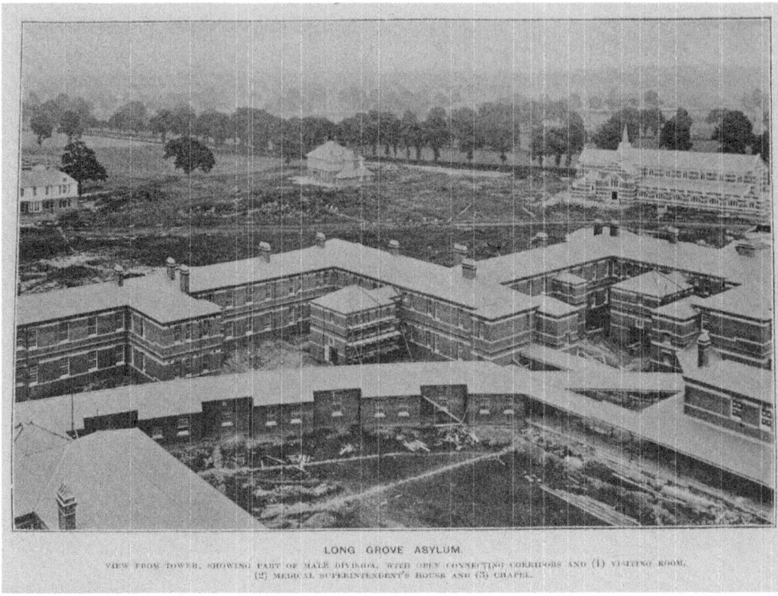

Fig. 5.5 Open Connecting Corridors at the Long Grove Asylum, Male Division. c.1906. LMA, LCC: 26.21. Asylums Committee Report, 1905–1906 (Reproduced with permission of London Metropolitan Archives, City of London)

but this was an unusual choice.[142] It may have been that White travelled to Maryland, but although he identified the Springfield Asylum, the state was better known for its Spring Grove asylum at Catonsville. Scull has detailed Medical Superintendent, George Henry Rohé's vociferous advocacy of sexual surgery as a cure for mental diseases at a time when 'medical opinion was moving more and more decisively in the opposite direction'.[143] Even before his death in 1899, however, an overview of the hospital facilities led the state Lunacy Commissioners to conclude that 'there is no better hospital for the treatment of State patients in

[142] LCC/MIN/710, Accommodation Sub-Committee Minute Book, 1896–1905, 19 May 1903.

[143] Scull, Andrew, 2006. *The Insanity of Place/The Place of Insanity: Essays on the History of Psychiatry*. Abingdon: Routledge: 169.

the Union'.[144] It was Rohé, in his role as the Medical Superintendent at Spring Grove, and as president of the Medical and Chirulogical Faculty of Maryland, who successfully lobbied for a second state asylum. Once approved, Rohé resigned his position at Spring Grove in May 1896 to oversee the building of the state's second purpose-built institution.[145] Rohé assisted with both the choice of location and the development of the plans for its construction and, in the years between its opening and Rohe's death in 1899, only chronic cases were admitted to the new asylum. It was after Rohe's successor Dr Clarke was appointed that the admission of acute cases was first tested, with 'several cases' and then extended. Only in 1900, were any specific blocks erected for the treatment of acute cases.[146]

In other ways too, Springfield appeared to be an unusual choice. It was isolated, the superintendent was 'at a loss' to how to keep the patients entertained, and occupying the patients in the Winter proved to be difficult. Moreover, the choice of Maryland largely ignored everything that had taken place in the intervening seven years. The time and effort that had gone into getting the funds for Smith to travel to other parts of Europe, along with the introductions and connections that were needed for him to meet with staff and to undertake tours of the various facilities, all appeared to be for nothing. Having said that, the final say on Maryland's suitability as a model of cheaper, better care for London was left to the assessment of both Stansfield and Smith. The convoluted attempts to explore asylums abroad had given their opinions a primacy that would not have happened without the original motion that pressed the Asylums Committee to look further afield than London's new boundaries.

In the end, while Stansfield (a member of the medical staff) and Smith (the engineer) remained convinced that the villa 'principle' was the right choice for London, they considered that its success depended 'upon the villa being designed for the special type of cases they have to

[144] *Tenth Report of the Lunacy Commission to His Excellency, the Governor of Maryland*. 1895. Baltimore: Sun Book and Job Printing Office: 7. Maryland State Archives. https://msa.maryland.gov/. Accessed 17 July 2019.

[145] Hurd, Henry M. 1916. *The Institutional Care of the Insane in the United States and Canada, Vol. II*. Baltimore: Johns Hopkins Press: 529, 534.

[146] Hurd, *The Institutional Care of the Insane in the United States and Canada*: 535–6.

accommodate and upon the suitable grouping of the villas. It is not possible, they continued to use the same arrangement of structure for all cases. The Maryland plans, Smith and Stansfield concluded, were 'an advance upon the barrack style of asylum common in England, in so far as it admits greater segregation with all its numerous advantages but beyond this we are not able to speak favourably of it'.[147] Once again, the issue related to London's specific needs to provide accommodation for acute, chronic and quiet cases and is perhaps indicative of the piecemeal way in which a Maryland style asylum sought to accommodate the former. As a result, the Accommodation sub-committee removed their support for the plan on 'account of the expense and difficulty of administration'.[148]

Going forward, it was Smith who was given the opportunity to design the institution that would become, the fifth on the Epsom estate and the eleventh for LCC. Ultimately known as West Park, Cochrane argues that by this time there had been time to commission a novel design, and while Smith received only a fifth of Hine's normal fee, his design was described as 'significantly more imaginative'.[149] In reality, the primary reason for Smith's appointment was his understanding of the 'practical requirements of the Committee', which was more than 'any outside architect could have' had.[150] Similarly, when, plans for what would become the Maudsley Hospital were underway, it was the Asylums Engineer who worked closely with the new Municipal Reform Councillors of Rowe, Easton and White and it was they who visited the Munich Psychiatric Clinic which was under the directorship of Kraepelin. Significantly, it was not expected that the Engineer would consult with Mott on any of the plans he produced.[151]

[147] LCC/MIN/710, Accommodation Sub-Committee Minute Book, 1896–1905, 24 November 1903.

[148] Ibid.

[149] Cochrane, Humane, Economical and Medically Wise: 265. Smith was allowed an assistant but, significantly, was only paid once the plans were approved by the Commissioners in Lunacy.

[150] LMA, LCC/MIN/711, Accommodation Sub-Committee Minute Book, 1905–1908, 3 July 1906.

[151] LMA, LCC/MIN/712, Accommodation Sub-Committee Minute Book, 1908–1910, 27 April 1909, 18 June 1909.

Once the Municipal Reformers were in power, Smith's work paused while they placed a moratorium on all large-scale capital projects and focussed on the nascent plans for what would become the Maudsley Hospital (see Chapter 4).[152] When it did resume, the influence of their attempts to reduce public spending were clear. The Municipal Reform dominated Asylums Committee's instruction to use cheaper building materials and to spend less on decorative items meant that the estimated cost was £30,320 cheaper than its immediate predecessor at Long Grove, and also £57,913 cheaper than the costs estimated by the Progressive led Committee in 1904.[153] At different times in the progress of the asylum, the Commissioners in Lunacy wrote to LCC to Committee to suggest that costs might have been lower still, citing estimates for what would be the sixth Lancashire Asylum at Whalley but, as Smith pointed out, both rates of pay for workmen and the price of materials were higher in the capital.[154] Indeed, the Progressives had predicted at the very beginning of the twentieth century, that future institutional provision would be more expensive because of these increased costs, making the Municipal Reform savings all the more stark.[155]

Conclusions

It is easy to see why Colonel Ford's 1896 motion requesting the Asylums Committee to work towards a better and less expensive way of dealing with pauper lunatics was approved in the Council chamber. However, this 'holy grail' of health care specifically, and public spending more generally, was mediated by a number of key factors. In the first place, it was the changes brought about by the LGA that enabled Ford to first suggest a trip abroad and then garner the appropriate levels of support that compelled the Asylums Committee to consider international examples of care. The emphasis on cash *and* care was the key difference between Ford and Brudenell Carter but we should not be

[152] LMA, LCC/MIN/711, Accommodation Sub-Committee Minute Book, 1905–1908, 16 July 1907.

[153] LMA, LCC/MIN/713, Accommodation Sub-Committee Minute Book, 1910–1912, 23 May 1911.

[154] Ibid: 28 November 1911.

[155] LMA, LCC/18.6, London County Council Minutes of Proceedings, January–April 1901, 30 April 1901.

fooled into thinking that the outcome for either of them was very different. Exploring transnational systems meant a discussion within the wider council about the costs of sending personnel abroad and whether this constituted value for money. This tells us something about the funding of transnational discussions but even this was subject to the debates about how public money should be spent. In the end, and after several lengthy debates at committee and council level, only one member of the administrative team in the form of the Asylums Engineer was granted the money to go abroad. This partly explains why it took so long for the report to move forward but then so too does the attempt to explore other options such as Receiving Houses. For the time being, calling in witness statements and reports from people who had already surveyed institutions abroad meant that there was at least evidence to help consider the management of lunacy that was taking place beyond London and beyond Great Britain. The reality here, however, was that the Council may have prevented those individuals from travelling abroad at the expense of the rate-payers but it did not prevent them from shaping future services. Thus, it was key individuals on the Asylums Committee who were able to pick and choose which aspects of expert and other opinion they were prepared to accept.

McDougall was apt to talk up LCC's strategy in relation to what he saw but this had to be framed within the rhetoric which focussed on the immediate and pioneering impact of the new administration. It is this that helps to explain the will to exchange ideas transnationally. Participating in both medical and municipal networks enabled the Council to reiterate the strengths of their asylum management on an international scale. The findings of Stansfield and, even of Mott, reiterated the medical will to arrest the growth of lunacy by focussing on acute services but this was pretty much the way that medical views were developing anyway. With this in mind, it is difficult to see what, other than giving key individuals a voice, the reports on international consultation contributed in terms of new ideas or directions. The Springfield Asylum appeared to offer that all-elusive model but, even here, it is telling that plans to replicate it were first dropped and then amended so that it might better suit London's needs. Municipal networks were important here but the civic pride in existing services meant that there were always limits to what would be deemed to be an acceptable paradigm. In the meantime, the piecemeal additions to the existing stock at places like Bexley and Long Grove allowed the Asylums Committee and the Council to carry on stressing the innovative ways in which they were apparently moving the administration of asylums forward. Individuals within the medical profession may have wished to have moved towards a separate system of acute care, but that ambition was constrained by the politics of the party confident in its own vision of mixed care. Whatever Ford had envisaged, the chief outcome of his motion was the maintenance of the status quo with the future of London's policy in the hands of key individuals. Significantly, the resolution to find a better and less expensive of dealing with London's insane population appears to show that the shape of future institutional provision was open to discussion. In reality, the Asylums Committee mediated the aspirations of the medical profession for acute services, and the demands of the Commissioners to provide adequate accommodation for chronic cases in line with its own views of how that would best serve London. The next chapter will show how these factors were affected by a shifting landscape of views about migrants and foreign nationals.

CHAPTER 6

The Politics of Difference

Introduction

The formation of LCC coincided with the economic distress of the 1880s, which, in turn, had prompted large-scale migrations to London. Those making their way to the capital travelled nationally and internationally and included those looking for work in the wake of agricultural depression and Jewish migrants escaping the pogroms of Eastern Europe and Russia.[1] The influx of large numbers of people was reflected in what Davies has described as the decade's '*causes celebres*' of housing and employment conditions,[2] but it was to impact on the housing of lunatics too. In line with other aspects of LCC policy, the rhetoric around the Progressives and their treatment of foreign lunatics was wholly positive. One such example was Sidney Webb, who wrote, in 1895, that

> to quote only one of the many instances of the thought that is now lavished on these unfortunates in our midst, the latest innovation is the appointment of an interpreter, able to converse in five foreign tongues. There is, it should be explained, no system of repatriation of lunatics, and many foreigners are accordingly doomed to remain permanently in our London asylums. Some of these can neither speak nor understand a word

[1] Davies, Local Government 1850–1920: 51.

[2] Ibid.

R. Ellis, *London and its Asylums, 1888-1914*,
Mental Health in Historical Perspective,
https://doi.org/10.1007/978-3-030-44432-7_6

of English, and it is a kindly thought of the Asylums Committee to seek in some slight degree to mitigate the awful mental loneliness of confinement in a foreign land by, at any rate, providing some means of occasional communication.[3]

Within a relatively recent and developing historiographical trend, scholars have teased out the incidences and causes of the confinement of 'foreigners' such as these, and to place them within wider socio-medical and legal frameworks. How 'foreign lunacy' was defined was dependent on individual national contexts. Studies have explored the exportation and mediation of dominant theories of classification and control into colonial settings, as well as the experience of particular groups of migrants, such as the Irish in English, American and Australian institutions.[4] In addition, recent edited collections have sought to further expand our understanding of migration and (mental) health. Individual chapters have drawn on a wide range of primary sources that has included personal correspondence, poems and novels, but the introduction and interpretation of legislation continues to be important.[5] Alison Bashford has provided an overview of how lunatics, idiots and imbeciles became subject to international border controls, whereas Suzuki's work on Japan is just one example of how laws passed in the early twentieth century were mediated at a local level.[6] In her study of modern-day immigration in New Zealand, Lynne Briggs has shown how the acceptance, or otherwise, of

[3]Webb, *The Work of the London County Council*: 6.

[4]See, for example, Ernst and Mueller, *Transnational Psychiatries, Social and Cultural Histories of Psychiatry in Comparative Perspective, c.1800–2000*. See also Mahone, Sloan, and Vaughan. 2007. *Psychiatry and Empire*. Basingstoke: Palgrave Macmillan.

[5]McCarthy, Angela and Coleborne, Catharine. 2012. *Migration, Ethnicity and Mental Health, International Perspectives 1840–2010*. New York: Routledge: 1–14. See also Chapters 4–9 in Harper, Majorie (ed.). 2016. *Migration and Mental Health: Past and Present*. London: Routledge. Littlewood, Roland and Lipsedge, Maurice. 1982. *Aliens and Alienists: Ethnic Minorities and Pyschiatry*. London: Penguin.

[6]Bashford, Alison. 2013. Insanity and Immigration Restriction. In *Migration, Health and Ethnicity in the Modern World*, eds. Catharine Cox and Hilary Marland, 14–35. Basingstoke: Palgrave Macmillan. Suzuki, A. 2012. Between Two Psychiatric Regimes: Migration and Psychiatry in Early Twentieth-Century Japan. In *Migration, Ethnicity and Mental Health, International Perspectives 1840–2010*, eds. Angela McCarthy and Catharine Coleborne, 141–56. New York: Routledge.

different immigrant groups can be 'conditioned, created or constrained by political circumstances'.[7] Often, however, the exact nature of those political circumstances in historical settings remains opaque. The aim here is to frame Webb's rhetoric within the rising tensions in relation to immigrants that culminated in, first, a Royal Commission on Alien Immigration, and then the passing of the Aliens Act in 1905.

The national 'Khaki election' of 1900 had seen a Liberal Party divided into pro- and anti-war factions and the Conservative Party swept to victory. Although there is some debate about the exact impact of imperialist rhetoric on the result of the election, one outcome was an increase in the number of restrictionist MPs, particularly in London's East End, who pressured the new Government for immigration reforms.[8] As David Feldman has pointed out, the Act 'was passed for London; or more precisely one part of it – the East End, and was designed to reduce Jewish immigration'.[9] While these concerns were not solely political, the passing of the Aliens Act was indicative of the political response to them and was to represent a watershed moment for both London and Great Britain. For the first time, legislation was introduced to limit immigration and the free movement of people into the country, and this was to act as the foundation for future legislation, regulation and restriction.[10]

With London at the heart of this shifting and contested landscape this chapter will add to the understanding of immigration and the reception of alien lunatics. It considers how political, as well as social and medical debates impacted on the treatment of foreign lunatics in the capital. In particular, Webb's rhetoric on the positive changes instigated by the Progressive regime seems to suggest an understanding of, and a will to meet the different needs of foreigners in London's asylums.

[7] Briggs, Lynne. 2012. The impact of Migration on the Mental Health of Refugee Women in Contemporary New Zealand. In *Migration, Ethnicity and Mental Health, International Perspectives 1840–2010*, eds. Angela McCarthy and Catharine Coleborne, 178–92. New York: Routledge: 184.

[8] Pellew, Jill. 2007. The Home Office and the Aliens Act, 1905. The Historical Journal 32:2: 369–85, 372. Windscheffel, *Popular Conservatism in London*: 181–90.

[9] Feldman, David. 1989. The Importance of Being English: Jewish Immigration and the Decay of Liberal England. In *Metropolis London: Histories and Representations Since 1800*, eds. David Feldman and Gareth Stedman Jones, 56–84. London: Routledge Revivals: 56.

[10] Feldman notes that some trade unionists turned 'anti-immigrant' in the face of the defeats of new unionism and the breakdown of labour organisation among immigrant groups. Feldman, The Importance of Being English: 56.

This chapter will analyse how this understanding of 'difference' worked in practice and how it was affected by the wider political currents relating to immigration. This chapter, more than any of the preceding ones, places patients at the heart of the analysis but it picks up on the familiar themes of rhetoric, finance and London's place at the heart of an increasingly networked global economy. To understand this here, the chapter will first frame London's place as a magnet for migrants from other parts of the UK, as well as the rest of the world, within a timeframe that pre-dates the introduction of the LGA. It will then consider the cost implications of the care of foreign lunatics and how that was affected by the ramping up of anti-alien sentiment, especially after the Municipal Reformers seized control of the Council following the 1907 election. In the sections that follow there will be an analysis of casebooks and related materials to demonstrate how and why the Aliens Act and existing lunacy legislation were used to deport individuals. Finally, attention will be turned to the role of LCC in its negotiations with local agencies and governmental departments at home and abroad as it sought to extend the scope of those who might be deported. Using quantitative data relating to foreign lunatics and their repatriations it, along with some case studies of those individuals affected, this chapter will show that any concerns about immigration generally, and particular groups specifically, were reductive. It will argue that the Municipal Reform dominated administration engaged less with debates about the 'low status' of immigrants and focussed simply on the catch-all title of 'foreign lunatic' in a bid to first limit the need for another large institution and then to manage its costs.

LCC and Foreign Lunatics

Webb's brief overview of the 'kindly thought' given to foreign lunatics is important, not least because the appointment of an 'interpreter attendant' at Colney Hatch in 1892 had very practical implications.[11] As Leonard Smith has pointed out, 'where the patient was foreign and did not speak good English, the authorities had the additional difficulty of trying to ascertain the degree of irrationality and this must have added to the sense that such patients were disturbed and excitable'.[12] Indeed, in

[11] LMA, LCC 26.21. Medical Superintendents Report, Colney Hatch: 13 April 1893.

[12] Smith, L.D. 1998. Insanity and Ethnicity: Jews in the Mid-Victorian Lunatic Asylum. *Jewish Culture and History* 1:1: 27–40, 31.

his description of a visit to Bethlem, Robert Gardiner Hill, an early advocate of 'non-restraint' in asylums, wrote that

> Some foreigners appeared to be fastened behind iron gates or in cages — jabbering and making an unearthly noise. Many of the patients were very ferocious, the hubbub and noise being almost deafening. At St Luke's Hospital the same state of things existed.[13]

In her study of twentieth-century diversity, Wendy Webster has shown how 'jabbering' was used as a sometimes pejorative term to describe a 'common alien sound' and there is evidence of that here too.[14] The Colney Hatch Visitors book, for example, revealed that when a Guardian of the Hackney Union visited the asylum to visit Sylvia R, he simply noted that he 'failed to elicit any information, she being unable to speak English'.[15] And, while the medical officer at Colney Hatch recognised Samuel R.'s muttered responses to questions, which could 'of course' be partly accounted for by language, he was, nevertheless, sure that the reason for it was 'chiefly mental defect'.[16]

In this context, there must have been frustration on the part of those described as insane, especially when even those supposedly acting as their advocates could not understand what they had to say or what they needed. The appointment of an interpreter who, according to Webb, spoke five languages, had obvious potential but, here, he was referring to one institution and that was Colney Hatch. Reverend Henry Hawkins, the Asylum's chaplain, described the 'mixed multitude' gathered within the asylum walls from its opening in 1851 to the then present day in 1901. Inmates hailed from 'probably every English county' along with 'natives of "Wild Wales", Caledonia, stern and wild, of the Sister Isle, of France, Belgium, Holland, Italy, Norway, Russia, Japan, *not* (within recollection) from China, though members of the embassy once paid a visit'.[17] The international flavour of Colney Hatch's inmate population reflected London's appeal to migrants.

[13] Hill, Robert Gardiner. 1870. *Lunacy: Its Past and Its Present*. London: Longmans.

[14] Webster, Wendy. 2018. *Mixing It: Diversity in World War Two Britain*. Oxford: Oxford University Press: 170.

[15] LMA, H12/CH/A6/1, Colney Hatch Visitors Book, 24 April 1891.

[16] LMA, H12/CH/B13/60, Colney Hatch Male Case Book, April–September 1907.

[17] Hawkins, *Some Notes on the History of the Colney Hatch Asylum, 1849–1901*: 21.

Beyond their language skills, there were cultural issues to consider too and for Jewish patients at least, there were some other interventions. In 1895, the Chairman of the Visitation Committee of the United Synagogue wrote to the Asylums Committee expressing his thanks for the arrangements that had been made for the Jewish patients to be supplied with Kosher meat.[18] Similarly, the Reverend Isaac Samuel the visiting Jewish Minister at Colney Hatch, expressed the warm thanks of the Chief Rabbi stating that the 'patients fully realise the importance of the boon conferred upon them.[19] As the minutes record, the sub-committee at that asylum spent an additional £119 on Kosher meat plus an additional £280 on a special kitchen, £40 on utensils and £69 on wages and emoluments a for special cook.[20]

Of course, not everyone saw Colney Hatch in such positive terms and even in the 1850s it had a reputation in some sections of the medical profession for being overgrown and unmanageable.[21] Its reputation in the popular imagination was fearsome and some people chose to end their lives rather than contemplate time as an in-patient.[22] As was shown in an earlier chapter, such views were often challenged by other stakeholders who stressed the positives of LCC Asylums, especially when contrasted with other, privately funded alternatives. Even then, Colney Hatch was not showcased in the same ways that some of LCC's later asylums were (see Chapter 5). Either way, LCC continued a policy of concentrating Jewish lunatics at Colney Hatch that had begun when the United Synagogue secured the agreement of the Middlesex magistrates to do so in 1872.[23] This had followed similar successes in agreeing to special arrangements at the Whitechapel Workhouse and the London hospital.

[18] LMA, LCC/MIN/567, 1894–1897, 15 October 1895.

[19] LMA, LCC 26.21. Report of the Colney Hatch Sub-committee: 1 May 1896.

[20] LMA, LCC/MIN/567, 1894–1897, 9 July 1895.

[21] Allmond, Liberty and the Individual: 33.

[22] John S. an insurance collector committed suicide after two 'unendurable' years. 'I have gone day by day, worse and worse', he wrote in his final note to his wife, 'till I can only see Colney Hatch before me, and sooner than go there I will end it.' Anon. 1896. A Dread of Colney Hatch. *Daily Mail*, 5 September. Similarly, an optician, William M., left a note that read 'Goodbye mother and sister. Forgive me. It is better than Colney Hatch. My head is dead', before hanging himself. Anon. 1902. Better than Colney Hatch. *Daily Mail*, 26 April.

[23] Smith, Insanity and Ethnicity: 36–7.

More broadly, Hawkins wrote with pride of the various religious denominations at Colney Hatch, including the 240 Jews looked after by a Reader and a lady visitor of their own Faith, and considerately treated in the preparation of food according to the customs of their religion. 'Consignments of unleavened biscuits, oranges &c, at Passover season [and] Jewish pastries from time to time', he continued, 'are tokens that are kindly considered'.[24] Such examples are indicative of something more than the preparation of food, they also say something about an understanding of the role of faith and customs in everyday life. Administrative agreements may have impacted on medical understandings of individuals but, as Smith points out, 'the sight of a man praying fervently in Hebrew for hours on end was bound to perplex the attendant and medical officer. There would be little comprehension as to the degree of normality of the behaviour'.[25] In addition, he has shown that Jewish patients were often forced to eat non-Kosher meat and were often recorded as refusing food or at least perceived to have been being difficult about it.

Smith's work focussed primarily on the provincial cities of Manchester, Birmingham and Liverpool but he included a brief overview of the Colney Hatch Asylum, and the work of the Reverend A. L. Green, a minister who had visited Jewish patients, and 'complained bitterly' about the non-kosher food at a conference in 1877.[26] As the work of the United Synagogue indicates, this was not an issue limited to asylums. When Hannah H., a Jewish patient from Leeds, was transferred to the West Riding Asylum, it was noted by the attendant of the Leeds Union Infirmary that she sometimes refused to take her food.[27] Similarly, the evidence to suggest that Rachel S., a 19-year-old Jewish patient, was a fit person for an asylum included her refusal to take food at the Mile End workhouse.[28] In this case, Rachel was described by the workhouse attendant as 'striking and biting at everyone' while the medical practitioner who signed her reception order 'found her in the padded room'. When I approached her, he wrote, 'she kicked at me and showed fright' and, in this respect, it is easy to see Rachel's refusal to take food as part of a

[24] Hawkins, *Some Notes on the History of the Colney Hatch Asylum*: 21.

[25] Smith, Insanity and Ethnicity: 33.

[26] Smith, Insanity and Ethnicity: 34.

[27] WYAS, C85/3/6/204, Case Reference, 15599, 10 May 1915.

[28] LMA, H12/CH/B/46/63, Colney Hatch Female Reception Orders, 16451–16475: 16474.

wider frustration at her incarceration.[29] With these examples in mind, it is little wonder that the Commissioners in Lunacy pressed for all Jewish patients under LCC care to be sent to Colney Hatch, as they did when they saw four persons professing to be of the Jewish faith at the Hanwell Asylum.[30]

In 1892–1893, Colney Hatch received 46 patients from the other LCC asylums, the majority of which were Jewish after the decision was again made to send all such patients in future.[31] This still did not mean that all Jewish patients necessarily went to Colney. As the Asylums Clerk explained,

> As far as possible vacancies at any particular asylum are allotted to those cases which arise in districts nearer to that asylum. This shortens the journey for the patient, and probably is more convenient to the friends who visit. All Jewish patients, however, are received at Colney Hatch Asylum where special arrangements for their religious needs have been made. When a lunatic is to be admitted who is known to have been an inmate of one of the London county asylums, wherever possible a vacancy is allotted at the asylum where he was treated previously. This secures continuity of treatment.[32]

If there was a special reason, because of reasons of health, or because of a request from one of their friends', then Jewish patients might be sent to or remain in one of London's other asylums.[33] This might mean easier access to a particular asylum, more visits from family members or the Poor Law Guardians, but it also meant that the special arrangements made at Colney Hatch for kosher food or religious ministrations were unavailable.

P. J. Waller suggests that 100,000–150,000 Jewish settlers made it to Great Britain in the period between 1881 and 1914.[34] As the architect

[29] Ibid.

[30] LMA, LCC 26.21. Report of the Hanwell Asylum Sub-committee for the Year Ending: 31 March 1890.

[31] LMA, LCC 26.21. Medical Superintendents Report, Colney Hatch: 13 April 1893.

[32] Keene, H.F. 1907. *Memorandum as to the Procedure with regard to the Admission and Discharge of Patients*. London: LCC.

[33] LMA LCC/MIN/572, Signed Minutes, June 1904–November 1905, 14 November 1905.

[34] Waller, *Town, City and Nation*: 26.

George H. Bibby intimated in 1895, the weight of immigrant numbers in the capital and 'in the great asylums of London, meant that the obvious difficulty of providing for the various kinds of religious ministrations are less than in the provinces'.[35] A recent study of institutions in Scotland has shown that there were no specialist food preparation facilities provided. Any pastoral support or contact with a Rabbi had to be facilitated through 'weekend passes' whereby patients were allowed temporary leave.[36] With this in mind, London's treatment of Jewish patients appears to be progressive, even if that pre-dated the Progressive administration of LCC. Some caution has to be exercised here, especially when Colney Hatch's mixed reputation is taken into account. Moreover, when the Council of the United Synagogue wrote to the Asylums Committee to ask if a Jewish Minister would be appointed to visit asylums other than Colney Hatch, they declined explaining they felt that they had done all that could be 'reasonably expected of them in way of special provision for Jewish patients'.[37] Similarly, one local newspaper drew a link to the dietary requirements of Jewish patients and the rising costs of asylum accommodation. 'Even the Jews go mad sometimes', explained the *Shoreditch Observer*, and at 'Colney Hatch the victualling bill is increased by the provision of special food for Jewish patients, the average price of Kosher meat being 2s per stone higher than the ordinary meat for other patients'.[38] Thus, while there was some investment in some services, there were limits to how far this would go and this helps to explain why specialist services were limited to Colney Hatch. Such concerns reflected the ongoing importance of the rates and there can be little doubt that some initiatives were linked to the wider rationalisation of services that was taking place from 1888 onwards (see Chapter 2).

In 1899 Nathanial (N. W.) Hubbard, who would later act as the Chairman of the Asylums Committee, pushed to extend Colney Hatch's

[35] Bibby, George H. 1895. *The Housing of Pauper Lunatics*. London: Drake, Driver and Leaver Ltd.: 30.

[36] Sarg, Cristin M. 2017. Scottish-Jewish 'Madness'? An Examination of Jewish Admissions to the Royal Asylums of Edinburgh and Glasgow, c.1870–1939. Unpublished PhD thesis, University of Glasgow: 290.

[37] LMA LCC/MIN/572, Signed Minutes, June 1904–November 1905, 14 November 1905.

[38] Anon. 1906. London County Asylums. *Shoreditch Observer, Hackney Express and Bethnal Green Chronicle*, 13 October.

role and moved that, as far as possible, all alien lunatics should be sent there. Medical Superintendents were instructed that, within 14 days of the admission of any alien lunatics who could not speak English, they were to communicate with the Central Office so that that the clerk might obtain the services of an interpreter to facilitate such a move.[39] In reality, the pressures of space meant that this was impossible to achieve without a significant re-orientation of LCC's admissions procedures. When the Commissioners in Lunacy visited Colney Hatch in May 1897, they directly questioned the figures that suggested there were vacancies for one man and three women on the grounds that the wards were overcrowded from the squeezing in of extra beds.[40] At Cane Hill in 1905 there was 60 'in excess of the proper numbers', while at Claybury there was a 'considerable excess' of 53 male and 133 female patients meaning beds were being made up in corridors and passages.[41] At Hanwell in the following year, the Commissioners described an 'excess' of 99 men and 144 women on the numbers that should have been in the institution.[42] Each of these cases of overcrowding meant that the concentration of one particular group in one asylum was always going to be difficult.

Figures from 1908 (Table 6.1), reveal that every one of LCC's asylums maintained significant minorities of foreign-born lunatics and this was reflected in London's other asylums too. Caroline Bressey's work on people of colour in the City of London Asylum has similarly emphasised the diversity of London in the nineteenth century.[43] For LCC, Colney Hatch may have had the largest population of foreign lunatics (38%) but that meant that majority (62%) were distributed across London's other nine institutions.

London was not the only place in Great Britain to have a number of alien lunatics within its institutions. Indeed, Liverpool, Leeds and Birmingham all had significant numbers of aliens who claimed poor law

[39] LCC/MIN/568, Signed Minutes, 1897–1899, 14 March 1899.

[40] LCC 26.21. Report of the Commissioners in Lunacy, Colney Hatch: 10 May 1897.

[41] *Fifty-Ninth Report of the Commissioners in Lunacy*, 1905: 338, 340.

[42] *Sixtieth Report of the Commissioners in Lunacy*, 1906: 343.

[43] Bressey, C. 2011. The City of Others: Photographs from the City of London Asylum Archive. *Interdisciplinary Studies in the Long Nineteenth Century*: 13. https://www.19.bbk.ac.uk/. Accessed 24 July 2019.

Table 6.1 The distribution of Alien Lunatics in LCC Asylums, 1908

Asylum	*Male*	*Female*	*Total*
Banstead	13	12	25
Bexley	48	8	56
Cane Hill	15	3	18
Claybury	26	21	47
Colney Hatch	105	121	226
Hanwell	25	21	46
Horton	31	42	73
Long Grove	52	23	75
The Manor	–	23	23
The Colony	1	–	1
Total	316	274	590

Source LMA LCC/MIN/711 Housing and Treatment of Lunatics, 1908–10, 24 March 1908

relief.[44] Moreover, the Royal Commission on Alien Immigration listed the cities of Birmingham, Cardiff, Leeds, Liverpool, Manchester and Sheffield, as cities, along with London, that sent Aliens to asylums via their various Poor Law Unions.[45]

Those in port cities complained of a more transient issue, as in the case of Hull in 1880 when a German woman was found wandering about the docks in a state of insanity. The large numbers *en route* to the United States meant that the city regularly received ships of emigrants from Germany, Sweden and Norway. 'There is a strong suspicion', reported one local newspaper, 'that the poor creatures are sent out of their country to avoid the costs of their maintenance' leaving the rate-payers of Hull to bear the financial burden.[46]

As early as 1893, Colonel Thomas Sandys, the Conservative MP for Bootle, asked the Home Secretary in the House of Commons if he was aware that the United States policy of refusing immigrants on the grounds of pauper lunacy meant that the steamships returned them and then 'let them loose' on Liverpool docks. To be sure, the United States saw a growth of 'nativist' sentiment in this period, culminating in legislation

[44] Anon. 1903. Aliens and Poor Law Relief. *Manchester Guardian*, 4 April.

[45] HMSO. 1903. *Royal Commission on Alien Immigration, Vol. III*. London: Wyman & Sons: 36. https://parlipapers.proquest.com/parlipapers. Accessed 24 July 2019.

[46] Anon. 1880. German Lunatics in England. *The Sheffield and Rotherham Independent*, 20 April.

to restrict the immigration of certain groups. While it is unclear just how many had been refused entry to America and were then returned to Liverpool, Sandys sought clarification on whether other port towns suffered the same fate. More specifically, he noted that the maintenance of alien pauper lunatics cost the ratepayers of the borough of Bootle £350 per annum and he asked the Home Secretary if he 'would include provisions to remedy this grievance in the proposed measure to prevent the immigration of pauper aliens'.[47] Similarly, in 1904, the Lancashire Asylums Board noted that it had 134 alien lunatics in its county institutions, of which, Germans, Russians, Jews, Swedes and Italians were said to predominate.[48] Mr Shelmerdine, a representative of Liverpool on the Board pressed for them all be shipped back to their native countries on the grounds that they were costing the county almost £7,000 per annum but Dr Rhodes (see previous chapter) pointed out that many alien lunatics had homes and families in England, and that returning foreign lunatics was a game 'that two could play'.[49] Nevertheless, in the debate that followed, it was argued that it was unfair that Lancashire ratepayers bore the burden of so many alien lunatics being 'dumped down' in Liverpool.[50] The debate ended when it was pointed out that medical superintendents did all they could to send aliens back to their countries of origin.

Figures produced shortly afterwards revealed that London was the third largest immigration port in terms of passenger numbers behind Hull and Dover.[51] Immigration Ports were the top 15 places in the country that received regular traffic from continental Europe and further afield but there were 70–80 other places where aliens sometimes landed and these were known officially as non-immigration ports because of the relatively low numbers involved.[52] On the face of it,

[47] Anon. 1892. House of Commons. *The Times*, 27 May.

[48] Anon. 1904. Aliens in Lancashire Asylums. *Manchester Guardian*, 26 August.

[49] Ibid.

[50] Ibid.

[51] HMSO. 1906. Aliens Act, 1905. Part 1, First Annual Report of HM Inspector London for the Year 1906. https://parlipapers.proquest.com/parlipapers. Accessed 24 July 2019.

[52] Along with London the Immigration Ports Consisted of Cardiff, Dover, Folkestone, Grangemouth, Grimsby, Harwich, Hull, Leith, Liverpool, Newhaven, Newcastle, North Shields, South Shields and Southampton. Aliens Act, 1905. Part 1, Fifth Annual Report of HM Inspector London for the Year 1910 (HMSO, London, 1911): 33–4. HMSO. 1906. Aliens Act, 1905. Part 1, First Annual Report of HM Inspector London for the Year 1906. https://parlipapers.proquest.com/parlipapers. Accessed 24 July 2019.

this seems to suggest, that London had a far more enlightened policy when it came to the treatment of aliens but, again, there had always been limits to what the county authorities were prepared to pay for. Under the Lunatics Amendment Act of 1853, the maintenance of pauper lunatics was the legal and financial responsibility of the parish from where they were sent—in other words the Poor Law. If 'settlement' could not be determined, then the individual became the financial responsibility of the County and this included all costs involved in conveying them to the asylum, their care and their burial, removal or discharge.[53] As a result, asylum authorities, both before and after the passing of the 1888 LGA, worked hard to determine the origins of any patients arriving at their institutions without the appropriate settlement details.

In some cases, as in the case of James M., from Illinois in the United States who, after investigation, was found to have spent three years in St Pancras, it was possible to find details of settlement.[54] In such cases, the key was finding some other local authority that would pay the costs of treatment. This tended to be easier with English cases and, to a lesser extent, with Scottish and Irish cases. In 1888, for example, the Middlesex magistrates had 46 applications for orders on the County Rate. With six cases pending, nine of those 'successfully resisted' were English cases and followed detective work by the Middlesex Clerk of the Peace which involved talking with patients in a bid to find out more about their life histories. This necessarily included costs of travel and out of pocket expenses for the Clerk and 'county agents', amounting in this case to a little over £17. This was dwarfed, however, by the yearly savings on maintenance for the nine cases which was estimated to be £225 4s 6d and a potential saving of £4,880 6s 6d on their future long-term care.[55] Of the orders made on the County, three were English, five were Irish and five were 'Scotch' and the remaining eighteen were all foreigners. This included a 'South American' found to be insane on the arrival of his ship in the West India Dock and a Swede, a 'Finlander' and a native

[53]LMA LCC/CL/PH/01/276, Suggestions for Regulations as to Asylum Finance, LCC, 1889.

[54]LMA LCC/ 26.21. Annual Reports for LCC Asylums Committee for 1889–1892, the First Annual Report of the Asylums Committee of the London County Council, for the year ending 31 March 1890.

[55]LMA, MS/SP/1888/01/061. 1888. Twenty Third Annual Report of the Clerk of the Peace in Respect of Pauper Lunatics Chargeable to the County, 19 January.

of Guernsey who were all connected with ships lying in one of London's Docks. By 1905, the number of foreigners adjudicated to the County of London had risen to 89; 56 of which came from places other than England, Ireland or Scotland.[56]

Immigration, Degeneration and Disease

Immigration had never been a one-way process and the Jewish Board of Guardians, formed in London in 1859, had been facilitating the repatriations of Jews from Eastern Europe from at least 1882.[57] Nevertheless, much of the rhetoric focussed on in-migration and, in the 1880s, the Conservative press warned Londoners that Home Rule for Ireland would lead to an influx of Irish peasants.[58] Often, accounts of the campaign against alien immigration in this period focussed on the parts played by its impact on the labour market and the 'displacement' of native-born inhabitants, but there were other perceived threats to consider too.[59] The arrival of some Russian émigrés, including Peter Kropotkin had prompted fears of social unrest and perhaps even revolution.[60]

In 1893, the *Lancet* made the case for excluding all foreign nationals on three grounds—moral, sanitary and economic, and David Feldman suggests that the focus of the 'immigrant question' shifted from 'the domestic to the imperial consequences of poverty'.[61] In particular, where there had once been concern from across the political spectrum for the impact of immigrants on public health, sweated labour and poverty,

[56] H12/CH/A3/8. The Sixteenth Annual Report of the Asylums Committee and Sub-committees of Banstead, Bexley, Cane Hill, Claybury, Colney Hatch, Hanwell, Horton The Manor, Epileptic Colony and Long Grove, 1905.

[57] In addition to helping with emigration and repatriation, the Board's roles included maternity provision, sanitary inspection, apprenticeship schemes and convalescent homes. See Reeves, Carole Anne. 2001. Insanity and Nervous Diseases Among Jewish Immigrants to the East of London, 1880–1920. Unpublished PhD thesis, University of London: 81.

[58] Windscheffel, *Popular Conservatism in London, 1868–1906*: 57.

[59] Harris, Bernard. 1999. Pro-alienism, Anti-alienism and the Medical Professions in Late-Victorian and Edwardian Britain. In *Race, Science and Medicine, 1700–1960*, eds. Waltraud Ernst and Bernard Harris, 189–217. London: Routledge: 207–8.

[60] Shpayer-Makov, The Reception of Peter Kropotkin in Britain, 1886–1917: 373–90.

[61] Harris, Pro-alienism, Anti-alienism and the Medical Professions: 208. Feldman, The Importance of Being English: 57.

there was a move to link the low status of immigrants with Britain's imminent international decline.[62] Fears about the growing economic might of the United States and Germany, and defeats of the British army in the early stages of the Boer War (1899–1902) were compounded by a conviction in some quarters that the physical health of the nation's population was in decline.[63] Within this discourse, immigrants were seen as bringing down the stock of the nation but also, in lowering wages or displacing workers, they made it difficult for the native population to prosper in the face of falling standards of living.[64]

The links between this, the poverty of the East End, and the perceived degeneration that went with it, were key drivers in the Progressive demands for social intervention, but for the medical press one of the chief concerns was the existence of high rates of physical disease among immigrant populations.[65] While the Medical Superintendent reported outbreaks of influenza, and scarlet and enteric fevers at the Colney Hatch Asylum, however, he did not seek to lay the blame for this on foreign lunatics within his asylum.[66] One explanation for this may have been the fact that most medical writers viewed Jews to be as healthy as the populations around them, if not healthier, but not everyone agreed. In a study of the prevalence of tuberculosis in London Asylums, Mott found that the Jewish population at Colney Hatch, most of whom were aliens, were more likely to die from it, but, he concluded, there was no evidence to suggest that staff in any of the asylums were likely to contract it from the patients.[67] Moreover, while the 1903 Royal Commission on Alien Immigration recommended that the immigration of certain classes of aliens should be subject to state control, one of its members,

[62] Feldman notes that some trade unionists turned 'anti-immigrant' in the face of the defeats of new unionism and the breakdown of labour organisation among immigrant groups. Feldman, The Importance of Being English: 58.

[63] Harris, Pro-alienism, Anti-alienism and the Medical Professions: 195–6. Feldman, The Importance of Being English: 59.

[64] Ibid.: 59. For concerns about the fitness and efficiency of the nation see also Pick, *Faces of Degeneration*.

[65] Griffiths, Were There Municipal Networks in the British World: 195–6.

[66] See, for example, LCC 26.21. Medical Superintendents Report, Colney Hatch: 13 April 1893.

[67] F.W. Mott cited in *Sixty-Third Report of the Commissioners in Lunacy*, 1909: 78. For a detailed overview see Reeves, Insanity and Nervous Diseases Among Jewish Immigrants: *passim*.

Kenelm E. Digby, offered a number of reservations noting at the outset of the Report, that there was little evidence to suggest that immigrants from Eastern Europe should be excluded. Digby was the Home Office's permanent Under Secretary who, along with Lord Rothschild, represented two of the Commission dissenting voices.[68] It has been proved, he argued, 'that there is very little illness amongst these immigrants, and that they are not found to have introduced any infection or contagious diseases. There is little or no evidence that lunatics come over with them …' and their health 'appears to be superior to that of the native population'.[69]

Digby was responding to prevalent medical views and while 'the medical press was concerned about the existence of high rates of physical disease, it is arguable that the most alarming statistics were those relating to insanity'.[70] The *BMJ* concluded that in Prussia and Bavaria, Jews were twice as likely to be insane than 'native' Germans. Smith has shown that the apparent predisposition to lunacy of Jews and the responses to it were a point of concern for Jewish community organisations and the Jewish Press from the 1860s.[71] Fredcrick Mott, LCC's pathologist would later claim that it was inborn factors and their degenerative effects that meant Jews were more liable to insanity than Christians on account of their neurotic temperament. Clearly, there were debates taking place in medical and other circles about the foreigners in London's asylums but to understand the political response to this, it is important to understand the impact of both the Aliens Act *and* the result of the 1907 County Council election.

[68] Those offering opposing views were the 'restrictionists'. Alfred Lytlleton, Major Evans-Gordon, Henry Norman, and W. Vallance. See Pellew, The Home Office and the Aliens Act: 372.

[69] HMSO. 1903. *Royal Commission on Alien Immigration, Vol. I*. London: Wyman & Sons: 45. https://parlipapers.proquest.com/parlipapers. Accessed 24 July 2019. For further evidence of more positive views on the health of Jewish immigrants see Harris, Pro-alienism, Anti-alienism: 203–7.

[70] Harris, Pro-alienism, Anti-alienism and the Medical Professions: 195–6.

[71] Smith, Insanity and Ethnicity: 28–9.

London County Council, Alien Lunatics and the Burden on the Rates

As part of discussions about whether a new asylum was needed, it was John McDougall who again raised the issue of housing *all* foreign lunatics at Colney Hatch in February 1908.[72] The Asylums Committee passed the issue to the Special (Housing and Treatment of Lunatics) sub-committee to consider. Given its focus on the pressure it was receiving from the Commissioners in Lunacy to build the eleventh asylum, and also the initial plans for the proposed mental hospital that would become the Maudsley, the matter was adjourned and was only considered at a later meeting in May.[73] Meanwhile, the Clerk was able to report on the number of aliens across London's stock of asylums and on the arrangements made to interpret for them. As can be seen in Appendix 5, there was a significant minority of patients who were unable to communicate in English. With limited services outside of Colney Hatch, medical superintendents reported a variety of informal interpretation means including the use of other patients as well as medical staff and attendants.

The evidence presented in Appendix 5 suggests that the number of patients unable to communicate in English was low but there are limits to the veracity of some of the information provided. Jacob C., a Hebrew, for example, was admitted to Colney Hatch on 10 July 1907 and remained there well beyond the date of the information collection exercise in Appendix 5. On reception at Colney Hatch, he was spoken to in German by two separate medical men and it was noted that while he professed to understand, they could not get any information. Later in his case notes, it is reported at different times that he did not speak English and the only things he could understand were swear words.[74] In other cases, there is evidence of a failure to identify a particular language and, whatever the Appendix 5 may suggest, there was some exasperation on the part of the medical staff with this. Abraham A., for example, who was admitted in November 1907, was described as speaking in a 'foreign tongue' and being 'unable to understand the simplest directions – e.g.,

[72]LMA, LCC/MIN/574, Signed Minutes, February 1907–1908, 11 February 1908.

[73]LMA, LCC/MIN/711, LCC/MIN/711, Accommodation Sub-committee Minute Book, 1905–1908, 24 March 1908, 26 May 1908.

[74]LMA, H12/CH/B13/60, Colney Hatch Male Case Book, April–September 1907: 50.

"raise your arm"'.[75] Reeves has concluded that patients were frustrated with linguistic as well as cultural barriers and simply 'switched off'[76] but evidence such as this tells us something about the limitations of the Progressive rhetoric that stressed the positive and inclusive nature of its support and care services. Even so, after the consideration of the report, there was a reiteration of the desire to send all alien lunatics to Colney Hatch.[77] As ever, the practical application of this policy was driven, in part at least, by the availability of space across all of London's institutions but the refocussing of attention on alien lunatics was to be about more than just the rationalisation of services at Colney Hatch.

Beyond these investigations, the views of imperial London's place within the world appeared to be unconnected to the management of the capital's asylums. The Municipal Reformers were 'closely aligned with the Conservative Party and, as a corollary, to its wider protectionist policy of Imperial preference'.[78] After 1907, the new Municipal Reform dominated LCC privileged British goods in their purchasing policy and paid good wages in, for example, clothing contracts as part of an attempt to attract the working class to the benefits of protectionism.[79] The LMS, in light of the economic distress faced by London's unemployed, reiterated a long-standing commitment to support British goods and manufacturing. It stated

> That in all works carried out by the Council, preference would be given to local workmen; that when British and foreign companies tendered for public works, then preference would be given to the former; and that British materials were to be used on public works as far as possible.[80]

[75] LMA, H12/CH/B13/61, Colney Hatch Male Case Book, October 1907–June 1908: 30.

[76] Reeves, Carole Anne. 2001. Insanity and Nervous Diseases Among Jewish Immigrants to the East of London, 1880–1920. Unpublished PhD thesis, University of London: 321.

[77] LMA, LCC/MIN/711, LCC/MIN/711, Accommodation Sub-committee Minute Book, 1905–1908, 26 May 1908.

[78] Ball and Sunderland, *An Economic History of London:* 411.

[79] Ibid.

[80] LMA, CLC/088/MS19527, London Municipal Society, Minutes of Council Meetings, 24 November 1909.

The impact of this policy on the Asylums Committee was to be limited. In November 1908, it was noted that some of the sample brooms and brushes received by its central office appeared to be made abroad and a resolution that, in future, only those wholly or partly made in the United Kingdom were to be accepted.[81] More important was the decision to place a moratorium on the building of the eleventh asylum.

Although Goodrich, the new Municipal Reform Chairman of the Asylums Committee, argued that another asylum was not necessary, McDougall, one of his Progressive predecessors, countered that it took five years to build an asylum which in time would see another 2000 patients (approximately) ready to be admitted.[82] Within this context, attention was turned to the numbers of foreign lunatics. Following a request from Dr John Davies (Municipal Reform), the clerk provided statistical evidence of the foreign nationals in London asylums.[83] At that point, the clerk identified 590 individuals in LCC's ten institutions, which he categorised into 30 nationalities or groups. Within this categorisation there were some broad groupings that included 'negro' and 'South American'. Far and away the largest groups were 'Russian', of which there were 174, and Germans of whom there were 164. The vast majority of Russian patients (163), were in Colney Hatch whereas the German patients were distributed more evenly across LCC's asylum stock. The other groups to reach double figures were French 57, Italian 34, Swiss 14, Austrian 18, Dutch 19, Turk, 13 and 'Unknown', 15.[84] Of the total, 181 had been in an asylum less than one year, and only 11 had been in the country for less than one year.

The aim of this census activity was to work out which, if any, foreign nationals could be 'repatriated' under the 1905 Aliens Act. The wording of the Act had been influenced by existing legislation in other parts of the world, which had sought to define those deemed to be 'undesirables'. Acts in New Zealand (1873), Newfoundland (1872) and

[81] LMA, LCC 18.6, London County Council, Minutes of Proceedings, July–December 1908: 17 November 1908.

[82] LMA, PH/Ment/3/5, Newspaper Cuttings, 'Local Government Journal', 16 May 1908.

[83] An update on the census a year later revealed that the number had risen to 620. LMA, LCC/MIN/574, Signed Minutes, February 1907–1908, 10 December 1907. LMA, PH/Ment/3/5, Newspaper Cuttings, 'Local Government Journal', 14 November 1908.

[84] LMA, LCC/MIN/574, Signed Minutes, February 1907–1908, 11 February 1908.

the USA (1891) all targeted persons liable to become a charge on public finances and that included lunatics.[85] Along with the 1905 Act, these were aimed at the Immigration Ports and ascertaining which individuals had been in the country for one year was important to LCC for this reason. As Henry Rowe (Municipal Reform), the successor to Goodrich as the Chairman of the Asylums Committee explained, a pauper lunatic could not be deported unless he became chargeable to the poor rate within a year of him landing in this country.[86] Section 3 of the Aliens Act enabled the Home Secretary to make an expulsion order for an alien, if such a person had been within three months of proceedings being taken been in receipt of any such parochial relief that disqualified a person for the parliamentary franchise. 'As maintenance in an asylum as a pauper lunatic constitutes poor relief', pointed out the Asylums Committee, 'we have directed that steps shall be taken under this section with a view to the deportation where possible, of alien pauper lunatics admitted into the London County Asylums'.[87]

Significantly, deportations, rather than investigations into the settlement of foreign lunatics began under the rule of the Municipal Reformers who set in train a new set of administrative procedures in relation to new arrivals.[88] This change in policy is further emphasised by the fact that Boards of Guardians in Liverpool, Cardiff and Glasgow had already started to deport certain lunatics under the Aliens Act but that was the limit at that point. Even the London Boards had not explored this as an option.[89] At Claybury, the medical staff were reactive and, because of the action being taken with a view to deporting alien patients, Medical Officers began to try and ascertain whether any of the new admissions came from foreign shores. There can be little doubt that this was linked to the 'considerable overcrowding' there and the Asylums Committee moved that this should be replicated across all of its asylums

[85] Bashford, A. and Gilchrist, C. 2012. The Colonial History of the Aliens Act. *The Journal of Imperial and Commonwealth History* 40:3: 409–37.

[86] LMA, PH/Ment/3/5, Newspaper Cuttings, 'Local Government Journal', 16 May 1908.

[87] The Act also applied to those found to be wandering without means or those found to be living under insanitary conditions due to overcrowding. LMA, LCC 18.6, London County Council, Minutes of Proceedings, January–March 1908, 11 February 1908.

[88] LMA, LCC/MIN/574, Signed Minutes, February 1907–1908, 12 November 1907.

[89] Ibid.

with any foreign nationals reported to the central office for further action.[90]

Although informed by the consideration of an eleventh asylum, the immediate catalyst for this action was said to be a visit to London by Dr Colin of the Ville Juif Asylum in Paris. During his visit, Colin had told some members of the Asylums Committee that is was the practice to remove British subjects back to Britain from France, with the assistance of the British Consul. The Asylums Clerk made enquires at the Foreign Office, and staff there reported that it had no such knowledge of the practice but there was a desire on their part to deport all foreign lunatics where possible.[91] 'I understand that HM Inspector under the Aliens Act is willing to render the Committee any assistance in this power', noted the Clerk, and when it was intimated that the whole cost of deportation would be paid by the Home Office, the Committee resolved to take up this offer.[92]

It had been the unemployment of the 1880s and the riots that went with it that saw the first suggestions for a restriction on immigration. While Feldman has argued that the impact of immigration on 'sweating' was overstated by Liberals, Tories and trade unionists, it is possible to see broad party political ideals coalescing around the issue as time progressed.[93] Alex Windscheffel, for example, has traced restrictionist rhetoric back to the general elections of 1892 and 1895 with links drawn by Conservative candidates between immigrant labour and unemployment, low wages and overcrowding.[94] Similarly, Geoffrey Alderman, has shown that on a national level, the Liberal Party's opposition to the Aliens Bill and the Aliens Act, saw an upturn in the votes cast for it by Jewish voters.[95] This was the case in Leeds where the sitting MP and brother of the Prime Minister, Gerald Balfour, received a 'hostile reception'

[90] LMA, LCC/MIN/575, Signed Minutes, March 1908–February 1909, 10 March 1908.

[91] LMA, LCC/MIN/574, Signed Minutes, February 1907–February 1908, 12 November 1907.

[92] LMA, LCC/MIN/574, Signed Minutes, February 1907–February 1908, 12 November 1907.

[93] Feldman, The Importance of Being English: 58.

[94] Windscheffel, *Popular Conservatism in London*: 76–7.

[95] Alderman, Geoffrey. 1998. *Modern British Jewry*. Oxford: Clarendon Press: 191–2.

from the 'Leeds Jews [who] apparently banded together to vote for the Liberal candidate'.[96]

For those in the Liberal Party, the protectionist element of any restrictions on movement attracted criticism on the grounds that it was unpalatable to free-traders and 'also offended another sacred principle in the canon of Liberal beliefs; the principle of asylum'.[97] It has been said that the Liberal Party opposition to the Aliens Act, 'became a means of rediscovering identity' for the party.[98] As Bernard Harris points out, such an understanding of the opposition to restrictions on immigration offers important evidence of a more positive attitude to aliens. Indeed, by the time the Asylums Committee was taking the decision to explore the use of the Aliens Act to deport lunatics from its institutions, the Liberal Party under Prime Minister Sir Henry Campbell-Bannerman had taken control of the country following the 1906 general election. Both Campbell-Bannerman's, and his Home Secretary, Herbert Gladstone's, opposition to the Aliens Act make the suggestion that there was a desire to deport all lunatics where possible, unusual to say the least.

Election literature at the time of the 1906 general election satirised Liberal policy as a pudding of unpalatable, and with the inclusion of John Bull, unBritish ingredients (Fig. 6.1). Included in the 'recipe' was 'Alien Paupers' and this stemmed from Campbell-Bannerman's longer-term opposition to the imposition of restrictions on immigration. On the third reading of the Aliens Bill, as leader of the opposition to Arthur Balfour's Conservatives, he had voted against it on the grounds that 'the man most likely to make a good citizen has no chance to come into this country unless he has money in his pocket. But the worthless man, the scamp, the lazy man can come if he has money in his pocket'.[99] This was an issue raised by some members of the Independent Labour Party too who attacked the Balfour government's moves to restrict immigration on similar grounds. 'To His Majesty's Government, the alien question is a matter of locality – and money', wrote one member.

[96] Anon. 1906. The General Election. *The Times*, 9 January.

[97] Harris, Pro-alienism, Anti-alienism and the Medical Professions: 193-4.

[98] John Garrard cited in Pellew, The Home Office and the Aliens Act, 1905: 372.

[99] Sir Henry Campbell-Bannerman cited in McMahon, Aoife. 2016. *The Role of the State in Migration Control*. Boston: Brill Nijhoff: 52.

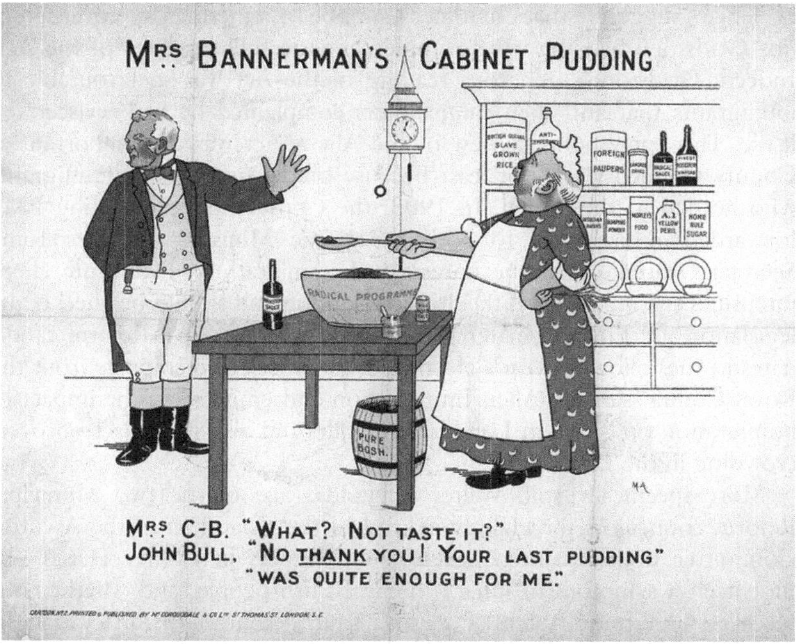
MRS BANNERMAN'S CABINET PUDDING
SLAVE GROWN RICE
FOREIGN PAUPERS
RADICAL PROGRAMME
PURE BOSH.
MA
MRS C-B. "WHAT? NOT TASTE IT?"
JOHN BULL. "NO THANK YOU! YOUR LAST PUDDING"
"WAS QUITE ENOUGH FOR ME."

Fig. 6.1 M.A. c.1906. 'Mrs Bannerman's Cabinet Pudding'. London: McCorquodale and Co. Ltd. London School of Economics, London. COLL MISC 0519/4 (Reproduced with permission of the London School of Economics under a Creative Commons Attribution-NonCommercial-ShareAlike [CC BY-NC-SA 3.0] license)

'If you are a Chinaman you are welcome in South Africa', he continued, 'and if you are a millionaire you are equally welcome in Park Lane, but if you are a Jewish tailor fying [*sic*] from injustice and persecution, you are not welcome in London at all … It is the duty of the working men of this country to prevent the perpetration of any such injustice'.[100]

More important in this context was the role of Gladstone who described the Aliens Act as a 'policy of his predecessors'.[101] All the

[100] Snell, H. n.d. *The Foreigner in England, the Problem of Alien Immigration*. Keighley: Wadsworth & Co.: 3.

[101] Glover, David. 2012. *Literature, Immigration and Diaspora in fin-de-siècle England, a Cultural History of the 1905 Aliens Act*. Cambridge: Cambridge University Press: 187.

evidence suggests that neither Campbell-Bannerman's government nor Gladstone had the will to implement the full measures of the Act. Indeed, Gladstone's generous reading of the Act was so favourable to immigrants that anti-alien campaigners complained he had 'eviscerated it'.[102] This party political view of the Aliens Act was also important at County Council level, not least because of the numbers of immigrants who headed to the capital. In 1903, the Conservative-supporting LMS forwarded a resolution to both the Prime Minister and the Home Secretary stating 'That the unrestricted immigration of destitute aliens intensifies the municipal difficulties of London and should be checked by legislation'.[103] Election materials produced for Municipal Reform candidates in the following year's election drew on selected snippets from the Royal Commission on Alien Immigration and emphasised the impact of immigration on crime in London generally, and also its impact on overcrowding in the East End.[104]

More specifically still, Walter Reynolds, one of the two Municipal Reform councillors for Hampstead, asked the Chairman of the Asylums Committee if the maintenance of alien paupers in Colney Hatch was 'not itself a symptom of lunacy in the British people, and whether our so-called Free-trade system was not a fruitful sources of lunacy (laughter)'.[105] While the immediate response to this was that individuals could not be repatriated unless they received poor relief within a year of their arrival, the numbers of alien lunatics in London's asylums were significant. In 1907, across London's metropolitan unions, 192 alien 'persons of unsound mind' were sent to a lunatic or imbecile asylum and another 74 were identified who had not been sent to an institution. These figures represented more than the combined totals for the principal towns and cities in the rest of England, Wales and Scotland.[106]

[102] Julius, Anthony. 2010. *Trials of Diaspora, a History of Anti-semitism in England*. Oxford: Oxford University Press: 276.

[103] LMA, CLC/088/MS19526, London Municipal Society, Minutes of Annual General Meetings, 14 December 1903.

[104] London Municipal Society. 1904. *London County Council Election, 1904: Facts and Arguments for Conservative Speakers and Candidates*. London: London Municipal Society.

[105] Anon. Our Alien Lunatics. *Daily Mail*, 13 May.

[106] Leeds and Manchester sent 32 and 31 aliens to asylums, respectively. HMSO. 1906. Aliens Act, 1905. Part 1, Second Annual Report of HM Inspector London for the Year 1907. https://parlipapers.proquest.com/parlipapers. Accessed 24 July 2019.

Clearly, there were wider medical concerns expressed about immigrants but the moves to repatriate these individuals was informed by the wider cost-cutting policies of the Municipal Reformers after the 1907 election. In reporting to the Council, the Asylums Committee stated that 'We need hardly point out the desirability of relieving the rates as far as possible, of the burden imposed upon them by reason of the maintenance imposed on them'.[107] Such attempts to remove 'burdensome' alien lunatics were welcomed by the Finance Committee, reflecting, as was shown in Chapter 3, the shared vision of the Municipal Reformers on public spending across the Council and its Committee.[108] The measures were also welcomed by the Commissioners in Lunacy who wrote of their hope that the repatriation of pauper lunatics, if successful, would do much to relieve the burden on the ratepayers of the County of London. For the Commissioners, it was the Government that was the driving force but there support was on the grounds that any such repatriations were in the interests of the lunatics themselves.[109]

In May 1908, a new census of alien lunatics revealed that there were 620 of them in London's asylums, of whom 232 were in Colney Hatch.[110] At this point, Sir Arthur Fell wrote to the Secretary of State for the Home Department to ask if he was aware of that fact, and that 'interpreters have to be provided for them, as they are mostly Russian Jews; and will he say how these aliens came to be admitted under the Aliens Act and whether there is a power to send them back to their country of origin'.[111] As the Conservative MP for Great Yarmouth, Fell was unconnected with LCC. Nevertheless, in line with the tropes apparent in the debates leading up to the introduction of the Aliens Act, Fell questioned what more could be done to exclude 'those who compete

[107] LMA, LCC 18.6, London County Council, Minutes of Proceedings, January–March 1908, 11 February 1908.

[108] LMA, LCC 18.6, London County Council, Minutes of Proceedings, November–December 1908, 22 December 1908.

[109] LMA, LCC 26.21, The Twenty-First Annual Report of the Asylums Committee of the London County Council, for the year ending 31 March 1910. The National Archive [Hereafter TNA], HO 144/970/B32798: ALIENS: Repatriation of Alien Lunatics, B32798/14.

[110] Anon. 1908. Our Alien Lunatics. *Daily Mail*, 13 May.

[111] TNA, HO 144/970/B32798: ALIENS: Repatriation of Alien Lunatics, B32798/24.

with the workers in the East End on London'.[112] However, in this case, his primary interest was in the steps that could be taken to deport those who had become a financial burden.[113]

In the follow up to Fell's questions, it was revealed that there had been 87 alien females and 96 alien males admitted to LCC asylums since the Aliens Act came into force on 1 January 1906 and up to 15 May 1908. Gladstone responded to Fell, describing his claims that they had been admitted under the Aliens Act as 'unfounded'. Of the 183 described by Keene, 112 had been in the country before January 1906 and only in 16 cases had they arrived since. Put simply, these people had been living and presumably working in London for a longer period than Fell had envisaged. Gladstone reiterated his power to only order expulsion, 'if a certificate is obtained from the court under Section (1) (b) of the Act'.[114] This section related specifically to those landing at a port and, if they were a lunatic or an idiot and likely to 'become a charge on the rates or otherwise a detriment to the public'.[115] There is some sense here of the anti-alien sentiment that was fomenting in relation to the treatment of lunatics after the passing of the Aliens Act but, as Gladstone explained, 'advantage is taken of this power in all proper cases'.[116] This caveat helps to explain the limitations of the Act. The majority of those in London's asylums had been in the country much longer than the twelve months demanded by the legislation and there was no power to apply it retrospectively. This was not the end of the issue, however, and to understand how these things were interpreted at a local level, there needs to be an understanding of how LCC used the legislation but also how it worked creatively in its attempts to expel individuals.

[112]Aliens in the East End of London, HC Deb 21 June 1906. Vol 159 c365. Historic Hansard. https://api.parliament.uk/historic-hansard/index.html. Accessed 24 July 2019.

[113]In 1906, Fell raised concerns about a deaf and dumb alien who was allowed into the country because it was impossible to establish his origins. Aliens Act, HC Deb 20 March 1906. Vol 154 c218. Historic Hansard. https://api.parliament.uk/historic-hansard/index.html. Accessed 24 July 2019.

[114]TNA, HO 144/970/B32798: ALIENS: Repatriation of Alien Lunatics, B32798/24.

[115]Aliens Act, 1905. 5 Edw. 7. Ch.13.

[116]TNA, HO 144/970/B32798: ALIENS: Repatriation of Alien Lunatics, B32798/24.

The Aliens Act, the Deportation of Lunatics and the Importance of Existing Legislation

At first, the number repatriated by LCC was relatively low. In the very first sweep, there was one male German and one Swiss woman with another four summons waiting to be heard.[117] By December 1909, the Asylums Committee reported that 18 lunatics had been repatriated under the Aliens Act and, again, the Finance Committee welcomed their continuing attempts to relieve the burden of such persons.[118] In the following year, a further 13 were repatriated under expulsion orders in the year ended 31 March 1910 and by August 1911, the number deported under the Act had reached 59.[119] This did not include a further 12 individuals who had been deported without the certificate being necessary, with another 8 cases still pending.

The prosecution of such cases demanded the services of a council solicitor with proceedings being heard before a magistrate. If the magistrate agreed to award a certificate for deportation under the Aliens Act, the case was passed to the Home Secretary to authorise the preparation of an expulsion order. In 1907–1908, for example, twelve applications had been granted by the presiding magistrate, but expulsion orders had been made by the Secretary of state in only five instances. He had declined to issue an order with a further six cases still under his consideration.[120] Where lunatics were summonsed to appear in court, they had to be physically fit and, somewhat ironically, mentally able to stand trial.[121] Patients could also apply for an adjournment so that they could acquire legal assistance. It is unclear how many took this opportunity but given that many of them were new to the country and were often poor it

[117] LMA, LCC 18.6, London County Council, Minutes of Proceedings, January–March 1908, 11 February 1908.

[118] LMA, LCC 18.6, London County Council, Minutes of Proceedings, December 1909, 14 December 1909.

[119] LMA, LCC 18.6, London County Council, Minutes of Proceedings, October–November 1910, 22 November 1910.

[120] LMA, LCC 26.21, Report of the Superintendent of the Colney Hatch Asylum for the year ending 31 March 1908.

[121] LMA, LCC/MIN/574, Signed Minutes, February 1907–1908, 11 February 1908.

seems unlikely that there would be either an understanding of the legal system or the financial wherewithal to make this likely.[122]

Hearings usually took place in the Bow Street Police Court as they did in the case of 'The Council v. Alexander H.', a Finnish seaman who had arrived in London aboard the SS Argyle from Christiana. Alexander was unable to attend and, after evidence was given in support of the Council's case, the magistrate 'intimated that he would issue his certificate to the Home Secretary recommending the expulsion of the alien'.[123] Shortly afterwards, with a missive from the Home Office, steps were taken to deport him to Russia under Section 77 of the 1890 Lunacy Act which stipulated that any three visitors of an asylum could order the discharge of a patient, even if that patient had not been cured. Of the thirteen people deported in the year ending 31 March 1910, four were escorted only as far as the English coast but it was more usual for them to be accompanied home. In Alexander's case, the Medical Superintendent reported that he had many volunteers from the attendant staff to travel with him.[124] By May of 1907, he had been deported to Hango in Finland with two attendants who left on the 15 May and returned on the 29 May. In the case of another seaman, Charli [*sic*] L., the removal to Gothenburg, also in line with Section 77 of the Lunacy Act, was expected to take one attendant seven days, which included travel, first to Grimsby to buy a ticket for the SS Aristo and then to Hull, to catch the boat.[125]

The two cases above were from the Bexley Asylum and the lack of extant case notes mean further consideration of the individuals involved is difficult. At Colney Hatch, the opposite is true and while the minute books do not appear to survive, some registers, reception orders and casebooks do. Even so, the evidence can be scant, particularly in relation to female patients. It is clear, however, that women were also deported under Section 77, as in the case of Louisa G. who was discharged relieved and deported to Germany in August 1909, and Mary K. who

[122] LMA, LCC/MIN/574, Signed Minutes, February 1907–1908, 11 February 1908.

[123] LMA, MIN/819/ Bexley Asylum Minute Book, July 1907–June 1908: 12 March 1908.

[124] LMA, LCC 26.21, The Twenty-First Annual Report of the Asylums Committee of the London County Council, for the year ending 31 March 1910. LMA, MIN/819/, Bexley Asylum Minute Book, July 1907–1908: 9 April 1908.

[125] LMA, MIN/819/, Bexley Asylum Minute Book, July 1907–1908: 9 April 1908.

was discharged recovered and deported to New York in June 1911.[126] Unfortunately, other more detailed evidence can be frustratingly absent. Where it does exist, it often reveals, again, the apparent importance of London as a port city and a point of disembarkation for foreign lunatics. This included Johanne V., a seaman, aged 28, from Holland. Johanne was a Protestant who apparently suffered from religious delusions but was otherwise in good health and during his short time in the asylum from April 1908 was described as quiet, orderly and employed. In August of the same year, he left the asylum in the charge of two attendants, headed for Amsterdam, where it was known that his father lived.[127] Simon O., aged 17, by contrast, had been convicted under an alias of Simon C. of stowing away aboard the SS Cestrian at Boston and sentenced to 21-days' imprisonment by Liverpool City Court for that offence and a further 21 days for wilful damage to the ship's fittings. It is likely that he headed to London because of a relative (an aunt) who was based in Mile End. On admission to Colney Hatch in December 1907, he was described as 'not so well mentally – owing to self-abuse and at different times he was said to be mischievous and troublesome'. In the Summer of 1908, he was sent in from the institution's summer fete after aggressively begging from visitors and the final entry before his discharge revealed that 'he can do nothing for himself, has to be dressed frequently wet and dirty'.[128] Despite being in a 'katatonic [*sic*] stupor', and therefore not 'mentally able', he was deported to Russia on 25 June 1910 under the Aliens Act. Simon had been Colney Hatch for over two years, and as a corollary, claiming parochial relief for that period too. The Aliens Act also allowed the deportation of those who had committed crimes but the evidence of why it took LCC so long, relatively speaking, to deport him is frustratingly absent.[129]

[126] LMA, H12/CH/B/003/006, Colney Hatch, Register of Female Patients, 1851–1914.

[127] LMA, H12/CH/B13/61, Colney Hatch Male Case Book, October 1907–June 1908: 103.

[128] LMA, H12/CH/B13/61, Colney Hatch Male Case Book, October 1907–June 1908.

[129] 'Under the Aliens Act, 1905, sec 1, leave to land can be withheld and sec 3 enables the Secretary of State to make an expulsion order requiring an alien to leave the United Kingdom, *inter alia*, … if it is certified to him by any court … that the alien has been convicted by that court of any misdemeanour or other offence for which the court has power to impose imprisonment without the option of a fine or an offence under par II of Sec 54 of the Metropolitan Police Act 1839 (note 2 &3 Vic c.47).' LMA, LCC/MIN/574, Signed Minutes, February 1907–1908, 12 November 1907.

The Aliens Act enabled the authorities to deport individuals in a way they had not done before, but this should not obscure the provisions of the existing lunacy legislation. In addition to Section 77 of the 1890 Lunacy Act, repatriation could also be governed by Section 71 which stated that it was only allowed where the family or friends of the patient desired removal and when the Secretary of State was convinced it would be of benefit.[130] In these cases, it is easy enough to see a role for families with individuals being discharged into their care. Betsy B., for example, was removed to Russia by her friends in December 1906.[131] After the Municipal Reformers came to power, Rachel S., a 19-year-old cigarette maker, was deported to Russia by authority of the Secretary of State under Section 71 and left Colney Hatch in the care of Myer S., and Rachel and Sally M., even though her address had been given as Mile End.[132] Similarly, Marie A. was removed by her husband to Germany following a warrant signed by the Secretary of State under Section 71. The supposed cause of Annie's insanity was said to be puerperal mania and her husband Frederick, a waiter who lived with her in William Street, St Pancras claimed that she blamed him for the death of their child. When Marie was released, it was Frederick who went with her to Germany.[133] For Margarita C., the extant records simply note that she was removed to Italy by her friends in December 1908.[134]

These cases, in particular, are significant because if the issue rested solely with finances, then the existing lunacy legislation offered families the opportunity to reclaim their kin and remain in the country. Under Section 79 of the 1890 Lunacy Act, those taking responsibility for their kin who were not 'cured', had to sign an official document, stating that the person concerned would 'no longer be chargeable to any Parish,

[130] LMA, LCC/MIN/574, Signed Minutes, February 1907–1908, 12 November 1907.

[131] LMA, H12/CH/B/003/003, Colney Hatch, Register of Female Patients, 1894–1898, H12/CH/B/003/006, Colney Hatch, Register of Female Patients, 1851–1914.

[132] LMA, H12/CH/B/46/63, Colney Hatch Female Reception Orders, 16451–16475: 16474.

[133] LMA, H12/CH/B/003/006, Colney Hatch, Register of Female Patients, 1851–1914. LMA, H12/CH/B/46/62, Colney Hatch Female Reception Orders, 16376: 16399: 16380.

[134] LMA, H12/CH/B/003/006, Colney Hatch, Register of Female Patients, 1851–1914.

Union, Liberty or County, and shall be properly taken care of and prevented from doing injury to her/himself or others'.[135]

It is possible that extended familial networks in countries of origin were behind some decisions to return home but, in other cases, pressure was exerted on some family members with some patients only discharged into the care of their friends on the understanding that they would return 'home'.[136] This included, Alexander M., who was described as a German Protestant and a carpenter and who also lived in Mile End with his wife and baby. Alexander arrived at Colney Hatch in January 1908 and in the final entry before he was discharged in August 1908, he was described as 'depressed and persecuted by voices who deny that his wife visits him and says that it is his sister'. Nevertheless, he left the asylum a few months later, leaving with an 'obstinate' bout of conjunctivitis 'on an undertaking from his wife with arrangements having been made for him to proceed back to his own country (Russia)' with no explanation of the confusion over his country of origin.[137] In other cases, the records reveal that people were discharged as 'relieved' and then deported with no reference to either the Aliens Act or the Lunacy Act.[138]

Return migration of people with lived experience of mental ill-health remains an under-researched area and the surviving evidence here says little about how the individuals being deported felt about the process.[139] Nor do they reflect on what the impact must have been on the people who remained on the wards after their peers had been removed but there were those who advocated for them. In a debate in Liverpool about the immigrants being 'dumped down' in the port, Dr Rhodes (see Chapter 5) pointed out that the matter sending people 'home' was not so clear cut as

[135] LMA, H12/CH/B/46/63, Colney Hatch Female Reception Orders, 16404: 16425: 16422.

[136] LMA, LCC 26.21, The Nineteenth Annual Report of the Asylums Committee of the London County Council, for the year ending 31 March 1908. LMA, LCC 26.21, The Twenty-First Annual Report of the Asylums Committee of the London County Council, for the year ending 31 March 1910.

[137] LMA, H12/CH/B13/61, Colney Hatch Male Case Book, October 1907–June 1908: 63.

[138] LMA, H12/CH/B/003/006, Colney Hatch, Register of Female Patients, 1851–1914, 29 April 1910, 10 October 1910, 26 November 1910.

[139] McCarthy and Coleborne, Mental Health, Migration and Ethnicity: 4.

many alien lunatics had lives and families in England.[140] This was certainly the case with Marco B., a 26-year-old piano action maker and Roman Catholic, who was admitted to Colney Hatch in June 1909. Although Marco had an impulse to commit suicide and was living with auditory hallucinations, it was noted that he was able to 'converse rationally on many points'. His language skills no doubt rested with the fact that, at the time of him being sent to the asylum he had lived in England for 22 years and had attended school there. The relative giving evidence on the reception order was his sister, and his father was listed as living in Clerkenwell. Despite this, and despite the fact that his symptoms showed no sign of abating, the case notes described him being 'transferred back to Italy'.[141] The same went for John W. an 18-year-old butcher who arrived at Colney Hatch in July 1907 via the St Giles Workhouse, having previously lived with his brother in Broad Street, Golden Square. John was described as melancholic who required 'some persuasion' to take his food and in November of the same year was described as untidy, unemployed, having faulty habits and interfering with other patients, which was becoming so troublesome it necessitated his removal. Although it was later noted that he had improved, his health was good and he was less interfering, the final entry in the casebook, recorded that he was deported to Warsaw.[142]

In John's case, it is unclear what, if any role his brother, or any other relative played but in other cases, the role of families appeared to be limited or even non-existent. It is highly likely that without the need for negotiation with family members or the ability to do so, it made the process of deportation easier. Ernest O., a Protestant from Germany who was apparently so violent that he was admitted to Colney Hatch under restraint, had no other family in England, and was deported to Germany within six months.[143] Annie A., 29 years old, and single was a cigarette maker who was admitted from the Whitechapel Union infirmary where she was described as 'strange and incoherent'. Annie had been admitted on 19 August 1907 and the asylum authorities wrote immediately to the relative listed on her reception order, an uncle, Mr Lavtasky of Queens

[140] Anon. 1904. Aliens in Lancashire Asylums, *Manchester Guardian*, 26 August.

[141] LMA, H12/CH/B13/63, Colney Hatch Male Case Book, February–October 1909: 83.

[142] LMA, H12/CH/B13/60, Colney Hatch Male Case Book, April–September 1907: 52.

[143] LMA, H12/CH/B13/63, Colney Hatch Male Case Book, February–October 1909: 72.

Road Clapham. The aim of the letter in such cases, alien or otherwise, was to inform relatives of the locus of their kin and to inform them of the times they could visit and the rules associated with it. Unfortunately, the letter was returned unopened a week later. In the interim, the asylums authorities contacted the Whitechapel Union, who has already returned her watch and ring, to ask them for the whereabouts of her 'pass-port'. While no other details are recorded it was noted in the Female Register that she was discharged relieved and deported to Russia in January 1908.[144]

Whatever had been the focus of the Aliens Act, its operation by the Asylums Committee was not limited to those that had been identified as 'problematic' in the debates leading up to its passing. Indeed, despite Kenelm Digby's reservations, the Royal Commission on Alien Immigration had recommended the regulation of some groups, including those from Eastern Europe and such views were prevalent in various official reports.[145] The report of His Majesty's Inspector under the Aliens Act, avoided any discussion of 'polemical matters' but, in line with the origins of the Aliens Act and its focus on Jewish Immigration from Russia, a survey of the first five years of the Act divided immigration into two key groups. The first was the majority of Russian immigrants of the Jewish faith who were engaged in three main industries of tailoring, cabinet-making and boot making. It was noted that, in the main, most of these individuals travelled to stay with relatives or friends who may have been settled in the country for some time. The Aliens Act had an impact on these groups and, while in 1906, the numbers making their way through the port of London, mainly to the East End was 7425 by 1910 it had fallen to 2463. The other, second group was of a 'miscellaneous' kind and included those passing through the cross-channel ports. The numbers here also looked to be falling but it was unclear if it was

[144]LMA, H12/CH/B/003/006, Colney Hatch, Register of Female Patients, 1851–1914, 27 January 1908.

[145]HMSO, 1903 *Royal Commission on Alien Immigration, Vol. I.* London: Wyman & Sons: 36. https://parlipapers.proquest.com/parlipapers. Accessed 24 July 2019.

quite the 'genuine decrease' that was happening in London with Russian immigrants.[146]

This division of immigrant groups into (Russian) Jews, and then everyone else, was mirrored in the Superintendent's annual report for Colney Hatch. In 1908, he noted that during the previous twelve months, 146 Jewish patients (72 men and 74 women) had been admitted and the total in the asylums was 421, an increase of 65 on the previous year. In the same period, 56 (31 men and 25 women) aliens were admitted and the total number in the asylum was 234 (115 men and 119 women). Of this figure, 167 (77 men and 90 women) were Jewish patients of Russian nationality, and the Superintendent noted that many of them were of a 'very low type'.[147]

In terms of medical attitudes, as Bernard Harris has pointed out, with the vast majority of Jewish immigrants being poor, and it can be difficult to separate attitudes to race from attitudes to poverty.[148] At Colney Hatch, however, the two were often conflated and a patient admitted in 1895 was listed in the case notes as 'Unknown Man' because it proved to be impossible to get any personal or other details from him. His description as both 'a short dark man, thick set of foreign type' and 'a Russian Jew' on admission was indicative of stereotypical profiling.[149] This may have also been the case with Victoria K. who had been originally identified as a 'Jewess' but at some point during her stay, this had been scratched out after a note on the file was made indicating that the Doctor had said that her religion should be changed to Roman Catholic. Even so, she was discharged as 'recovered' and deported to Hamburg in September 1909, revealing that in terms of the monies to be saved from the repatriation of lunatics, gradations of race became

[146]Along with London the Immigration Ports consisted of Cardiff, Dover, Folkestone, Grangemouth, Grimsby, Harwich, Hull, Leith, Liverpool, Newhaven, Newcastle, North Shields, South Shields and Southampton. HMSO. 1911. Aliens Act, 1905. Part 1, Fifth Annual Report of HM Inspector London for the Year 1910. https://parlipapers.proquest.com/parlipapers. Accessed 24 July 2019.

[147]LMA, LCC 26.21, Report of the Superintendent of the Colney Hatch Asylum for the year ending 31 March 1908.

[148]Harris, Pro-alienism, Anti-alienism and the Medical Professions: 194–5.

[149]H12/CH/B13/43A, Colney Hatch Male Case Book, October 1895–April 1896, 10 December 1895.

Table 6.2 Nationalities of individuals deported from LCC Asylums, 1909

Nationality	N
German	14
Russian	10
Dutch	6
Austrian	5
American	5
Italian	5
French	4
Swiss	3
Finnish	2
Swedish	1
Norwegian	1
Greek	1
Chinese	1
Roumanian [*Sic*]	1
Total	59

Source LMA, LCC 18.6, London County Council, Minutes of Proceedings, October–November 1911, 24 October 1911

much less important.[150] As the Superintendent of Colney Hatch concluded, 'An endeavour is now being made to effect the repatriation of *all* alien patients who have been only a short time in the country'.[151]

Table 6.2 reveals the destinations of those deported by LCC's Asylums Committee in the first few years of the Aliens Act. On the one hand, this reflects the cosmopolitan nature of the people involved and is further evidence, if it was needed, of London's status as a magnet for immigrants from around the world. On the other hand, it is indicative of how the issue of deportation had become reductive for politicians. This additional evidence emphasises the fact that the attempts to reduce spending on a new asylum had become straightforwardly entwined with anti-alien sentiment. Rather than focussing on this 'type' or that 'type' of immigrant, as official and medical reports still tended to do, it merely focussed on the fact that these were foreigners who were no longer a

[150] LMA, H12/CH/B/003/006, Colney Hatch, Register of Female Patients, 1851–1914.

[151] My emphasis. LMA, LCC 26.21, Report of the Superintendent of the Colney Hatch Asylum for the year ending 31 March 1908.

burden on the rates—even where their maintenance costs were covered by the Poor Law Unions.

Despite this, one key criticism of the Municipal Reformers, was, that for all their rhetoric, they failed to significantly reduce expenditure, and it was the same here.[152] The number of foreign nationals affected by increased attempts to deport them represented a significant minority of all patients. It is difficult to know how many were 'encouraged' to return home using the provisions of existing lunacy legislation but only 10% of the aliens identified in London's asylums were deported under the auspices of the Aliens Act (see Table 6.2). Of the 59 cited, the Home Secretary had vetoed the proposed deportation of another 14 cases providing some evidence, at least, that the new Liberal government was not simply deporting individuals in all cases. Another four patients in this period had died before an order could be effected and one patient had been removed to a private asylum.[153]

Deportations, Negotiations and International Diplomacy

The evidence above has to be mediated by the fact that LCC did not always act alone, either in the UK or abroad. The Public Control Department of the Council 'rendered valuable assistance' to immigration officers appointed under the Aliens Act to the cases of young immigrant women who arrived in London with letters from native employment agencies offering them work.[154] This was in addition to the support from voluntary agencies, such as the Jewish Association for the Protection of Girls and Women, which worked primarily in the East End of London. They were concerned with prostitution and other groups focussing on 'social purity' worked in other parts of the country.[155] These organisations were

[152] Ball and Sunderland, *An Economic History of London*: 411.

[153] LMA, LCC 18.6, London County Council, Minutes of Proceedings, October–November 1911, 24 October 1911.

[154] The Public Control Department had a wide remit and employed 'about a hundred inspectors at work administering Acts over the metropolis which the Council had to enforce'. Its work was aimed at the 'individuals who would inflict injury or injustice on the community'. Anon. 1892. *Three Years Good Work*: 24.'

[155] Bartley, Paula. 2000. *Prostitution, Prevention and Reform in England, 1860–1914*. London: Routledge: 171.

not always looking to deport individuals and the Jewish Association, which had been formed in 1885, had expressed concerns that in some countries, young Jewish women were 'driven to vice through physical and mental distress'.[156] In such cases they lobbied against deportation on the grounds that those sent back would be at the mercy of border guards who might be unsympathetic to their plight and, possibly even anti-Semitic.

By contrast, Carol Reeves has shown that the Jewish Board of Guardians had no hesitation in funding the repatriation of patients released from Colney Hatch 'on trial', even though they had not been officially discharged, on the grounds that their anti-social behaviour had become an embarrassment to the local community.[157] In addition to the cases above, Tseng F. Y., a Buddhist, was discharged as recovered in April 1910 after seven months in Colney Hatch and apparently left to go back to China. This was welcomed by the Chinese Legation in London who described him 'as not a desirable person to have in England' and asked for advice on the best means for prosecuting deportation.[158] In these cases, parochial and provincial authorities could elicit support from the Foreign Office, who in turn would liaise with the Home Office. The Town Clerk for Tynemouth sought such support to repatriate Pedro N. to Spain and parochial authorities abroad also had a role to play.[159]

In the years immediately following the passing of the Aliens Act, there were several attempts to agree on diplomatic accords at a governmental level. James Moran and Lisa Chilton have explored how foreign states contested notions of lunacy using English in the nineteenth century but in this case there was an attempt to formalise agreements at the level of the state.[160] These usually came via the UK's Foreign Office and, in 1908, the Home Department received a missive from Sir Edward Grey, the Foreign Secretary, to explain that the French Embassy in London

[156] Ibid.

[157] Reeves, Insanity and Nervous Diseases Among Jewish Immigrants: 76.

[158] LMA, H12/CH/B13/63, Colney Hatch Male Case Book, February–October 1909: 125.

[159] TNA, HO 45/10360/154554 LUNACY: Repatriation of Lunatics—Arrangements Between Great Britain and Spain, 22 May 1907.

[160] Moran, J. and Chilton, L. 2016. Mad Migrants and the Reach of English Civil Law. In *Migration and Mental Health*, ed. Majorie Harper, 149–70. London: Routledge: 159–65.

was willing to reach an agreement in regard to the repatriation of French and English pauper lunatics.[161] Grey's biographer has shown that he wanted Britain to have closer relations with France and this may have piqued his interest.[162] Research into the matter by the Foreign Office showed that by 1904, agreements existed with France, Germany, Italy, Austria and the Netherlands, even if the nature of them was not 'precisely ascertainable'.[163] It was clear, however, that they focussed on the retention of lunatics, rather than their expulsion. Civil Servants at the Foreign Office considered any such agreement to have come to an end with the introduction of the Aliens Act and opened discussions so that arrangements for mutual Anglo-French repatriations might be made.[164] The Home Department was important here and, via information collected by the Commissioners in Lunacy, passed the details of individuals in asylums, along with any contact details of living family and/or friends, to the Foreign Office.[165]

The Foreign Office was primarily concerned with British nationals abroad, but after much negotiation with the French authorities, The Scottish Office, the Irish Government, the LGB and the Commissioners in Lunacy, any agreement reached an impasse. The Home Department, felt that it would not be a good policy to upset the existing arrangements whereby the United Kingdom and the principal European countries maintained each other's pauper lunatics.[166] The Home Department's stance rested on two key factors. The first of these was the issue of asylum and, in response to Grey, Gladstone's Office re-emphasised that the Aliens Act enabled the facilitation of deportation but that did not make it obligatory. The Secretary of State, the letter to Grey stated,

[161] TNA, HO 45/10560/169330 LUNACY: France and United Kingdom. Repatriation of Pauper Lunatics, 26 August 1908.

[162] Robbins, K. 2011. Grey, Edward, Viscount Grey of Fallodon. *Oxford Dictionary of National Biography*. https://www.oxforddnb.com/. Accessed 4 July 2019.

[163] TNA, HO 144/970/B32798: ALIENS: Repatriation of Alien Lunatics, B32798/20.

[164] Ibid.

[165] See, for example, TNA, FO 369/36: Russia, Code 238, Files 176–18279: 375.

[166] TNA, HO 45/10560/169330 LUNACY: France and United Kingdom. Repatriation of Pauper Lunatics, 28 October 1911.

> does not think it would be right to enforce the expulsion from the country of an alien lunatic, who with his family and friends had lived in England for many years and would practically be a stranger in his own country; and the reverse would hold good, for it would not be desirable to repatriate to England a British Lunatic whose long residence in a foreign country had made him for all practical purposes a native of that country.[167]

The second issue was a practical one that related to the numbers of British nationals in foreign asylums, compared with the numbers of foreigners in British asylums. Even after 1905, His Majesty's Inspector under the Aliens Act wrote to the Home Office to once again highlight the issue of lunatics who had been refused entry into the United States, being 'dumped' in Britain's ports. 'England [sic] has no grievance against America expelling her undesirable aliens but England's position in the line of traffic renders her particularly open to be damaged by American expulsions…'.[168] The reference here was to the UK's geographical place in migrations to the United States from continental Europe, with migrants making their way into the country through ports such as London and Hull and then travelling, often via the railways, to a point of departure such as Liverpool.[169] Indeed, the concerns raised here mirrored the debate that had taken place in that city and, along with the issue of many aliens having family in England, Dr Rhodes argued that many more Englishmen were being maintained in foreign asylums.[170] While the Municipal Reform dominated LCC may have complained about the impact of foreign nationals, discussions between the Home Department and the Commissioners in Lunacy revealed that there were 817 foreign nationals in the asylums in England and Wales, while reports from the State Board of Insanity for Massachusetts alone suggested that they had treated 1500 British lunatics between 1904 and 1906.[171]

[167] TNA, HO 144/970/B32798: ALIENS: Repatriation of Alien Lunatics, B32798/14.

[168] TNA, HO 45/10360/154559 ALIENS: Repatriation of Insane or Helpless Aliens from U.S.A. 5 August 1907.

[169] Panayi, Panikos. 2010. *An Immigration History of Britain: Multicultural Racism Since 1800*. London: Routledge: 53.

[170] Anon. 1904. Aliens in Lancashire Asylums. *Manchester Guardian*, 26 August.

[171] TNA, HO 45/10360/154554 LUNACY: Repatriation of Lunatics—Arrangements Between Great Britain and Spain, 2 March 1908.

Attempts by LCC to similarly identify and remove Scottish and Irish lunatics were also vetoed by the LGB. 'We are therefore reluctantly compelled to refrain from taking any further action', concluded the Committee, 'and such lunatics must continue to be a charge upon the London ratepayers as they cannot be removed upon adjudication'.[172] Similarly, when in 1910 the Asylums Committee wanted to ramp up the deportation of other groups, the Clerk wrote to the Under Secretary of State for the Colonies asking for some arrangement to be put in place for the repatriation of 'colonials'.[173] This was particularly problematic for LCC because everyone born in the British Empire was considered to be British and were, therefore, beyond the scope of the Aliens Act.[174] After receiving a response, the Clerk warned the Committee that there probably more London Lunatics in the Colonies than 'colonials' in London Asylums, which would potentially mean more lunatics rather than fewer.[175] Without state-sponsored help in these cases, LCC continued to conduct its own longer-term negotiations, as was the case of Canadian, Thomas K. Thomas had arrived at Liverpool as a steerage passenger on the SS Sagamore in November 1912 and was admitted to Bexley Asylum in the following month. From February 1913, the Clerk of Asylums Committee had been in correspondence with Canadian Authorities as well as the White Diamond Steamship Company to discuss the terms of his deportation.[176] It was the 'Department of the Interior, Government of Canada Emigration Branch' who facilitated discussions with the Province of New Brunswick, which, in turn, agreed to receive Thomas at its provincial Hospital for the Insane. These longer-term discussions help to explain why he was not deported until 1915.[177]

As such, the decision to seek and carry out expulsions remained in the hands of parochial authorities and the Home Department and Foreign Office were only involved where the transfer of individuals came within their purview. One example of this was the British subjects held in the

[172] LMA, LCC 18.6, London County Council, Minutes of Proceedings, July–October 1908, 14 July 1908.

[173] LMA, LCC/576, Signed Minutes, March 1909–July 1910, 9 November 1909.

[174] I am grateful to Wendy Webster for this information.

[175] LMA, LCC/576, Signed Minutes, March 1909–July 1910, 8 February 1910.

[176] LMA, LCC/MIN/580, Asylums and Mental Deficiency Minute Book, November 1914–July 1915, 27 July 1915.

[177] Ibid.

Egyptian Abbassia Asylum, which came to the notice of the Foreign Office following contact from His Majesty's Consular Officers in the country. The asylum was described as 'insufficient' for the care of British nationals and with British steamship companies refusing to transport lunatics or demanding prohibitive rates to do so, assistance was sought to explore alternative ways to repatriating them. Only after negotiations between the Commissioners in Lunacy, the Home Department, the Foreign Office and the War Office was the use of army transports authorised which enabled British Nationals to return home.[178] In other cases, the local decisions to expel individuals from the UK continued to vex some national agencies. Also in 1910, the government of the Netherlands complained via diplomatic channels to the Foreign Office that the deportation of Dutch nationals by LCC, was in breach of an earlier agreement in which 'it was agreed that each country would take charge of lunatic subjects of the other, and found within its territory'.[179] This was to be followed by complaints from the French government about the expulsion of pauper lunatics from the Channel Islands of Jersey and Guernsey.[180] It was these very local decisions, including those by LCC, that led to some national agreements. An Anglo-German agreement was reached in 1913 after the German Government been described as 'making all manner of difficulties in regard to cases of German pauper lunatics whom we try to expel in in pursuance of certificates under the Aliens Act'.[181] Similarly, a final note on the files relating to an Anglo-French agreement suggested that 'French lunatics are now about the only ones we cannot get rid of', while another note in another hand added 'Yes, but they did not like the shape which the draft took and they have been smothering it'.[182] Either way, any such agreements did not replace existing, local processes or lead to blanket deportations.

[178]TNA, HO 45/10659/212622, Repatriation of British and Maltese Lunatics from Egypt, 1911–1912.

[179]TNA, HO 144/970/B32798: ALIENS: Repatriation of Alien Lunatics, B32798/36.

[180]TNA, HO 45/10560/169330 LUNACY: France and United Kingdom. Repatriation of Pauper Lunatics, 28 October 1911.

[181]TNA, HO 45/10995/167955: MENTAL HEALTH: Repatriation of Foreign Lunatics. Anglo-German Agreement, 1913, 16755:1.

[182]TNA, HO 45/10560/169330 LUNACY: France and United Kingdom. Repatriation of Pauper Lunatics, 26 January 1914.

This, no doubt, was due to the number of foreign lunatics in London's asylums but it was for this reason that in 1913, the Home Office signalled its intention to shift the burden of expulsion from national to local funds. The Home Secretary, who by that time was Reginald McKenna, stated that the principal effect of deportation was to relieve local rates, and as a corollary, felt, that the local authority when called upon should pay up to one-half in those cases that cost more than £15.[183] The Asylums Committee responded saying that the proposals may hinder or prevent future repatriations. By this time the total number of alien lunatics deported by LCC had risen to 68 and 28 of them had cost more than £15 per person. Given the Liberal government's treatment of the Aliens Act, it is no surprise that the McKenna would not move on the issue but the Asylums Committee's threats of a moratorium on future deportations proved to be hollow. Indeed, they immediately set about negotiations with the Finance Committee, which, in turn, applied to the LGB for sanction under the Local Authorities (Expenses) Act, 1887, to cover the expenditure of one-half of the cost of the repatriation of a female patient to Hungary.[184] The costs of these cases could differ enormously, depending on where individuals were being deported to, but this did not prevent the policy of repatriations from continuing. The deportation of Mier G., for example, involved negotiation with the United States' authorities, who arranged to meet him on arrival, payments to attendants to travel with him across the Atlantic and estimated costs of £36, of which the Council was expected to pay half.[185] In December 1913 *The Times* reported that estimated costs of removing three alien lunatics would be £92, £23, and £34 with costs to the Council of £46, £11 10s, and £17, respectively. With rising costs, the Finance Committee pushed the Asylums Committee to claim the costs of deportation from the Poor Law Guardians, via the LGB. This, once again, emphasised the role of settlement but it was intimated that, if this could not be agreed, then any deportations would cease. In the end, it was the outbreak of war in 1914 that curtailed attempts

[183] LMA, LCC/578, Signed Minutes, March 1912–October 1913, 25 February 1913.

[184] Ibid.

[185] LCC costs were sanctioned by the Local Government Board under the Local Authorities (Expenses) Act, 1887. LMA, LCC/MIN/580, Asylums and Mental Deficiency Minute Book, November 1914–July 1915, 24 November 1914.

to deport individuals to Europe, as in the case of Gustav L. who had been scheduled to return to Russia.[186] Thus, at the very end of the period covered by this book, there was a debate about whether the costs of deportation represented value for money or not. As the Municipal Reform dominated Asylums Committee minutes record, the relatively 'small and definite' liability of deportation compare very favourably with the 'considerable and indefinite liability' of ongoing institutional treatment.[187]

Conclusions

While there has been a developing interest in the treatment of foreign nationals in asylums around the world, the impact of the United Kingdom's 1905 Aliens Act has received little attention. Generally speaking, as Harris points out, 'the development of medical attitudes to anti-alienism was also influenced by a wide range of other factors, including the persistence of anti-Semitism, the rise of Social Darwinism, the fear of national and racial decline, and the belief that the influx of foreign immigrants threatened the foundations of Britain's nascent welfare state'.[188] These factors go some way to explaining the stereotypical descriptions of foreigners in the Colney Hatch casebooks. More importantly, this chapter has emphasised the importance of political views in driving policy on the maintenance of alien pauper lunatics in London's asylums.

To be sure, there were some continuities across the period and, whatever Sidney Webb may have claimed about the positive impact of the Progressive administration, the apparently benign interventions on behalf of Jewish patients, for example, did not simply begin and end with the election victory of 1889. Given the shared focus of all candidates on value for money, there had always been some limits to what aliens might expect in terms of their asylum experience. Indeed, concerns about the costs of the treatment of foreign lunatics were being expressed by politicians and commentators in places other than London long before the introduction of the Aliens Act

[186] LMA, LCC/MIN/580, Asylums and Mental Deficiency Minute Book, November 1914–July 1915, 24 November 1914.

[187] LMA, LCC/MIN/580, Asylums and Mental Deficiency Minute Book, November 1914–July 1915, 26 January 1915.

[188] Harris, Pro-alienism, Anti-alienism and the Medical Professions: 207–8.

in 1905. Even though some on the political left had supported anti-immigrant measures, in London the most vocal of critics were in the Municipal Reform party and those allied to it. Their election victory in 1907 allowed them to exclude alien paupers in a way that had not been done before in the capital, and it was this that acted as the catalyst for change. By this time, the terms 'deport' and 'repatriate' were used interchangeably, and it was only in the negotiation of an Anglo-German agreement that any references to the expelling of individuals were replaced with 'repatriation'.[189] This was an obvious attempt to somehow soften the language that would have been little comfort to those forcibly removed, especially those such as Marco B. who had been in the UK for most of his childhood, and all his adult life.

The limits of the Aliens Act, along with a central Liberal Government that lacked the inclination to implement it, meant that the numbers directly affected in LCC asylums were small. This does not necessarily reflect its wider impact. Unfortunately, the case notes do not record how those made doubly vulnerable by their alien status, and their perceived parlous mental state felt about deportation, how they reacted to it, or how they were received when they returned 'home'. Nor does it consider the impact on those who remained on the wards. In terms of numbers too, the figures are somewhat clouded by the ongoing references to the provisions of 1890 Lunacy Act. This Act had offered the authorities a longer-term opportunity to deport individuals, so long as it was in their best interests. The evidence here shows that, after 1907, some people were encouraged to return 'home' and that was followed by a series of failed attempts to repatriate even more individuals. The failure to reach an agreement with the 'colonies', or to reach an agreement with the LGB for the expulsion of Scottish and Irish paupers only serves to shine a light on the motivations of the 'new' Asylums Committee. Politicians, as well as the press, and those in the medical professional had all raised concerns about the potential for immigrants to have a deleterious effect on public order, public health and the public purse. In this case, the moves by LCC to deport individuals were indiscriminate and

[189]TNA, HO 45/10995/167955: MENTAL HEALTH: Repatriation of Foreign Lunatics. Anglo-German Agreement, 1913, 16755:5.

were intimately connected with the decision to postpone the building of London's eleventh asylum. As such, it is easy to see the connections with broader political outlooks but also frame that within the Municipal Reform approach that sought to arrest the public spending. With this in mind, it seems unlikely that the Progressives, had they remained in power, would have adopted the same approach.

CHAPTER 7

Conclusions

It is easy to see the twin issues of well-being and mental ill-health as something that affect us all and, as a result, as non-contentious areas of policy that are somehow above the grubby world of party politics. Commenting on the passing of LCC's Hospitals into the hands of the NHS in 1948, for example, the Chairman of LCC, Walter Owen stated that:

> 'our natural feelings of regret at the passing of this service is tempered by the knowledge that we have given into capable hands a hospital organisation in London second to none in the world in size and efficiency and in the humanitarian purpose it has achieved.'[1]

Such comments look back to those early suggestions that emphasised the limited control that LCC had on its then nascent Asylums Committee. They also look forward to the all-party parliamentary groups that seek to wrestle with the apparently inexorable demand for mental health services in the twenty-first century. What this book has shown, by contrast, is the significant impact that democratic politics had on the finances, management and mismanagement of asylums and their treatment regimes.

[1] London County Council, *LCC Hospitals: A Retrospect*: 10.

R. Ellis, *London and its Asylums, 1888-1914*,
Mental Health in Historical Perspective,
https://doi.org/10.1007/978-3-030-44432-7_7

To be clear, this has not been an attempt to turn the clock back to those 'dry as dust narratives' that failed to include the interrelations between asylums and the world beyond their walls.[2] Instead, it has shown that by extending the scope of analysis into the wider social and political affairs of London, it has placed the management of asylums within a complex web of issues that help to explain the development of its services. A forensic analysis of the committee records pertaining to London as a municipality, rather than case studies of its individual asylums alone, illuminates their place in the consciousness of politicians and the political class in this period. Methodologically too, extending the analysis to (party) political tracts and election materials, helps to explain the motivations of decision-makers, even if they often remain frustratingly anonymous in terms of their lives outside of those sources.

The 1890 Lunacy Act compelled local authorities to build and manage institutions, just as the 1845 Act had done before it. In doing so it draws our attention to the ways in which the post-1888 authorities facilitated, rather than negotiated or interpreted such legislation. In reality, the introduction of the LGA, brought party political scrutiny to the management and treatment of madness for the first time. What followed in London was periods of political dominance, by first the Progressive Party and then the Municipal Reformers, which fundamentally impacted on the administration of lunacy. In this respect, we can, again, look forward to the twentieth and twenty-first centuries and an understanding that mental health policies do not appear in a (party) political vacuum. Instead, the direction of services was and is defined in the liminal space that exists in the obligation to provide services, but it is one that is framed by wider ideologies and the priorities that stem from them. It is within this space that we can see the interpretation of national legislation at a local level and politicians were not, and are not, mere ciphers in this process.

This is not to claim that the party was king because party loyalties were not as clearly defined as they have been in later periods. Nevertheless, election victories and majorities in the council chamber allowed parties those all-important first steps of choosing the Chairman of committees, and then packing those committees with individuals of similar political views or shared values. Here, we have to be careful because even in the committee rooms, people did not vote on

[2] Ignatieff, Total Institutions and Working Classes: 168.

straightforward party political lines. Whatever election and other materials might have said, there was not a single unified vision for the management of London, or its asylums. This was partly because of the breadth of opinion that existed with those parties and because, as this book has shown, all too often the ways in which councillors voted were affected by a myriad of other issues. Personal and local interests, along with the careful spending of public money were mediating factors for all councillors who had to face their electors every three years. Nevertheless, the driving force for key initiatives came from individuals with an interest in pushing forward their own agendas and it was people like McDougall, Cooper and Collins who were able to draw on wider party-based support when 'outsiders', such as Brudenell Carter were not. Moreover, while the Progressives broadly supported the inclusion of women on the Council, not least because of their potential roles in the care of female lunatics, its party structures and processes for their nomination as candidates did not make this immediately achievable.

Often, the administration of the capital's lunatic population depended on a series of small steps, tortuous at times, starting with the Asylums Committee or one of its sub-committees. Support in these places allowed initiatives to be further tested in the Council Chamber, even if that process could take months and years as plans and initiatives were passed up through the hierarchical committee structure, debated at each point, and then passed back down again for adoption, revision or rejection. This emphasises the importance of the Council's committee structure, but it also highlights the role played by attendance. It was only those councillors who attended committee meetings that could hope to shape policies but, once again, rather than being separate from the political landscape, the management of asylums was seen as central to it. Indeed, party election literature from both sides reveals that issues relating to asylums, including committee attendance, were rarely top of the agenda when it came to political campaigns but the fact that it featured there at all, reveals its importance to wider political discourse and debate.

Significantly, the treatment of what today would be called vulnerable individuals was used as an important context in attacks on opposing parties and their policies. Such attacks were not limited to the Council Chamber or the committee rooms used by the Asylums Committee. Debates and disagreements spilled out into the pages of the press. The representations of what passed for good work was coloured by the politics of those newspapers, with the *Spectator* and the

Star offering key examples of Conservative and Liberal views, respectively. The fact that *The Times* reported only on the work of one County Council (London) meant that the work of its Asylums Committee featured in the national press but, beyond this visibility, we should not presume that in terms of the management of madness, London was exceptional.

In his lectures to the Collège de France in 1973 and 1974, Michel Foucault explored the strategies of power that gave rise to discourses of truth. For him, the locus of this power was very much focused on psychiatry and its domain within the 'battlefield' that was the asylum.[3] This limits our understanding of the impacts of a shifting political landscape, and fails to take into account how politicians sought to define their own truths. Hyperbole and excoriation of asylum management—in particular relating to treatment of patients, good or otherwise, were nothing new. However, this period saw a shift away from a focus on individual asylums and their staffs to broader attacks on the wider politically-based management structure that was the Council. The decision to remove beer is one obvious example here and, although it was implemented mainly as a result of John McDougall, it was nevertheless co-opted, presented and seen as a Progressive policy, and was praised and condemned in equal measure on those terms. Similarly, as this book has shown, asylums were often represented as sites of 'mismanagement' or probity by the Council, depending on the political lens through which they were viewed. Both parties marshalled evidence that enabled them to conduct attacks on both the management of asylums specifically and the management of London, more generally.

More importantly, the management and administration of asylums became useful ammunition in the fundamental debates surrounding the provision of welfare and whether that represented good value for money or not. Here, of course, we need to be attentive to the critiques of important figures in the History of Psychiatry, such as Foucault and Andrew Scull. Both have highlighted the social and economic factors in the genesis of institutional responses to madness, and the dominance of bourgeois ideologies in their development. Nevertheless, the levels of investment in policies on health were determined both by financial capacity and the will to intervene in key areas. In the run-up to

[3] Foucault, Michel. 2008. *Psychiatric Power: Lectures at the Collège de France, 1973–1974*. Basingstoke: Palgrave Macmillan: 7, 93.

the introduction of the LGA and in its aftermath, the Liberal and the Conservative parties had very different visions for the management of the capital. The Progressives regarded 'municipal activity as the best solution for social problems' but the extension of government into a range of key areas was to draw the ire of the Moderates and Municipal Reformers.[4] As Davies points out, the 'partisan dichotomy' between both parties on the adoption of 'advanced, activist driven, municipal programmes' was evident in the Progressives aspirations to control public services and their corresponding rejection of municipal enterprise.[5] It was these issues that marked the clear water between the parties and influenced key decision-making in this period, and the management of asylums cannot be separated from it.

Melling and Forsythe have shown the developing strength of the Finance Committee in Devon in the period after the passing of the LGA. There is some sense of that here and as well as the lunacy legislation, the operation of the Council and its Asylums Committee was governed by an increasing number of rules and regulations in the form of its Standing Orders. Nevertheless, without a consideration of party politics in this period, it is easy to see mental health as a series of purely administrative and internecine disputes. In London, a more stringent financial regulation of the Asylums Committee only really came with a change in the majority administration in 1907 when it, the Finance Committee, and the whole Council was dominated by the Municipal Reformers.

With the election victory of 1907 came other key changes too, which saw Municipal Reformers attempts to limit the size of (local) government and spending and, as a corollary, drive down the rates. Ultimately, they managed to stabilise the rate at 1s 5d but they failed to significantly reduce expenditure. In the interim, their attempts to rein in public spending affected the management of asylums as attempts were made to squeeze budgets. With this in mind, it would be easy to suggest that the period of Progressive rule was a golden age for asylums and their staff and patients, but this was clearly not the case. Imperialistic notions of London's place in the world directly affected the treatment of those vulnerable individuals, and politicians, as well as medical professionals, were seduced by the rhetoric of eugenics and segregation.

[4] Porter, *London: A Social History*: 332.

[5] Davies, Local Government 1850–1920: 52–3.

As a propagandist, Sidney Webb was just one of the political commentators who did an excellent job of talking up both the Progressive-dominated LCC and, *inter alia,* its Asylums Committee. Other key stakeholders involved in the management of madness, such as Poor Law Officials and the Commissioners in Lunacy, were apt to point out the shortcomings in care and, by implication, some of the rhetoric that stressed only the positives of their administration. Ongoing issues of overcrowding and abuse at London's asylums show the limits of political claims but there is evidence that for some patients, things changed for the worse after 1907. In this case, we can see the impact in the reductions in budgets that led to more beds being squeezed into already overcrowded wards, and reductions to maintenance budgets that must have impacted on individual asylum environments. Then, there was the targeting of foreign patients and, again, there is a link here to politicians' broader world views. Recent debates in the UK about EU nationals and Commonwealth citizens in the wake of the Windrush scandal are just two examples of how easy it is for settled status to become disrupted by political and economic concerns. In the case of the Aliens Act, fears about the apparently parlous state of the Empire and the impact that undesirable aliens were having on the general stock of the nation had a direct impact on the treatment of patients. Linking this to attempts to reduce spending after 1907 meant, that while individual experiences of care may not have changed, the chances of foreigners being deported in this period greatly increased—even if they had been living in Great Britain for a significant amount of time.

None of this means that experts were not important or that patients and their families were unable to resist the asylum or use it for their own purposes. However, while the expertise of staff such as the Asylums Clerk and the Asylums Engineer was procedural, in other cases the opinion that politicians allowed themselves to be influenced was mediated on how far those opinions matched their own political and personal ambitions in each case. It is telling that when Clifford Smith was tasked with the design of the eleventh asylum for London, it was on the grounds that he understood, more than any external architect, the 'practical requirements of the [Asylums] Committee'.[6]

[6]LMA, LCC/MIN/711 Accommodation Sub-Committee Minute Book, 1905–1908, 3 July 1906.

Studies of modern-day services have highlighted the dominance of western definitions of mental ill-health and their apparent universal portability to other geographies and cultural contexts.[7] In the period that LCC was formed, medical opinion remained divided on how pauper lunatics should be best treated and divided on how lunacy should be prevented. It is this understanding that helps to explain why the medical press often despaired of some of the decisions made by the Council. They, and medical staff within LCC structures such as Stansfield, may have pushed for more investment in acute services but there were always limits to how far politicians were prepared to go with that. This narrative may help to explain why this period that has often been seen as a time of stagnation, retrenchment and retreat, and why its institutions were described by Scull as 'Museums of Madness'. Cochrane too has followed this narrative and has seen the initial discussions and development of the Maudsley Hospital as an aberration. Instead, he argues that the mainstream pre-occupation of the Asylums Committee was one of sequestration, but this was not the case.[8] The example of Receiving Houses is pertinent here, not just because it was hoped that they would bring about a reduction in the numbers accessing institutional care, but also because the Asylums Committee used this and other potential initiatives to postpone the building of other large-scale asylums. Understanding this in relation to the Progressive aspiration to affect the wider administration of London adds nuance to this, but it is clear both parties wanted to call a halt to the building of large-scale institutions. While they ultimately failed, the Progressives wanted to shift investment to acute and extra-institutional services, while the Municipal Reformers simply wanted to rein in spending across the board. During the era of Progressive dominance at least, we can see cheaper facilities being discussed for groups such as aged patients but we can also see these discussions being stymied on the grounds they did not 'serve all the interests', and did not meet the vision that placed LCC as world leader in care.

We already know what Poor Law Officials and the Commissioners in Lunacy thought of such views but to this we can add the patients themselves. Politicians may have claimed to advocate for the people in their care, but they were not really interested in their opinion. Even here, understanding their support is dependent on understanding two key

[7] Mills, China. 2014. *Decolonizing Global Mental Health: The Psychiatrization of the Majority World*. London: Routledge.

[8] Cochrane, Humane, Economical and Medically Wise: 265.

factors. The first of these is the ballot box and the triennial elections which meant that politicians always had an eye on the issue of the rates and how that might play out for the electorate. In this context, this was much more important than the patients themselves. Those whose care was paid for by the Poor Law found themselves excluded from the franchise and while this book has tried to include how patients responded to LCC's management of asylums, it has largely eschewed substantive analysis on the grounds that politicians were not interested in their individual responses. Again, the abolition of alcohol is a good example of this and while it was evidently not liked by the patients, and neither was it welcomed by all in the medical profession and within the Lunacy Commission, it did not stop the Progressives making political capital of the changes. In this respect, we can see the emergence of another group, namely party politicians, who claimed to advocate on behalf of the patients as part of their wider strategies for government. The co-opting of patients as part of party rhetoric marks another important shift in their roles in elections and electioneering.

This is not to say that, all of a sudden, these parties had plans and policies on mental health because they did not, and this brings us to a second key point. Whatever politicians, then and now, may claim about their responses to mental ill-health and its care and treatment, the responses to it were and are defined by how that fits within their broader world views. The fact that, at the time of writing, we are living in an age of austerity and we have seen a retrenchment in public funding brings the issues described above into sharp relief. What this book has clearly shown, however, it that we cannot hope to understand the historical development of services without an understanding of the politics and the ideologies of those involved. Whatever politicians may claim, their policies on mental ill-health are not 'non-contentious' and they are not apolitical.

Appendix 1: List of Officers and Staff at the Long Grove Asylum, 1907

Male officers	Medical staff (5)	Medical Superintendent
		First Asst. Medical Officer
		Second Asst. Medical Officer
		Third Asst. Medical Officer
		Fourth Asst. Medical Officer
	Clerk's office (3)	Clerk of the Asylum
		First Asst. Clerk
		Second Assistant Clerk (2)
	Stores (5)	Storekeeper
		First Clerk
		Second Clerk (2)
		Storekeeper's Boy
	Head attendants (4)	Head Day Attendant (3)
		Head Night Attendant
	Engineers office (2)	Foreman Engineer
		Engineers Stores Clerk
	Others (3)	Inspector
		Dispensing Chemist
		Farm Bailiff

(continued)

R. Ellis, *London and its Asylums, 1888-1914*,
Mental Health in Historical Perspective,
https://doi.org/10.1007/978-3-030-44432-7

Female officers	All (5)	Matron Head Night Attendant Workmistress Laundrymistress Head Day Attendant
Attendants	All (172)	Male (86) Female (86)
Additional staff	All (25)	Stores Porters (4) Gate Porters (2) Coal Porter (1) Laundryman (1) Baker (1) Butcher (1) Fireman (1) Tailor (1) Pigman (1) Labourers (5) Cowmen (2) Shoemaker (1) Carters (3) Asst. Gardener (1)

Source LMA, LCC/MIN/574, Signed Minutes, February 1907–February 1908, 14 May 1907

Appendix 2: The Asylums Committee After the 1907 Election

Name	*Additional*	*Party*	*Meetings (possible)*	*Meetings (attended)*	*Attendance (%)*
A.O. Goodrich (Chairman)	J.P.	MR	15	15	100.0
J. Davies	M.D., J.P.	MR	15	15	100.0
H.J. Greenwood		MR	15	15	100.0
T. Hunter		P	15	15	100.0
W.C. Johnson	J.P.	P	15	15	100.0
L. Salmon	(to 9 July 1907)	MR	5	5	100.0
E. Denny	Rev.	P	15	14	93.3
C. Jesson		P	15	14	93.3
H.R. Taylor (Vice Chairman)	J.P.	P	15	13	86.7
E.G. Easton	J.P.	MR	15	13	86.7
W. Haydon		MR	15	13	86.7
Sir John McDougall		P	15	13	86.7
E. White, J.P.	Alderman, from 1904*	MR	15	13	86.7
A. Pownall		MR	15	12	80.0
H.V. Rowe		MR	15	12	80.0

(continued)

R. Ellis, *London and its Asylums, 1888-1914*,
Mental Health in Historical Perspective,
https://doi.org/10.1007/978-3-030-44432-7

Name	*Additional*	*Party*	*Meetings (possible)*	*Meetings (attended)*	*Attendance (%)*
Lord Alexander Thynne		MR	15	12	80.0
P. Vosper		MR	15	12	80.0
F.S. Smith		L	15	11	73.3
G. Dew		L	15	10	66.7
The Earl of Kerry	MVO, DSO	MR	15	10	66.7
W.L. Dowton	J.P.	MR	15	9	60.0
G.K. Naylor	Alderman from 1907**	L	15	9	60.0
E.A.H. Jay	To 11 June 1907	MR	4	2	50.0
T. Chapman		S	15	7	46.7
W. Reynolds		MR	15	7	46.7
C.K. Murchison	To 12 November 1907	MR	9	4	44.4
The Viscount Lewisham		MR	15	6	40.0
W. Crooks	M.P.	P	15	4	26.7
G. Billings	J.P.	MR	15	3	20.0
W.W. Thompson	Alderman from 1904*	MR	15	3	20.0
F.L. Dove		MR	15	1	6.7
R.H. Montgomery		MR	15	1	6.7
W.S.M. Knight	From 19 July	MR	5	0	0.0
The RH Lord Michelham	From 8 October 1907. Alderman from 1907**	MR	7	0	0.0

MR—Municipal Reform, S—Socialist, P—Progressive, L—Labour
*'London County Council', *The Times*, 16 March 1904, p. 4
**'London County Council', *The Times*, 9 March 1907, p. 13

Appendix 3: Suggested Sites for a New Asylum, 28 February 1905

	Name of estate	*Locality*	*Miles from London*	*Nearest station*	*Miles from railway station*
1	Northaw Great Wood	Potters bar	16	Potters Bar	4
2	Carpenders Park	Pinner	15	Bushey	1½
3	Leggatts Farm	Watford	19	Watford	1
4	Little Bushey Estate	Bushey	16	Bushey	1½
5	Cross Farm	Bovingdon	25	Boxmoor	2
6	Bendrose Farm	Amersham	23	Chalfont	¾
7	Durrants Estate	Coxley Green, Rickmansworth	22	Watford	2¼
8	Roughwood Park	Chalfont	20	Chorley Wood	1
9	Naphill	West Wycombe	38	West Wycombe	2
10	Hazelemere	High Wycombe	35	High Wycombe	2

Source LCC/MIN/711 Accommodation Sub-Committee Minute Book, 1905–1908, 28 February 1905

R. Ellis, *London and its Asylums, 1888-1914*,
Mental Health in Historical Perspective,
https://doi.org/10.1007/978-3-030-44432-7

Appendix 4: Membership of LCC's Committee on a Hospital for the Insane, 1890

Committee member	*Affiliation*	*Membership of other LCC Committees*	*Other memberships listed*	*Member of the Asylums Committee, April 1890*
Francis Culling Carr-Gomm, J.P.	Progressive	None listed	Late Chairman of the Committee for the London Hospital	Yes
Robert Brudenell Carter FRCS	Moderate	Vice Chairman of the Sanitary and General Purposes Committee	Ophthalmic Surgeon to St George's Hospital	Yes
John Burns	Progressive	None listed	None listed	No
Captain Walter Haweis James RF	Moderate	Chairman of the Sanitary and General Purposes Committee	None listed	No

(continued)

R. Ellis, *London and its Asylums, 1888-1914*,
Mental Health in Historical Perspective,
https://doi.org/10.1007/978-3-030-44432-7

Committee member	*Affiliation*	*Membership of other LCC Committees*	*Other memberships listed*	*Member of the Asylums Committee, April 1890*
John Hutton	Progressive	Chairman of the Building Act Committee	Member of the Committee of the Royal Free Hospital; Vice Chairman of the London Temperance Hospital	Yes
(Dr? Listed as Mr) George Blundell Longstaff, MB, FRCP	Moderate	None listed	None listed	No
Philip Meadows Martineau, J.P.	Progressive	Chairman of the Asylums Committee	None listed	Yes

Source LCC/CL/PH/01/276, Report of the Committee on a Hospital for the Insane, LCC, 1890

Appendix 5: Alien Lunatics Unable to Communicate in English in LCC Asylums, 1908

Asylum	*Male*	*Female*	*Total*	*Difficulty, if any, as to interpretation*
Banstead	3	3	6	No difficulty … as there are several sensible persons among the patients and several of the medical staff are able to converse with them…
Bexley	9	1	10	No great difficulty … in the case of Europeans but with Eastern races there has been considerable difficulty….
Cane Hill	2	1	3	Both males are demented and unable to make their wants known … female has rudimentary knowledge of English but can…
Claybury	1	5	6	So far no difficulty…
Colney Hatch	29	48	77	All can make their wants known through the interpreter attendant except one male patients who speaks Spanish
Hanwell	–	–	–	None
Horton	4	14	18	Considerable difficulty occurs in some cases … Many of them are able to express themselves by signs in an intelligent manner. It is probable that a large number could not be understood by any interpreter owing to incoherence and language defects

(continued)

R. Ellis, *London and its Asylums, 1888-1914*,
Mental Health in Historical Perspective,
https://doi.org/10.1007/978-3-030-44432-7

Asylum	*Male*	*Female*	*Total*	*Difficulty, if any, as to interpretation*
Long Grove	13	16	29	None
The Manor	–	4	4	... [The] Medical Superintendent has always been able to find an interpreter among one of the remaining alien patients upon whom he can rely to give a correct translation
The Colony	1	–	1	Have to rely entirely upon signs ... often a matter of difficulty and results are unsatisfactory
Total				

Source LMA LCC/MIN/711 Housing and Treatment of Lunatics, 1908–1910, 26 May 1908

Bibliography

Archival and Manuscript Sources

Bishopsgate Institute

228/10. 1898. Fabian Society, Questions for London County Councillors.

229/12, Davies, A. Emil. 1937. *The LCC 1889–1937: A Historical Sketch*. London: Fabian Society.

229/14. 1905. Entente Municipale, Visit of the Municipal Council of Paris, to London.

230/4, Baumann, Arthur A. c.1890. The London County Council. *The Universal Review*: 493–502.

LH P4168. 1913. Women's Local Government Society, LCC Election, an Appeal to Women.

LH P2291. 1891. Fabian Society, Questions for London County Councillors.

P3008. 1890. Fabian Society, Questions for Reform Candidates.

P3422. 1913. Women's Local Government Society. Nineteen Reasons Why Women Are Wanted on London County Council.

British Library

Anon. 1901a. *The London County Council of 1895 and 1898*. London: Alexander and Shepherd.

Anon. 1901b. *London County Council Election 1901*. London: Alexander and Shepherd.

Anon. 1901c. *London County Council: A Letter to Women Electors*. London: Alexander and Shepherd.

R. Ellis, *London and its Asylums, 1888-1914*,
Mental Health in Historical Perspective,
https://doi.org/10.1007/978-3-030-44432-7

8139B22. c.1907. *The Daily Mail and the Fight for London: A Handbook to the London County Council Election Giving both Sides.*

Rhodes, J. Milson and Marshall, Edwin W. 1902. *Report on a Visit of Inspection to Colonies and Hospitals.* London: P.S. King and Son.

Guildhall Library

LMS72. 1910. London Municipal Pamphlets and Leaflets.

'LCC Election 1907', Copy of Manifesto issued 4 December 1906.

'The London County Council', Municipal Reform Leaflet A23.

'Municipal Reform and Model Management', Municipal Reform Leaflet A16.

'Why Was the Works Department Closed?', Municipal Reform Leaflet A7.

LMS106. 1898. *London County Council, Election 1898, Facts and Arguments.* London: London Municipal Society.

LMS107. 1904. *London County Council, Election 1904, Facts and Arguments.* London: London Municipal Society.

LMS108. 1910. *London County Council, Election 1910, Facts and Arguments Vol. 1.* London: London Municipal Society.

LMS110. 1913. *London County Council, Election 1913, Facts and Arguments.* London: London Municipal Society.

LMS116. 1912. Borough Council Elections 'Municipal Reform v Progressive Socialism'.

LMS122. 1908. London Municipal Pamphlets and Leaflets.

'The Progress of Municipal Reform', Municipal Reform Pamphlet 26.

'The Work of Municipal Reform in London, 1907–1909', Municipal Reform Pamphlet 37.

'The Progress of Municipal Reform—It's Your Money We Save', Municipal Reform Pamphlet 102.

LMS123. 1909. London Municipal Pamphlets and Leaflets, 'The Work of Municipal Reform in London, 1907–1909', Municipal Reform Pamphlet 37.

LMS124. 1909. London Municipal Pamphlets and Leaflets.

'What the Municipal Reform have done in Two Years!', Municipal Reform Leaflet 117.

'You Must Vote Again for Municipal Reform. Why?', Municipal Reform Leaflet 127.

GL LMS126. 1909. London Municipal Pamphlets and Leaflets.

'Rising rates', Municipal Reform Leaflet 136.

'How the Radical-Progressive Government Raises Your Rates', Municipal Reform Leaflet 140.

LMS127. 1909. London Municipal Pamphlets and Leaflets. 'The Progress of Municipal Reform', Municipal Reform Pamphlet 47.

LMS132. 1898. London Municipal Society. Election Leaflets and Pamphlets.

'Reckless Squandering of Ratepayers Money', Leaflet No. 41.

'Electors of London!', Leaflet No. 46.

'Squandering the Rates', Leaflet No. 55.

LMS133. No date (n.d.). London Municipal Society, Election Leaflets and Pamphlets.
'Truth Will Out!', Leaflet No. 12, Series A.
'Municipal Reform v Progressive Socialism', Leaflet No. 17.
PAM3462. 1911. *Sixteenth Annual Report of the London Reform Union for 1910*. London: London Reform Union.
PAM3472. 1898. Progressive Party Leaflets. 'Who Have Done London's Work?', Leaflet No. 9.
PAM3556. 1907.
'What the Progressive Party on the County Council has done for Temperance in London?', Leaflet No. 13.
'A Letter to Women Electors?', Leaflet No. 18.
PM 3438. 1907. Progressive Leaflets, London County Council Election 1907.
'The Progressives and Temperance Reform'. London: Progressive Election Committee.
'Eighteen Year's good Progressives Work for the People'. London: Progressive Election Committee.
SL:30:03. 1898. A Collection of Tracts.
London Municipal Society, 'Election 1898, Facts and Arguments', London Municipal Society.
Sir John Lubbock, 'On the Real Issues of the London County Elections', London: London Municipal Society.

House of Commons Parliamentary Papers

The annual reports of the Commissioners in Lunacy have been accessed via the House of Commons Parliamentary Papers website. https://parlipapers.proquest.com/parlipapers.
Copy of the Annual Reports of the Commissioners in Lunacy to the Lord Chancellor, from the Forty-third Report (1889) to the Sixty-fourth Annual Report (1910).

John Rylands Library

LCC. 1907. *Report of the Education Committee of the London County Council Submitting a Report of the Council's Officers on the Bathing Arrangements in Schools in Germany and Holland*. London: P.S. King and Son.

London Metropolitan Archives

ACC/1632/001, Minutes of the Progressist Party of the London County Council, 1890–1895.
ACC/1632/002, Minutes of the Progressive Party of the London County Council, 1895–1900.
ACC/3606/001, Election Literature and Newspaper Cuttings, 1906–1907.
BBG/423, St Olave's Union Committee Reports, 1892–1893.

BBG/514/001, Letters from Government Departments 1890–1892.
CLC/088/MS19526, London Municipal Society, Minutes of Annual General Meetings.
CLC/088/MS19528, London Municipal Society, Minutes Executive Committee Meetings.
GLC/DG/AE/ROL/82/001,
LCC Standing Orders, 1891–1893.
LCC Standing Orders, 1906–1907.
H12/CH/A3/2, The Eighth Annual Report of the Asylums Committee and Sub-committees of Banstead, Cane Hill, Claybury, Colney Hatch, Hanwell, The Heath and Horton Asylums, 1897.
H12/CH/A3/8, The Sixteenth Annual Report of the Asylums Committee and Sub-committees of Banstead, Bexley, Cane Hill, Claybury, Colney Hatch, Hanwell, Horton The Manor, Epileptic Colony and Long Grove, 1905.
H12/CH/A6/1, Colney Hatch Visitors Book.
H12/CH/B/003/002, Colney Hatch, Register of Female Patients, 1888–1894.
H12/CH/B/003/003, Colney Hatch, Register of Female Patients, 1894–1898.
H12/CH/B/003/004, Colney Hatch, Register of Female Patients, 1898–1902.
H12/CH/B/003/005, Colney Hatch, Register of Female Patients, 1903–1907.
H12/CH/B/003/006, Colney Hatch, Register of Female Patients, 1851–1914.
H12/CH/B13/43A, Colney Hatch Male Case Book, October 1895–April 1896.
H12/CH/B13/60, Colney Hatch Male Case Book, April–September 1907.
H12/CH/B13/61, Colney Hatch Male Case Book, October 1907–June 1908.
H12/CH/B13/63, Colney Hatch Male Case Book, February–October 1909.
H12/CH/B/46/62, Colney Hatch Female Reception Orders, 16376–16399.
H12/CH/B/46/63, Colney Hatch Female Reception Orders, 16451–16475.
LCC 18.6, London County Council, Minutes of Proceedings, January 1889–December 1915 (Multiple Volumes)
LCC 26.21, Annual Reports for LCC Asylums Committee (Multiple Volumes).
LCC/MIN/565, Signed Minutes, 1889–1892 to LCC/MIN/578 Signed Minutes, March 1912–October 1913 (14 Volumes)
LCC/MIN/580, Asylums and Mental Deficiency Minute Book, November 1914–July 1915.
LCC/MIN/710, Accommodation Sub-Committee Minute Book, 1896–1905.
LCC/MIN/711, Accommodation Sub-Committee Minute Book, 1905–1908.
LCC/MIN/713, Accommodation Sub-Committee Minute Book, 1910–1912.
LCC/MIN/714, Accommodation Sub-Committee Minute Book, 1912–1913.
LCC/MIN/747, Pathologist Sub-Committee Minute Book, 1892–1901.
LCC/MIN/748, Pathologist Sub-Committee Minute Book, 1901–1908.
LCC/MIN/759, Stansfield, T.E.K. Hereditary and Insanity.
LCC/CL/PH/01/276, Miscellaneous Printed Papers.

Asylums Finance. 1899. Suggestions of Lord Lingen, LCC.

Brudenell Carter, R. 1889. Committee on a Hospital for the Insane.

Bryan, F. 1905. Report of the Medical Superintendent on Dr Mott's Report on the Itch.

Cooper, G.J. and Mott, F.W. 1904. Interim Report on Medical Statistics, LCC.

Heath Asylum, Bexley. 1899. Report by the Clerk of the Council, LCC.

Keene, H.F. 1907. *Memorandum as to the Procedure with Regard to the Admission and Discharge of Patients.* London: LCC.

Keene, H.F. 1907. *Report of the Clerk in Connection with Question of the Need for Additional Accommodation.* London: LCC.

LCC. 1890. Report of the Committee on a Hospital for the Insane.

LCC. c.1904. *The Epileptic Colony, Ewell.* London: LCC.

Marsh, T.A. 1898. Scheme of London Asylums Committee for Providing Receiving Houses & c., Fulham Union.

McDougall, John. 1901. *Notes of a Visit Made in 1897 to Canadian and American Asylums.* London: P.S. King and Son.

Mott, F.W. 1896. *Housing of Lunatics.* London: LCC.

Partridge, R.W. 1893. Report of the Clerk. London: LCC.

Report of Sub-Committee appointed by Provisional Asylums Committee, 19 June 1889.

Report of the Special Sub-Committee appointed to Consider the appointment of a Pathologist, LCC, 1894.

Regulations as to Asylums Finance. 1899. LCC.

Smith, W.C.C. 1901. *Notes of a Visit to Continental and British Asylums.* London: LCC.

Stansfield, T.E.K. 1894. *Report on a Visit to Some American Asylums.* London: LCC.

Stansfield, T.E.K. 1896. Report to the Special Sub-Committee (Housing of the Insane) of the Asylums Committee.

Suggestions for Regulations as to Asylum Finance, LCC, 1889.

LCC/PH/Ment/3/5, Newspaper Cuttings.

LCC/PH/MENT/05/003, Minutes of Meetings of Asylum Officers, 1899–1915, 28 March 1899.

MS/SP/1888/01/061. 1888. Twenty Third Annual Report of the Clerk of the Peace in Respect of Pauper Lunatics Chargeable to the County.

London School of Economics

Coll. Misc. 904.

N.d. How to Reform London Government, Progressive Leaflet 20.

N.d. London Reform Union, Leaflet No. 57, 'What the County Council Has Done for Temperance Reform'.

N.d. London Reform Union, Leaflet No. 49, 'The Truth About the Works Department'.

1896. London Reform Union, Leaflet No. 74, 'The Truth About the Works Department of the London County Council'.
1896. London Reform Union. 'The County Council and the Vestries: The Two Partners in London Government'.
F35/41. c.1905. Radford, G.H. The Story of London County Council 1901–1904.
ILP/6/22/1/84504.
1913. J. Gilbert Dale Labour Candidate.
1913. London County Council, An Urgent Appeal to Ministers and Churches.
J2/210. Anon. 1909. *London Under the Moderates.* London: Alexander and Shepherd Ltd.
JS/57–60. c.1907. *Our London! What London Is and How It Is Governed.* London: Morning Leader Pamphlet Department.
LSE JS/57–60. Gilbert, J.D. 1909. *Two and a Half Years Record of the Moderate Party.* London: London Reform Union.
JS/203–211.
Anon. 1909. London Under the Moderates.
Webb, Sidney. 1895. Six Years' Work on the London County Council.

The National Archive
FO 369/36, Russia, Code 238, Files 176—18279.
HO 45/10360/154554, LUNACY: Repatriation of Lunatics—Arrangements Between Great Britain and Spain.
HO 45/10360/154559, ALIENS: Repatriation of Insane or Helpless Aliens from U.S.A.
HO 45/10512/130843, ALIENS: International Congress on Destitute Aliens.
HO 45/10560/169330, LUNACY: France and United Kingdom. Repatriation of Pauper Lunatics.
HO 45/10659/212622, Repatriation of British and Maltese Lunatics from Egypt, 1911–1912.
HO 45/10995/167955, MENTAL HEALTH: Repatriation of Foreign Lunatics. Anglo-German Agreement, 1913.
HO 144/970/B32798, ALIENS: Repatriation of Alien Lunatics.

West Yorkshire Archive Service
C85/1/12/5. 1890. Report of the Sub-Committee and Medical Superintendent of the West Riding Asylum for the Year 1889, West Yorkshire Printing Co., Wakefield.
WYAS, C85/1/13/5. Medical Director's Journal 1888–1894.

Legislation
Aliens Act, 1905. 5 Edw. 7. Ch. 13.
Local Government Act. 1888. 51 and 52, Vict., c. 41.

Newspapers and Periodicals
British Architect
British Medical Journal
Chelsea News and General Advertiser
Daily Chronicle
Daily Mail
Daily News
Journal of Mental Science
Journal of the Royal Institute of British Architects
London
London Argus
London County Council Staff Gazette
London Daily News
Manchester Guardian
Morning Post
Municipal Journal
Reynold's Newspaper
The Sheffield and Rotherham Independent
Shoreditch Observer, Hackney Express and Bethnal Green Chronicle
The Speaker
Spectator
The Standard
The Times
Universal Review
Westminster Review

Websites
Archive.org
Historic Hansard
Legislation.gov.uk
Maryland State Archives
Oxford Dictionary of National Biography
Royal College of Surgeons
UK Parliamentary Papers

Other Published Sources

Anon. 1892. *Three Years Good Work for the People*. London: National Press Agency.

Anon. 1907a. *London County Council Election 1907: Facts and Arguments for Municipal Speakers and Candidates*. London: London Municipal Society.

Anon. 1907b. *The Story of the London County Council*. London: George Edward Wright.

Anon. 1911. *Report and Special Report from the Select Committee on the Asylums Officers (Employment, Pensions, and Superannuation) Bill.* London: Wyman and Sons.

Bibby, George H. 1895. *The Housing of Pauper Lunatics.* London: Drake, Driver and Leaver Ltd.

Bibby, George H. 1896. *The Planning of Lunatic Asylums.* London: Bradley T. Batsford.

Bucknill, J.C. 1876. *Notes on Asylums for the Insane in America.* London: J&A Churchill.

Burdett, Henry C. 1891a. *Hospitals and Asylums of the World, Vol. I, History and Administration.* London: J&A Churchill.

Burdett, Henry C. 1891b. *Hospitals and Asylums of the World, Vol. II, Asylum Construction.* London: J&A Churchill.

Donald, Robert. 1901. *The London Manual for 1901.* London: Edward Lloyd Limited.

The Earl of Rosebery. 1894. *Municipal and Social Reform.* London: Liberal Publications.

Earle, Pliny. 1841. *A Visit to Thirteen Asylums in Europe.* Philadelphia: Dobson.

Firth, J.F.B. and Simpson, Edgar R. 1888. *London Government Under the Local Government Act, 1888.* London: Knight and Co.

Fox, George L. 1895. The London County Council and Its Work. *Yale Review*, May: 80–102.

Geake, Charles. 1899. *Appreciations and Addresses Delivered by Lord Rosebery.* London: John Lane.

Greene, Richard. 1889. The Care and Cure of the Insane. The Universal Review 4: 493–508.

Harris, Percy. 1913. *London and its Government.* London: J.M. Dent and Sons.

Hawkins, Rev Henry. 1901. *Some Notes on the History of the Colney Hatch Asylum, 1849–1901.* London: Potter, Batten and Davies.

Hill, Robert Gardiner. 1870. *Lunacy: Its Past and its Present.* London: Longmans.

Hine, George T. 1901. Asylums and Asylum Planning. *Journal of the Royal Institute of British Architects*, February: 161–84.

Hurd, Henry M. 1916. *The Institutional Care of the Insane in the United States and Canada, Vol. II.* Baltimore: Johns Hopkins Press.

Jephson, Henry. 2010. *The Making of Modern London, Progress and Reaction.* London: Bowers Brothers.

Lancashire Asylums Board. 1900. *Report of a Deputation Appointed Visit Asylums on the Continent.* Salford: W.F. Jackson and Sons.

London County Council. 1890. *A Review of the First Year's Work of the Council in a Series of Addresses Delivered by the Chairman, the Earl of Rosebery.* London: LCC.

London Municipal Society. c.1912. *The Municipal Reformers and Labour, London County Council Election 1913, Facts and Arguments for Municipal Reform Speakers and Candidates.* London: George Berridge and Co.

Snell, H. n.d. *The Foreigner in England: The Problem of Alien Immigration.* Keighley: Wadsworth and Co.

Stoddart, Jane T. 1900. *The Earl of Rosebery, K.G.: An Illustrated Biography.* London: Hodders and Stoughton.

Webb, Sidney. 1895. *The Work of the London County Council.* London: The London Reform Union.

Wilson, Woodrow. 1889. *The State: Elements of Historical and Practical Politics.* Boston: D.C. Heath and Co.

Secondary Sources

Alderman, Geoffrey. 1998. *Modern British Jewry.* Oxford: Clarendon Press.

Allderidge, Patricia. 1991. The Foundation of the Maudsley Hospital. In *150 Years of British Psychiatry, 1841–1991*, eds. G.E. Berrios and H. Freeman, 79–88. London: Gaskell.

Allmond, Gillian. 2017. Liberty and the Individual: The Colony Asylum in Scotland and England. *History of Psychiatry* 28:1: 29–43.

Andrews, Jonathan, Briggs, Asa, Porter, Roy, Tucker Penny and Waddington, Keir. 2013. *The History of Bethlem.* London: Routledge.

Arnold, Catharine. 2008. *Bedlam: London and its Mad.* London: Simon and Schuster.

Aspinwall, Bernard. 1984. *Portable Utopia, Glasgow and the United States, 1820–1920.* Aberdeen: Aberdeen University Press.

Ayers, Gwendoline M. 1971. *England's First State Hospitals and the Metropolitan Asylums Board 1867–1930.* London: Wellcome Institute of the History of Medicine.

Ball, Michael and Sunderland, David. 2001. *An Economic History of London, 1800–1914.* London: Routledge.

Barham, Peter. 2007. *Forgotten Lunatics of the Great War.* New Haven: Yale University Press.

Bartlett, Peter. 1999. *The Poor Law of Lunacy: The Administration of Pauper Lunatics in Mid-Nineteenth Century England.* London: Leicester University Press.

Bartlett, Peter and Wright, David. 1999. Community Care and Its Antecedents. In *Outside the Walls of the Asylum*, eds. Bartlett, Peter and Wright, David, 1–18. London: Athlone.

Bartley, Paula. 2000. *Prostitution, Prevention and Reform in England, 1860–1914.* London: Routledge.

Barton, Walter E. 1987. *The History and Influence of the American Psychiatric Association.* Washington, DC: American Psychiatric Association: 38–9.

Bashford, Alison. 2013. Insanity and Immigration Restriction. In *Migration, Health and Ethnicity in the Modern World*, eds. Catharine Cox and Hilary Marland, 14–35. Basingstoke: Palgrave Macmillan.

Bashford, Alison and Gilchrist C. 2012. The Colonial History of the Aliens Act. *The Journal of Imperial and Commonwealth History* 40:3: 409–37.

Bewley, Thomas. 2008. *Madness to Mental Illness a History of the Royal College of Psychiatrists*. Trowbridge: Cromwell Press: 45.

Briggs, Asa. 1990. *Victorian Cities*. London: Penguin.

Briggs, Lynne. 2012. The Impact of Migration on the Mental Health of Refugee Women in Contemporary New Zealand. In *Migration, Ethnicity and Mental Health, International Perspectives 1840–2010*, eds. Angela McCarthy and Catharine Coleborne, 178–92. New York: Routledge.

Butler, David and Butler, Gareth. 2011. *British Political Facts*. Basingstoke: Palgrave Macmillan.

Cannadine, David and Reeder David, eds. 1982. *Exploring the Urban Past, Essays in Urban History by H.J. Dyos*. Cambridge: Cambridge University Press.

Chambers, Paul. *Bedlam: London's Hospital for the Mad*. Birmingham: Ian Allan Publishing.

Chandler, J.A. 2000. *Explaining Local Government, Local Government in Britain Since 1800*. Manchester: Manchester University Press.

Cherry, Steve. 2013. *Mental Health Care in Modern England: The Norfolk Lunatic Asylum/St Andrews Hospital, 1810–1998*. Woodbridge: Boydell.

Clavin, Patricia. 2011. Introduction: Conceptualising Internationalism Between the World Wars. In *Internationalism Reconfigured, Transnational Ideas and Movements Between the Wars*, ed. Daniel Laqua, 1–15. London: I.B. Tauris.

Cochrane, David. 1988. Humane, Economical and Medically Wise: The LCC as Administrators of Victorian Lunacy Policy. In *The Anatomy of Madness, Vol. III, The Asylum and Its Psychiatry*, eds. W.F. Bynum, Roy Porter and Michael Shepherd, 247–72. London: Routledge.

Davies, John. 1988. *Reforming London: The London Government Problem, 1855–1900*. Oxford: Clarendon Press.

Davies, John. 1989. The Progressive Council, 1889–1907. In *Politics and the People of London: The London County Council 1889–1965*, ed. Andrew Saint, 27–48. London: Hambledon Press.

Davies, John. 2001. Local Government 1850–1920: The Metropolitan Board of Works and the London County Council. *London Journal* 26: 47–56.

Doyle, Barry M. 2001. The Changing Functions of Urban Government: Councillors, Officials and Pressure Groups, 1835–1950. In *The Cambridge Urban History of Britain*, eds. D.M. Palliser, Peter Clark and Martin J. Daunton, 287–313. Cambridge: Cambridge University Press.

Doyle, Barry M. 2015. *The Politics of Hospital Provision in Early Twentieth-Century Britain*. London: Routledge.

Dunbabin, J.P.D. 1965. Expectations of the New County Councils, and Their Realization. *Historical Journal* 8:3: 353–79.

Dutton, David. 2014. *A History of the Liberal Party Since 1900*. London: Palgrave Macmillan.

Eastoe, S. 2016. Idiocy, Imbecility and Society in Victorian England: Caterham Imbecile Asylum, 1867–1911. Unpublished PhD thesis, University of London, Birkbeck.

Ellis, Rob. 2001. A Field of Practise or Mere House of Detention. Unpublished PhD thesis, University of Huddersfield.

Ellis, Rob. 2008. The Asylum, the Poor Law and the Growth of County Asylums in Nineteenth-Century Yorkshire. Northern History 45:2: 279–93.

Ellis, Rob. 2013a. A Constant Irritation to the Townspeople. Local, Regional and National Politics and London's County Asylums at Epsom. *Social History of Medicine* 26:4: 653–67.

Ellis, Rob. 2013b. Asylums and Sport: Participation, Isolation and the role of Cricket in the Treatment of the Insane. *International Journal of the History of Sport* 30: 83–101.

Ernst, Waltraud. 2010. Practising "Colonial" or "Modern" Psychiatry in British India? Treatments at the Indian Mental Hospital at Ranchi, 1925–40. In *Transnational Psychiatries, Social and Cultural Histories of Psychiatry in Comparative Perspective, c.1800–2000*, eds. Waltraud Ernst and Thomas Mueller, 80–115. Newcastle: Cambridge Scholars Publishing.

Ernst, Waltraud and Mueller, Thomas. 2010. Introduction. In *Transnational Psychiatries, Social and Cultural Histories of Psychiatry in Comparative Perspective c.1800–2000*, eds. Waltraud Ernst and Thomas Mueller, ix–xxiii. Newcastle: Cambridge Scholars Publishing.

Ewen, Shane. 2009. Policing Party Politics in the Midlands, c.1900–1938. In *Urban Politics and Space in the Nineteenth and Twentieth Centuries, Regional Perspectives*, ed. B. Doyle, 64–79. Newcastle: Cambridge Scholars Publishing.

Ewen, Shane and Hebbert, Michael. 2007. European Cities in a Networked World During the Long 20th Century. *Environment and Planning C-Government and Policy* 25:3: 327–40.

Fee, Elizabeth and Porter, Dorothy. 1992. Public Health, Preventive Medicine and Professionalization: England and America in the Nineteenth Century. In *Medicine in Society*, ed. Andrew Wear, 249–76. Cambridge: Cambridge University Press.

Feldman, David. 1989. The Importance of Being English: Jewish Immigration and the Decay of Liberal England. In *Metropolis London: Histories and Representations Since 1800*, eds. David Feldman and Gareth Stedman Jones, 56–84. London: Routledge Revivals.

Fennell, Phil. 1996. *Treatment Without Consent: Law Psychiatry and the Treatment of Mentally Disordered People Since 1845*. London: Routledge.

Finn, M.A. 2012. The West Riding Asylum and the Making of Modern Brain Sciences in the Nineteenth Century. Unpublished PhD thesis, University of Leeds.

Foucault, Michel. 1991 (1967). *Madness and Civilization.* London: Routledge.

Foucault, Michel. 2008. *Psychiatric Power: Lectures at the Collège de France, 1973–1974.* Basingstoke: Palgrave Macmillan.

Fraser, Derek. 1976. *Urban Politics in Victorian England.* Atlantic Highlands, NJ: Leicester University Press.

Fraser, Derek. 1979. *Power and Authority in the Victorian City.* Oxford: Basil Blackwell.

Fraser, Derek. 1980. Politics and Society in the Nineteenth Century. In *A History of Modern Leeds*, ed. Derek Fraser, 270–300. Manchester: Manchester University Press.

Fraser, Derek, ed. 1982. *Municipal Reform and the Industrial City.* New York: Leicester University Press.

Frosch, William and Richardson, Diane. 2004. Pliny Earle MD, 1809–1892. *American Journal of Psychiatry* 161:11: 1989.

Garrard, John. 2003. Scandals: A Tentative Overview. In *Corruption in Urban Politics and Society, Britain 1780–1950*, eds. James Moore and John Smith 23–40. Aldershot: Ashgate.

Geddes Poole, Andrea. 2014. *Philanthropy and the Construction of Victorian Women's Citizenship.* Toronto: University of Toronto Press.

Gibbon, Gwilym and Bell, Reginald W. 1939. *History of the London County Council.* London: Macmillan and Co.

Gijswijt-Hofstra, M., Oosterhuis, H., Vijselaar, J. and Freeman, H., eds. 2005. *Psychiatric Cultures Compared: Psychiatric and Mental Health Care in the Twentieth Century Comparison and Approaches.* Amsterdam: Amsterdam University Press.

Gillespie, James. 1989. Municipalism, Monopoly and Management: The Demise of Socialism in one County, 1918–1933. In *Politics and the People of London: The London County Council 1889–1965*, ed. Andrew Saint, 103–26. London: Hambledon Press.

Glover, David. 2012. *Literature, Immigration and Diaspora in fin-de-siècle England: A Cultural History of the 1905 Aliens Act.* Cambridge: Cambridge University Press.

Gorsky Martin and Sheard, Sally, eds. 2006. *Financing Medicine: The British Experience Since 1750.* London: Routledge.

Grant, James. 1838. *Sketches in London.* London: W.S. Orr and Co.

Griffiths, John. 2009. Were There Municipal Networks in the British World c.1890–1939. *The Journal of Imperial and Commonwealth History* 37:4: 575–97.

Hamlett, Jane. 2015. *At Home in the Institution, Material Life in Asylums, Lodging Houses and Schools in Victorian and Edwardian England.* Basingstoke: Palgrave Macmillan.

Hammond, J.L. 1935. The Social Background, 1835–1935. In *A Century of Municipal Progress: The Last Hundred Years*, eds. Harold J. Laski, W. Ivor Jennings and William Robson, 37–54. London: George Allen & Unwin Ltd.

Hare, Edward. 1983. Was Insanity on the Increase? *British Journal of Psychiatry* 143: 439–55.

Harris, Bernard. 1999. Pro-alienism, Anti-alienism and the Medical Professions in Late-Victorian and Edwardian Britain. In *Race, Science and Medicine, 1700–1960*, eds. Waltraud Ernst and Bernard Harris, 189–217. London: Routledge.

Harrison, B. 1973. Pubs. In *The Victorian City: Images and Realities, Vol. 1*, eds. H.J. Dyos and M. Wolff, 161–90. London: Routledge and Kegan Paul.

Harrison, J.F.C. 1990. *Late Victorian Britain 1875–1901*. London: Fontana Press.

Hasluck, E.L. 1948. *Local Government in England*. Cambridge: Cambridge University Press.

Haward, Harry. 1932. *The London County Council from Within: Forty Years Official Recollections*. London: Chapman and Hall.

Hayes, Bob. 2007. Lancashire Public Asylum Provision: Regional Co-operation. Local Rivalry and Factional Interest, 1889–1914. In *Urban Politics and Space in the Nineteenth and Twentieth Centuries, Regional Perspectives*, ed. Barry Doyle, 80–98. Newcastle: Cambridge Scholars Publishing.

Hayward, Rhodri. 2010. Germany and the Making of 'English' Psychiatry: The Maudsley Hospital, 1908–1939. In *International Relations in Psychiatry*, eds. Volker Roelcke, Paul J. Weindling and Louise Westwood, 67–90. Rochester: University of Rochester Press.

Hennock, E.P. 1973. *Fit and Proper Persons: Ideal and Reality in Nineteenth Century Urban Government*. London: Edward Arnold.

Hide Louise. 2013. From Asylum to Mental Hospital: Gender, Space and the Patient Experience in London County Council Asylums, 1890–1910. In *Residential Institutions in Britain, 1725–1970*, eds. Jane Hamlett, Lesley Hoskins and Rebecca Preston, 51–64. London: Pickering and Chatto.

Hide, Louise. 2014. *Gender and Class in English Asylums, 1890–1914*. Basingstoke: Palgrave Macmillan.

Hollis, Patricia. 1987. *Ladies Elect: Women in English Local Government, 1865–1914*. Oxford: Clarendon Press.

Howe, Anthony. 1996. Towards the "Hungry Forties": free Trade in Britain, c.1880–1906. In *Citizenship and Community: Liberals, Radicals and Collective Identities in the British Isles, 1865–1931*, ed. Eugenio F. Biagini, 192–218. Cambridge: Cambridge University Press.

Hunter, Richard and Macalpine, Ida. 1974. *Psychiatry for the Poor: 1851 Colney Hatch Asylum—Friern Hospital 1973*. London: Dawsons of Pall Mall.

Ignatieff, Michael. 1983. Total Institutions and Working Classes: A Review Essay. *History Workshop Journal* 15: 167–73.

Inwood, Stephen. 2000. *A History of London*. London: Macmillan.

Jackson, Mark. 2010. Permeating National Boundaries. European Influences on the Emergence of 'Medico-Pedagogy' in Late Victorian and Edwardian Britain. In *International Relations in Psychiatry*, eds. Volker Roelcke, Paul J. Weindling and Louise Westwood, 30–47. Rochester: University of Rochester Press.

Jackson, W. Eric. 1965. *Achievement: A Short History of the LCC*. London: Longmans, Green and Co.

Jeyes, Samuel. 1906. *The Earl of Rosebery*. London: J.M. Dent and Co.

Jones, Edgar, Rahman, Shahina and Woolven, Robin. 2007. The Maudsley Hospital: Design and Strategic Direction, 1923–1939. *Medical History* 51: 357–78.

Jones, Kathleen. 1960. *Mental Health and Social Policy, 1845–1959*. London: Routledge and Kegan Paul.

Julius, Anthony. 2010. *Trials of Diaspora: A History of Anti-semitism in England*. Oxford: Oxford University Press.

Keith-Lucas, Bryan. 1977. *English Local Government in the Nineteenth and Twentieth Centuries*. London: The Historical Association.

Keith-Lucas, Bryan and Richards, Peter G. 1978. *A History of Local Government in the Twentieth Century*. London: George Allen & Unwin Ltd.

Laski, Harold J. 1935. The Committee System in Local Government. In *A Century of Municipal Progress: The Last Hundred Years*, eds. Harold J. Laski, W. Ivor Jennings and William Robson, 82–108. London: George Allen & Unwin Ltd.

Laski, Harold J., Jennings, W. Ivor and Robson, William, eds. 1935. *A Century of Municipal Progress: The Last Hundred Years*. London: George Allen & Unwin Ltd.

Lawrence, J. 1993. Class and Gender in the Making of Urban Toryism, 1880–1914. *English Historical Review* 108: 629–52.

Levene, Alysa, Powell, Martin, Stewart, John and Taylor, Becky. 2011. *Cradle to Grave: Municipal Medicine in Interwar England and Wales*. Bern: Peter Lang.

London County Council. 1949. *LCC Hospitals: A Retrospect*. London: Staples Press.

McCarthy, Angela and Coleborne Catharine. 2012. Mental Health, Migration and Ethnicity. In *Migration, Ethnicity and Mental Health, International Perspectives 1840–2010*, eds. Angela McCarthy and Catharine Coleborne 1–14. New York: Routledge.

McMahon, Aoife. 2016. *The Role of the State in Migration Control*. Boston: Brill Nijhoff.

Melling, Joseph. 1999. Accommodating Madness. New Research in the Social History of Insanity and Institutions. In *Insanity, Institutions and Society, 1800–1914*, eds. Joseph Melling and Bill Forsythe, 1–30. Abingdon: Routledge.

Melling, Joseph and Forsythe, Bill. 2006. *The Politics of Madness.* London: Routledge.

Melling, Joseph, Adair, Richard and Forsythe, Bill. 1997. A Proper Lunatic for Two Years: Pauper Lunatic Children in Victorian and Edwardian England. Child Admissions to the Devon County Asylum, 1845–1914. *Journal of Social History* 31:2: 371–405.

Melling, Joseph, Forsythe, Bill and Adair, Richard. 1999. Politics of Lunacy: Central State Regulation and the Devon Pauper Lunatic Asylum, 1845–1914. In *Insanity, Institutions and Society, 1800–1914*, eds. Joseph Melling and Bill Forsythe, 68–87. Abingdon: Routledge.

Mills, China. 2014. *Decolonizing Global Mental Health: The Psychiatrization of the Majority World.* London: Routledge.

Millward, Robert and Sheard, Sally. 1995. The Urban Fiscal Problem, 1870–1914: Government Expenditure and Finance in England and Wales. *The Economic History Review* 48:3: 501–35.

Mooney, Graham and Reinarz, Jonathan. 2009. Hospital and Asylum Visiting in Historical Perspective: Themes and Issues. In *Permeable Walls: Historical Perspectives on Hospital and Asylum Visiting*, eds. Graham Mooney and Jonathan Reinarz, 7–30. Amsterdam: Rodopi.

Moore, James R. 2006. *The Transformation of Urban Liberalism: Party Politics and Urban Governance in Late Nineteenth Century England.* Aldershot: Ashgate.

Moran, James E. and Chilton, L. 2016. Mad Migrants and the Reach of English Civil Law. In *Migration and Mental Health*, ed. Majorie Harper, 149–70. London: Routledge.

Moran, James E. and Topp, Leslie. 2006. Introduction. In *Madness, Architecture and the Built Environment*, eds. Leslie Topp, James E. Moran and Jonathan Andrews, 1–16. London: Routledge.

Murphy, Elaine. 2003. The Administration of Insanity in England 1800–1870. In *The Confinement of the Insane International Perspectives, 1800–1965*, eds. Roy Porter and David Wright, 334–49. New York: Cambridge University Press.

Murphy, Elaine. 2006. Workhouse Care of the Inane, 1845–90. In *Mental Illness and Learning Disability Since 1850*, eds. Pamela Dale and Joseph Melling, 24–45. London: Routledge.

Nevers, Jean-Yves. 2003. The "Iron Triangle" of Municipal Government: Trade Unions, Bureaucracy and Political Parties in a French Town (Toulouse, 1910–1970). In *Municipal Services and Employees in the Modern City: New Historic Approaches*, eds. Michèle Dagenais, Irene Maver and Pierre-Yves Saunier 159–76. Aldershot: Ashgate.

Novella, E.J. 2016. Travel and Professional Networks in the Origins of Spanish Psychiatry. *História, Ciências, Saúde-Manguinhos* 23:4: 1023–40.

Owen, David. 1982. *The Government of Victorian London, 1855–1889.* Cambridge, MA: Belknap Press.

Panayi, Panikos. 2010. *An Immigration History of Britain: Multicultural Racism Since 1800.* London: Routledge.

Pellew, Jill. 2007. The Home Office and the Aliens Act, 1905. *The Historical Journal* 32:2: 369–85.

Pennybacker, Susan. 1989. The Millennium by Return of post. Reconsidering London Progressivism, 1889–1907. In *Metropolis London, Histories and Representations Since 1800*, eds. David Feldman and Gareth Stedman Jones, 129–62. London: Routledge.

Pennybacker, Susan. 1995. *A Vision for London, 1889–1914: Labour Everyday Life and the LCC Experiment.* London: Routledge.

Philo, Chris. 1987. "Fit Localities for an Asylum": The Historical Geography of the Nineteenth-Century 'Mad Business' in England as Viewed Through the Pages of the Asylum Journal. *Journal of Historical Geography* 13:4: 398–415.

Pick, Daniel. 1989. *Faces of Degeneration: A European Disorder, c.1848–1918.* Cambridge: Cambridge University Press.

Porter, Roy. 1994. *London: A Social History.* London: Hamish Hamilton Ltd.

Porter, Roy and Wright, David. 2003. *The Confinement of the Insane: International Perspectives 1800–1965.* Cambridge: Cambridge University Press.

Powell, Martin. 1995. Did Politics Matter? Municipal Public Expenditure in the 1930s. *Urban History* 22:3: 360–79.

Reeves, Carole Anne. 2001. Insanity and Nervous Diseases Among Jewish Immigrants to the East of London, 1880–1920. Unpublished PhD thesis, University of London.

Reinarz, Jonathan and Wynter, R. 2014. The Spirit of Medicine: The Use of Alcohol in Nineteenth-Century Medical Practice. In *Drink in the Eighteen and Nineteenth Centuries*, eds. S. Schmid and B. Schmidt-Haberkamp, 127–40. London: Pickering and Chatto.

Rethink Mental Illness. n.d. APPG on Mental Health. https://www.rethink.org/get-involved/public-affairs/appg-on-mental-health. Accessed 3 July 2019.

Roelcke, Volker, Weindling, Paul J. and Westwood, Louise. 2010. *International Relations in Psychiatry.* Rochester: University of Rochester Press.

Saint, Andrew. 1989. Technical Education and the Early LCC. In *Politics and the People of London: The London County Council 1889–1965*, ed. Andrew Saint, 71–92. London: Hambledon Press.

Sarg, Cristin M. 2017. Scottish-Jewish 'Madness'?: An Examination of Jewish Admissions to the Royal Asylums of Edinburgh and Glasgow, c.1870–1939. Unpublished PhD thesis, University of Glasgow.

Saunier, Pierre-Yves. 2008. Introduction: Global City, Take 2: A View from Urban History. In *Another Global City: Historical Explorations into the Transnational Municipal Moment 1850–2000*, eds. Pierre-Yves Saunier and Shane Ewen, 1–18. Basingstoke: Palgrave Macmillan.

Schemeideback, Heinz-Peter. 2010. Inspecting Great Britain: German Psychiatrists' Views of British Asylums in the Second Half of the Nineteenth Century. In *International Relations in Psychiatry*, eds. Volker Roelcke, Paul J. Weindling and Louise Westwood, 12–29. Rochester: University of Rochester Press.

Schneer, Jonathan. 1999. *London 1900: The Imperial Metropolis*. New Haven: Yale University Press.

Scull, Andrew. 1984. Was Insanity Increasing: A Response to Edward Hare. *British Journal of Psychiatry* 144: 432–6.

Scull, Andrew. 1993. *The Most Solitary of Afflictions*. New Haven: Yale University Press.

Scull, Andrew. 2006. *The Insanity of Place/The Place of Insanity: Essays on the History of Psychiatry*. Abingdon: Routledge.

Scull, Andrew. 2009. *Hysteria: The Disturbing History*. Oxford: Oxford University Press.

Scull, Andrew. 2015. *Madness in Civilization: A Cultural History of Insanity from the Bible to Freud, from the Madhouse to Modern Medicine*. London: Thames and Hudson.

Sheard, Sally. 2006. Reluctant Providers? The Politics and Ideology of Municipal Hospital Finance 1870–1914. In *Financing Medicine: The British Experience Since 1750*, eds. Martin Gorsky and Sally Sheard, 112–29. London: Routledge.

Sheldrake, John. 1989. The LCC Hospital Service. In *Politics and the People of London: The London County Council 1889–1965*, ed. Andrew Saint, 187–98. London: Hambledon Press.

Shepherd, Anne and Wright, David. 2002. Madness, Suicide and the Victorian Asylum: Attempted Self-Murder in the Age of Non-restraint. *Medical History* 46: 175–96.

Shpayer-Makov, Haia. 1987. The Reception of Peter Kropotkin in Britain, 1886–1917. *Albion: A Quarterly Journal Concerned with British Studies* 19:3, 373–90.

Smellie, K.B. 1946. *A History of Local Government* London: George Allen & Unwin Ltd.

Smith, L.D. 1998. Insanity and Ethnicity: Jews in the Mid-Victorian Lunatic Asylum. *Jewish Culture and History* 1:1: 27–40.

Smith, L.D. 1999. The County Asylum in the Mixed Economy of Care. In *Insanity, Institutions and Society, 1800–1914*, eds. Joseph Melling and Bill Forsythe, 33–47. London: Routledge.

Stewart, John. 2005. The Finest Municipal Hospital Service in the World? Contemporary Perceptions of the London County Council's Hospital Provision, 1929–39. *Urban History* 32: 327–44.

Stokes, Wendy. 2011. Missing from the Picture: Women's Initiatives in English Local Government. In *Women and Representation in Local Government: International Case Studies*, eds. Barbara Pini and Paula McDonald, 95–108. London: Routledge.

Strange, Julie-Marie. 2005. *Death, Grief and Poverty in Britain 1870–1914.* Cambridge: Cambridge University Press.

Summerson, J. 1973. The Artifact. *The Victorian City: Images and Realities, Volume 1*, eds. H.J. Dyos and M. Wolff, 311–32. London: Routledge and Kegan Paul.

Suzuki, Akihito. 1995. The Politics and Ideology of Non-restraint: The Case of the Hanwell Asylum. *Medical History* 39: 1–17.

Takabayashi, Akinobu. 2017. Surviving the Lunacy Act of 1890: English Psychiatrists and Professional Development During the Early Twentieth Century. *Medical History* 61:2: 246–69.

Taylor, Barbara. 2015. *The Last Asylum: A Memoir of Madness in Our Times.* Chicago: University of Chicago Press.

Taylor, Jeremy. 1991. *Hospital and Asylum Architecture in England 1840–1914.* London: Mansell.

Taylor, Jeremy. 2007. The Architect and the Pauper Asylum in Late Nineteenth-Century England. G.T. Hine's Review of Asylum Space and Planning. In *Madness, Architecture and the Built Environment*, eds. Leslie Topp, James E. Moran and Jonathan Andrews, 263–81. London: Routledge.

Thomson, Mathew. 1993. Social Policy and the Management of the Problem of Mental Deficiency in Inter-war London. *London Journal* 18: 129–42.

Thomson, Mathew. 1998. *The Problem of Mental Deficiency, Eugenics, Democracy and Social Policy in Britain c.1870–1959.* Oxford: Clarendon Press.

Tomes, Nancy. 1988. The Great Restraint Controversy: A Comparative Perspective on Anglo-American Psychiatry in the Nineteenth Century. In *The Anatomy of Madness, Vol. III, The Asylum and Its Psychiatry*, eds. W.F. Bynum, Roy Porter and Michael Shepherd, 191–225 London: Routledge.

Topp, Leslie. 2007. The Modern Mental Hospital in Late Nineteenth-Century Germany and Austria: Psychiatric Space and Images of Freedom and Control. In *Madness, Architecture and the Built Environment*, eds. Leslie Topp, James E. Moran and Jonathan Andrews, 241–62. London: Routledge.

Turner, John, et al. 2015. The History of Mental Health Services in Modern England: Practitioner Memories and the Direction of Future Research. *Medical History* 59: 599–624.

Tyler, Paul. 2007. *Labour's Lost Leader: The Life and Politics of Will Crook.* London: Tauris Academic Studies.

Walk, Alexander. 1976. Medico-Psychologists, Maudsley and the Maudsley Hospital. *British Journal of Psychiatry* 128: 19–30.

Walkowitz, Judith R. 1992. *City of Dreadful Delight: Narratives of Sexual Danger in Late-Victorian London*. London: Virago.

Waller, P.J. 1983. *Town, City and Nation: England 1850–1914*. Oxford: Clarendon Press.

Wallis, J. 2015. *Investigating the Body in the Victorian Asylum*. London: Palgrave.

Walton, John. 1985. Casting Out and Bringing Back in Victorian England: Pauper Lunatics, 1840–40. In *The Anatomy of Madness, Vol. II, Institutions and Society*, eds. W.F. Bynum, Roy Porter and Michael Shepherd, 132–46. London: Tavistock Publications.

Ward, Stephen V. 2000. Re-examining the International Diffusion of Planning'. In *Urban Planning in a Changing World: The Twentieth Century Experience*, ed. Robert Freestone, 40–60. London: E. & F.N. Spon.

Weightman, Gavin and Humphries, Steve. 1985. *The Making of Modern London, 1845–1914*. London: Sidgewick and Jackson.

Westwood, Louise. 2006. Separatism and Exclusion. Women in Psychiatry. In *Mental Illness and Learning Disability Since 1850*, eds. Pamela Dale and Joseph Melling, 91–111. London: Routledge.

Windscheffel, Alex. 2007. *Popular Conservatism in London, 1868–1906*. Woodbridge: Boydell Press.

Wohl, A.S. 1977. *The Eternal Slum: Housing and Social Policy in Victorian London, Studies in Urban History, Vol. 5*. London: Edward Arnold.

Woodhouse, Diana. 2001. *The Office of Lord Chancellor*. Oxford: Hart Publishing.

Wright, David. 1997. Getting Out of the Asylum: Understanding the Confinement of the Insane in the Nineteenth Century. *Social History of Medicine* 10: 137–55.

Yanni, Carla. 2007. *The Architecture of Madness: Insane Asylums in the United States*. Minneapolis: University of Minnesota Press.

Yeomans, Henry. 2014. *Alcohol and Moral Regulation: Public Attitudes, Spirited Measures and Victorian Hangovers*. Bristol: Policy Press.

Young, Ken. 1975. *Local Politics and the Rise of Party: The London Municipal Society and the Conservative Intervention in Local Elections, 1894–1963*. Leicester: Leicester University Press.

Young, Ken and Garside, Patricia L. 1982. *Metropolitan London, Politics and Urban Change, 1837–1981: Studies in Urban History Vol. 6*. London: Edward Arnold.

Index

R. Ellis, *London and its Asylums, 1888-1914*,
Mental Health in Historical Perspective,
https://doi.org/10.1007/978-3-030-44432-7

M

The manufacturer's authorised representative in the EU is Springer Nature Customer Service Centre GmbH, Europaplatz 3, 69115 Heidelberg, Germany. If you have any concerns regarding our products, please contact ProductSafety@springernature.com

Printed and bound by CPI Group (UK) Ltd, Croydon, CR0 4YY

30/09/2026

02225459-0010